HANDBOOK OF COSMETIC SKIN CARE

Series in Cosmetic and Laser Therapy
Published in association with the *Journal of Cosmetic and Laser Therapy*

Already available

1. David J Goldberg
   Fillers in Cosmetic Dermatology, ISBN 9781841845098
2. Philippe Deprez
   Textbook of Chemical Peels, ISBN 9781841842954
3. C William Hanke, Gerhard Sattler, Boris Sommer
   Textbook of Liposuction, ISBN 9781841845326
4. Paul J Carniol, Neil S Sadick
   Clinical Procedures in Laser Skin Rejuvenation, ISBN 9780415414135
5. David J Goldberg
   Laser Hair Removal, Second Edition, ISBN 9780415414128
6. Benjamin Ascher, Marina Landau, Bernard Rossi
   Injection Treatments in Cosmetic Surgery, ISBN 9780415386517
7. Avi Shai, Robert Baran, Howard Maibach
   Handbook of Cosmetic Skin Care, Second Edition, ISBN 9780415467186

Forthcoming

8. Jenny Kim, Gary Lask
   Comprehensive Aesthetic Rejuvenation: A Regional Approach, ISBN 9780415458948
9. Neil Sadick, Paul Carniol, Deborshi Roy, Luitgard Wiest
   Illustrated Manual of Injectable Fillers, ISBN 9780415476447
10. Paul Carniol, Gary Monheit
    Aesthetic Rejuvenation Challenges and Solutions: A Global Perspective, ISBN 9780415475600
11. Neil Sadick, Diane Berson, Mary Lupo, Zoe Diana Draelos
    Cosmeceutical Science in Clinical Practice, ISBN 9780415471145
12. Anthony Benedetto
    Botulinum Toxins in Clinical Dermatology, Second Edition, ISBN 9780415476362
13. Robert Baran, Howard Maibach
    Textbook of Cosmetic Dermatology, Fourth Edition, ISBN 9781841847009
14. David J Goldberg, Alexander L Berlin
    Disorders of Fat and Cellulite, ISBN 9780415477000
15. Ken Beer, Mary Lupo, Vic Narurkar, Wendy Roberts
    Cosmetic Bootcamp Primer, ISBN 9781841846989

HANDBOOK OF COSMETIC SKIN CARE

SECOND EDITION

EDITED BY

AVI SHAI MD
*Department of Dermatology, Soroka University Medical Center,
Ben-Gurion University, Beer-Sheva, Israel*

HOWARD I. MAIBACH MD
*Department of Dermatology, University of California, San Francisco
School of Medicine, San Francisco, California, U.S.A.*

ROBERT BARAN MD
Nail Disease Center, Cannes, France

Line illustrations provided by Michal Yerushalmi-Rahamim

informa
healthcare

© 2009 Informa UK Ltd

First published in the United Kingdom in 2009 by Informa Healthcare, Telephone House, 69-77 Paul Street, London EC2A 4LQ. Informa Healthcare is a trading division of Informa UK Ltd. Registered Office: 37/41 Mortimer Street, London W1T 3JH. Registered in England and Wales number 1072954.

Tel: +44 (0)20 7017 5000
Fax: +44 (0)20 7017 6699
Website: www.informahealthcare.com

All rights reserved. No part of this publication may be reproduced, stored in a retrieval system, or transmitted, in any form or by any means, electronic, mechanical, photocopying, recording, or otherwise, without the prior permission of the publisher or in accordance with the provisions of the Copyright, Designs and Patents Act 1988 or under the terms of any licence permitting limited copying issued by the Copyright Licensing Agency, 90 Tottenham Court Road, London W1P 0LP.

Although every effort has been made to ensure that all owners of copyright material have been acknowledged in this publication, we would be glad to acknowledge in subsequent reprints or editions any omissions brought to our attention.

Although every effort has been made to ensure that drug doses and other information are presented accurately in this publication, the ultimate responsibility rests with the prescribing physician. Neither the publishers nor the authors can be held responsible for errors or for any consequences arising from the use of information contained herein. For detailed prescribing information or instructions on the use of any product or procedure discussed herein, please consult the prescribing information or instructional material issued by the manufacturer.

A CIP record for this book is available from the British Library.
Library of Congress Cataloging-in-Publication Data

Data available on application

ISBN-13: 978 0 41546 718 6
ISBN-10: 0 4154 6718 7

Distributed in North and South America by
Taylor & Francis
6000 Broken Sound Parkway, NW, (Suite 300)
Boca Raton, FL 33487, USA

Within Continental USA
Tel: 1 (800) 272 7737; Fax: 1 (800) 374 3401
Outside Continental USA
Tel: (561) 994 0555; Fax: (561) 361 6018
Email: orders@crcpress.Com

Book orders in the rest of the world
Paul Abrahams
Tel: +44 (0) 207 017 4036
Email: bookorders@informa.com

Composition by Aptara®, Inc.
Printed and bound in India by Replika Press Pvt Ltd.

Contents

Contributors ix
Notes for the Reader xi
Acknowledgments xii

1. Cosmetics and Cosmetic Preparations: Basic Definitions 1
   Avi Shai, Robert Baran, and Howard I. Maibach

2. Skin Structure 4
   Avi Shai, Robert Baran, and Howard I. Maibach

3. Principles in the Preparation of Medical and Cosmetic Products 14
   Sima Halevy and Avi Shai

4. Skin Moisture and Moisturizers 24
   Avi Shai, Howard I. Maibach, and Robert Baran

5. Skin Cleansing 34
   Avi Shai and Howard I. Maibach

6. Creams and Liquid Emulsions for Facial Cleansing 41
   Avi Shai, Howard I. Maibach, and Robert Baran

7. Facial Cleansing Masks 43
   Avi Shai, Howard I. Maibach, and Robert Baran

8. Skin Aging and Its Management 46
   Avi Shai, Howard I. Maibach, and Robert Baran

9. Acne 58
   Alex Zvulunov

10. Sun and the Skin 77
    Dafna Hallel-Halevy

11. Networks of Blood Vessels on the Skin 92
    Moshe Lapidoth

12. Cellulite 98
    Ron Yaniv

13. Injection Lipolysis: A New Method of Body Contouring 102
    Franz Hasengschwandtner

14. Inflammation, Dermatitis, and Cosmetics 106
    Arieh Ingber and Avi Shai

15. **Skin Tumors** 115
    Avi Shai and Daniel Vardy

16. **Active Ingredients in Cosmetic Preparations** 131
    Gil Yosipovitch

17. **Retinoic Acid** 143
    Avi Shai, Howard I. Maibach, and Robert Baran

18. **α-Hydroxy Acids** 148
    Ron Yaniv and Stanley Levy

19. **β-Hydroxy and Polyhydroxy Acids** 155
    Stanley Levy, Avi Shai, and Howard I. Maibach

20. **Bleaching and Bleaching Preparations** 158
    Avi Shai, Robert Baran, and Howard I. Maibach

21. **Astringents** 166
    Avi Shai, Robert Baran, and Howard I. Maibach

22. **Preparations Used in Dermatology** 168
    Marcelo H. Grunwald

23. **Liposomes** 175
    Alex Zvulunov

24. **Chemical Skin Peeling** 179
    Josef Shiri

25. **Laser and Light Treatments in Dermatology and Their Cosmetic Applications** 187
    Moshe Lapidoth

26. **Fillers and Soft Tissue Augmentation** 193
    Ines Verner and Christopher Rowland Payne

27. **Cosmetic Use of Botulinum Toxin** 201
    Ines Verner and Christopher Rowland Payne

28. **Mesotherapy** 207
    Evangeline B. Handog and Encarnacion R. Legaspi-Vicerra

29. **Camouflaging Skin Lesions and Other Disfiguring Conditions** . . . 212
    Victoria L. Rayner

30. **Hair Structure and Its Care** 220
    Emilia Hodak

31. **Shampoo** 229
    Avi Shai, Robert Baran, and Howard I. Maibach

32. **Hair Conditioners** 237
    Itzchak Shelkovitz-Shilo

33. Methods for Temporary Hair Removal *Zehava Laver*	*241*
34. Permanent Hair Removal: Electrolysis *Zehava Laver*	*249*
35. Nails *Marina Landau and Robert Baran*	*257*

Appendix 1. *Applying Cosmetic Preparations to the Face and Neck* 266
Appendix 2. *Camouflaging Disfiguring Conditions* 268
Appendix 3. *Fragile Nails* 271
Appendix 4. *Glossary* 273

Index 283

Contributors

Robert Baran
Nail Disease Center
Cannes
France

Marcelo H. Grunwald
Professor of Dermatology
Ben-Gurion University
Senior Dermatologist
Department of Dermatology
Soroka University Medical
 Center
Beer-Sheva
Israel

Sima Halevy
Professor of Dermatology
Ben-Gurion University
Chairman, Department of
 Dermatology
Soroka University Medical Center
Beer-Sheva
Israel

Dafna Hallel-Halevy
Lecturer, Ben-Gurion
University
Senior Dermatologist
Department of Dermatology
Soroka University Medical Center
Beer-Sheva
Israel

Evangeline B. Handog
Vice-Chair, Department of Dermatology
Asian Hospital and Medical Center
Philippines

Franz Hasengschwandtner
Network Lipolysis - Scientific & Medical
 Director
Medical Director of Spa-Clinic and Therapy
 Center
Bad Leonfelden
Austria

Emilia Hodak
Professor of Dermatology
Tel Aviv University
Senior Dermatologist
Department of Dermatology
Rabin Medical Center
Petah-Tikva
Israel

Arieh Ingber
Professor of Dermatology
The Hebrew University
Chairman, Department of Dermatology
Hadassah Medical Center
Jerusalem
Israel

Marina Landau
Senior Dermatologist
Department of Dermatology
Ichilov Medical Center
Tel Aviv
Israel

Moshe Lapidoth
Senior Dermatologist
Head of Laser Center
Rabin Medical Center
Petah-Tikva
Israel

Zehava Laver
Senior Dermatologist
General Health Fund
Tel Nordau
Tel Aviv
Israel

Encarnacion R. Legaspi-Viverra
Consultant, Dr. Victor R. Potenciano
 Medical Center
Philippines

Stanley Levy
Adjunct Clinical Professor of
  Dermatology
University of North Carolina School
  of Medicine
Chapel Hill, North Carolina,
  and Director of Medical Affairs
Revlon Research Center
Edison, New Jersey,
USA

Howard I. Maibach
Department of Dermatology
University of California
San Francisco School
  of Medicine
San Francisco, California
USA

**Christopher Rowland
  Payne**
Consultant Dermatologist
The London Clinic
Devonshire Place
London
UK

Victoria L. Rayner
Dermatology Associate
University of California
Director of Training
Center of Appearance & Esteem
  Training Institute
San Francisco, California
USA

Avi Shai
Department of Dermatology
Soroka University Medical Center
Ben-Gurion University
Beer-Sheva
Israel

Itzchak Shelkovitz-Shilo
Senior Dermatologist
Sheba Medical Center
Tel Hashomer
Israel

Josef Shiri
Senior Dermatologist
Chairman, Tel Aviv Institute of Dermatology
General Health Fund and Sheba
  Medical Center
Tel Hashomer
Tel Aviv
Israel

Daniel Vardy
Professor of Dermatology
Ben-Gurion University
Senior Dermatologist
Beer-Sheva
Israel

Ines Verner
Senior Dermatologist
Department of Dermatology
Tel Hashomer University Hospital
  & Clinic of Dermatology and Aesthetics
Kiriat Ono
Israel

Ron Yaniv
Senior Dermatologist
Sheba Medical Center
Tel Hashomer
Israel

Gil Yosipovitch
Professor of Dermatology
Department of Dermatology,
  Neurobiology and Anatomy, and
  Regenerative Medicine
Wake Forest University Health Sciences
Winston-Salem, North Carolina
USA

Alex Zvulunov
Senior Lecturer, Ben Gurion
  University
Senior Pediatrician and Dermatologist
Pediatrics Dermatology Unit
Schneider Children's Medical Center
Petah-Tikva
Israel

Notes for the Reader

This book provides a clear and easily understandable review of the topics presented, while maintaining a purely scientific approach, conforming to data supported by scientifically researched criteria. The book relies on common, accepted knowledge in the field of dermatology, as it appears in the conventional dermatology textbooks and peer reviewed journals [such as those cited on Medline (PubMed), a computerized database of medical journal articles].

Sections of the text are highlighted in boxes—these present a more detailed explanation and discussion of some of the topics, and are intended for the more advanced reader.

Readers are advised to read first the introductory chapter on skin structure, as this provides definitions of several basic terms such as "epidermis" and "dermis," which are used throughout the book.

Many of the chapters discuss common skin problems and conventional skin treatments, such as bleaching of dark skin spots and peeling. These chapters are intended to broaden the reader's knowledge regarding the wide range of available regimens, and not to encourage readers to diagnose and treat skin disorders requiring the advice of a dermatologist.

The editors welcome corrections and suggestions for the next edition of the book.

Acknowledgments

The authors wish to thank the following for their valuable help and contribution to this text: Professor Reuven Bergman, Professor Sima Halevy, and Professor Michael David for reviewing chapters in the book; Dr. Emanuela Cagnano for the figures on pages 5 (lower) and 81 (upper middle); Dr. Rodney Dawber (two illustrations on page 237); Elsevier for the illustrations on page 144 (reproduced from Olsen EA et al., Tretinoin emollient cream: A new therapy for photodamaged skin. *J Am Acad Derm* 1992; **26**:215–224), on page 151 (reproduced from Ditre CM et al., Effects of α-hydroxy acids on photoaged skin: A pilot clinical, histologic, and ultrastructured study. *J Am Acad Derm* 1996; **34**:187–195), and on page 152 (reproduced from Bergfeld W et al., Improving the cosmetic appearance of photoaged skin with glycolic acid. *J Am Acad Derm* 1997; **36**:1011–1013); Audra J. Geras and Novartis for the illustrations on pages 5 (upper), 8, 79, and 118 (lower); Dr. Marcelo H. Grunwald for the figure on page 125 (bottom right); Professor Axel Hoke for the figures on pages 94 and 96 (upper left); Dr. L. Kachko for the figures on pages 9 and 47 (upper A, B); Professor Ronald Marks for the illustrations on page 120 (upper and 123 (right), which are taken from his book, *Skin Disease in Old Age*, 2nd edition (Martin Dunitz, 1999); Dr. Bernardo Mosovich for the figure on page 122 (upper); Mr. Naftali Oron for his most valuable ongoing advice throughout the course of this project; Janssen Pharmaceutica for the illustration on page 234; Dr. AA Ramelet (two illustrations on page 95); RN Richards and GE Meharg, for the figures on pages 244, 250, 252, and 253, which are taken from their book, *Cosmetic and Medical Electrolysis and Temporary Hair Removal: A Practice Manual and Reference Guide*, Second edition (Medric Limited, 1997); Dr. Timothy J. Rosio (four illustrations on page 187 and 188); Professor Berthold Rzany for illustrations on pages 202 and 203; Professor Amiram Sagi for the figure on page 125 (upper right); Nikolaus J. Smeh for the figures on pages 134, 135 (upper), and 136, which are taken from his book, *Creating Your Own Cosmetics—Naturally* (Alliance Publishing House, 1995); Dr. Gil Yosipovitch for his initiative in this project; our particular thanks to Dr. Gary Zentner for his assistance with editing and preparation of the text; and the following contributors to Robert Baran and Howard Maibach (eds), *Textbook of Cosmetic Dermatology*, 2nd edition (Martin Dunitz, 1998) who have kindly allowed their material to be used.

Finally, our particular thanks to Dr. Gary Zentner for his assistance with editing and preparation of the text; to Dr. Gil Yosipovitch for his initiative in this project; to Professor Reuven Bergman, Professor Sima Halevy, and Professor Michael David for reviewing chapters in the book; to Dr. Alex Zvulunov for his assistance and for his contribution, stemming from a broad knowledge in medicine and dermatology, of the table on page 173–174; and to Mr. Naftali Oron for his most valuable ongoing advice throughout the course of this project.

Notes on the Second Edition
During the last decade, there have been vast and rapid changes in the field of cosmetics and skin care. In the making of this edition, the editors invested much effort in bringing this book up to the current level of knowledge by adding chapters on the latest developments and updating the entire text. The editors wish to thank Ms Kristina Hawthorne for her significant contribution in the preparation of this edition, and Miss Abigail Shai for her active participation in the proofreading process.

1 | Cosmetics and Cosmetic Preparations: Basic Definitions

Avi Shai, Robert Baran, and Howard I. Maibach

Contents Basic definitions • Definition of a cosmetic product • Classification of cosmetic preparations • The gray area between a drug and a cosmetic product

BASIC DEFINITIONS

Cosmetics deals with those aspects of the skin related to beauty. This profession concentrates on skin care, protecting the skin, and improving its appearance. The word "cosmetic" is derived from the Greek *kosmesis* (adorning), from *kosmeo* (to order or arrange).

A **cosmetician** is a person engaged in the field of cosmetics, whose work is directed toward the care, protection, and improvement in the appearance of the skin.

Dermatology refers to the medical specialty of diagnosing and treating diseases of the skin, hair, and nails.

A **dermatologist** is a physician specializing in the various aspects of skin disease.

The term **cosmetology** is relatively vague and cannot always be found in dictionaries. It refers to the scientific and investigative basis of cosmetics, with its biological, chemical, and medical ramifications.

The term **cosmetologist** is derived from the term "cosmetology." In its broad meaning, it refers to someone who specializes in the investigative aspects of cosmetics: he/she can be a chemist, a biologist, or a physician. However, this definition varies from one country to another. In some countries, such as the United States, it is a formal title subjected to the regulations of each individual state. To become a cosmetologist, one has to graduate from a school of cosmetics. In other countries, however, there is no recognized medical/professional specialty of cosmetology so, in practice, the title of "cosmetologist" may be used by anyone who decides to call himself/herself as such.

DEFINITION OF A COSMETIC PRODUCT

The U.S. Food, Drug and Cosmetic (FDC) Act defines cosmetics as:

(1) Articles intended to be rubbed, poured, sprinkled or sprayed on, introduced into, or otherwise applied to the human body or any part thereof for cleansing, beautifying, promoting attractiveness, or altering the appearance; and
(2) Articles intended for use as a component of any such articles except that such a term shall not include soap.

There is a significant difference between cosmetic products and drugs (including drugs intended for application to the skin), which the reader should be familiar with. Drugs are defined in the FDC Act as including:

articles intended for use in the diagnosis, cure, mitigation, treatment or prevention of disease in man ... articles (other than food) intended to affect the structure or any function of the body of man.

It follows from the above that a cosmetic product (not being a drug) is not meant to affect the structure or function of the skin. However, nowadays this strict definition is becoming more and more blurred.

CLASSIFICATION OF COSMETIC PREPARATIONS

Cosmetic preparations are classified in accordance with their function:

- those that improve appearance and beautify
- those related to skin care
- those related to skin protection

Improving Appearance and Beautifying
The aim of beautifying products is to impart a pleasant and attractive appearance by emphasizing those areas of the face or body that look better, in order to focus the observer's gaze on them. At the same time, an attempt is made to camouflage less attractive areas and correct skin lesions, if necessary. This category of cosmetic products includes various makeups, hair dyes, and nail polishes, etc.

Skin Care
Cosmetics are used to obtain and retain a smooth, soft and supple skin. Moisturizing and cleansing preparations belong to this category. Some have a protective effect.

Skin Protection
The aim of protective products is to shield the skin from the external effects of the sun, wind, cold, etc. Sunscreen preparations belong to this category. Moisturizers also have a protective effect on the skin. Soaps that contain antibacterial substances are also included in this category, since they do provide a certain degree of antibacterial protection to the skin.

THE GRAY AREA BETWEEN A DRUG AND A COSMETIC PRODUCT

In the past, the division between cosmetic products and drugs was clear cut. Nearly all cosmetics were no more (and did not usually claim to be anything other) than simple moisturizing, cleansing, or coloring products.
    Currently, the boundary between drugs and cosmetic products for skin care is becoming blurred. Many cosmetic products are marketed with statements such as:

- "Accelerates the renewal of cells"
- "Builds up supportive tissue in the skin"
- "Repairs sun damage to the skin"
- "Repairs skin aging"

    All of the above effects can only be achieved by drugs, since they relate to changes in the function and structure of the tissue.
    Sometimes the difference between a cosmetic product and a drug lies in the concentration of the active ingredient in the product. For example, in low concentrations, α-hydroxy acids function essentially as moisturizing agents; it is only in higher concentrations that they have any significant effect on the epidermis.
    Not only the border between cosmetic products and drugs is hazy but there is also a gray area between cosmetic treatments and dermatology. A cosmetician's treatment can alter the structure and function of the skin—for example, in the treatment of acne, or in the application of permanent makeup, etc. Therefore, some modern cosmetic products lie in an increasingly gray area and can almost be defined as medications. This fact confers a serious responsibility on those involved in cosmetic treatment, requiring them to have a fairly deep knowledge of the subject, and to exercise careful judgement when using the cosmetic products at their disposal.

Cosmeceuticals

The term "cosmeceuticals" was first popularized by the dermatologist, Professor Albert Kligman, in the mid 1980s. This term comprises a combination between the terms "cosmetics" and "pharmaceuticals" and refers to preparations between these two groups.

The need to reclassify the traditional approach originates from the FDC Act, defining drugs as compounds that affect the structure of the skin or its function, as opposed to cosmetic products.

According to FDC Act definitions, a cosmetic product is not supposed to change or affect the structure or function of body tissue. With the accumulation of more and more knowledge in the physiology and pharmacology of the skin, it has become evident that every cosmetic preparation and every compound, even the most simple, may alter the skin up to a certain extent. The degree of alteration merely depends on the concentration of each material and duration of exposure. It is clear, however, that not every cosmetic product can be regarded as a drug. There is an area between what can be considered purely a drug or purely a cosmetic. The term "cosmeceuticals" (or "active cosmetics") serves to define those products which may exert some beneficial effect on the skin but cannot be regarded as having a clear biological therapeutical effect, which would require them to be classified as drugs.

The classical products which may be regarded as cosmeceuticals are retinol preparations, which are less potent than tretinoin (the latter being a drug). Other products that may be regarded as cosmeceuticals are, for example, α-hydroxy acids, β-hydroxy acids, and certain bleaching agents.

The term "cosmeceuticals" remains controversial. It has not been accepted by all researchers. For the time being, it has no legal standing in most countries and has not been recognized by the FDA. In the cosmetics industry, it is used to indicate products that may have beneficial effects due to certain physiological activities. The term, therefore, has an additional marketing value.

2 | Skin Structure

Avi Shai, Robert Baran, and Howard I. Maibach

Contents Overview • Skin thickness • Functions of the skin
• Epidermis • Dermis • Subcutis: the layer of fat beneath the dermis

OVERVIEW

Familiarity with the structure and function of the skin is essential for a clear understanding of this book.

The skin, the largest organ in the human body, is composed of two layers: the epidermis and the dermis. Underneath the dermis lies the subcutis, which consists mainly of fat cells.

- **Epidermis**—The epidermis forms the outer layer. At the base of this layer, the cells continuously divide, forming new cells. As cells are made, they are pushed toward the surface by the newer cells underneath them, and eventually reach the keratinous layer. Finally, the outermost cells in the keratinous layer are shed.
- **Dermis**—The dermis forms the layer below the epidermis and is thicker than the epidermis. The dermis is mainly made up of collagen and elastin fibers. It also contains blood vessels, nerves, sensory organs, sebaceous glands, sweat glands, and hair follicles.
- **Subcutis**—This layer lies beneath the dermis and consists of fat cells.

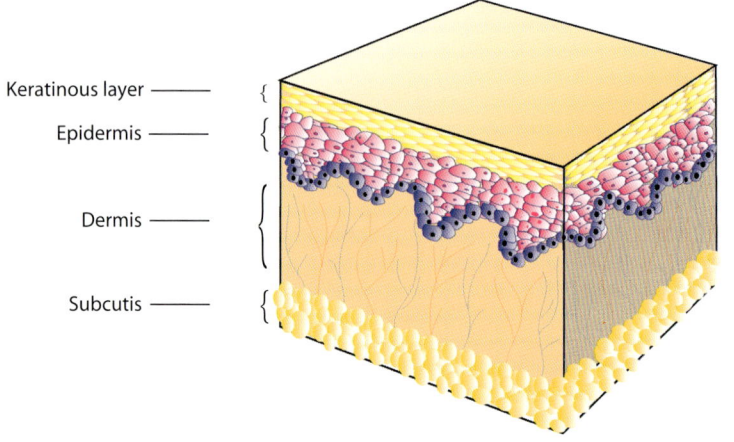

Structure of the skin.

SKIN THICKNESS

Skin thickness ranges from 1 to 4 mm. This thickness, and those of each of its layers, varies in different areas of the body.

The epidermis is generally thin. It is particularly so in the skin of the eyelids: approximately 0.1 mm. The epidermis is particularly thick in the soles and palms, where it is approximately 1 mm deep.

The dermis is up to 20 times as thick as the epidermis. It tends to be particularly thick on the back, where it can be approximately 3 to 4 mm.

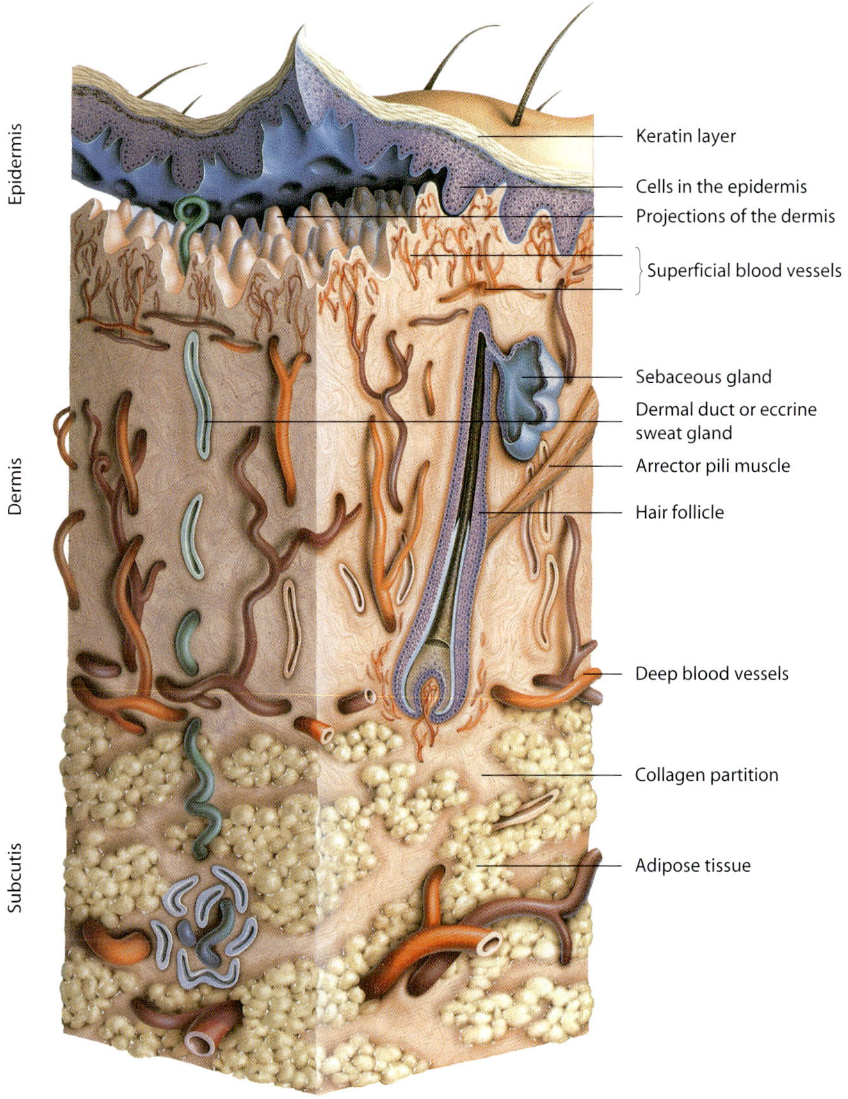

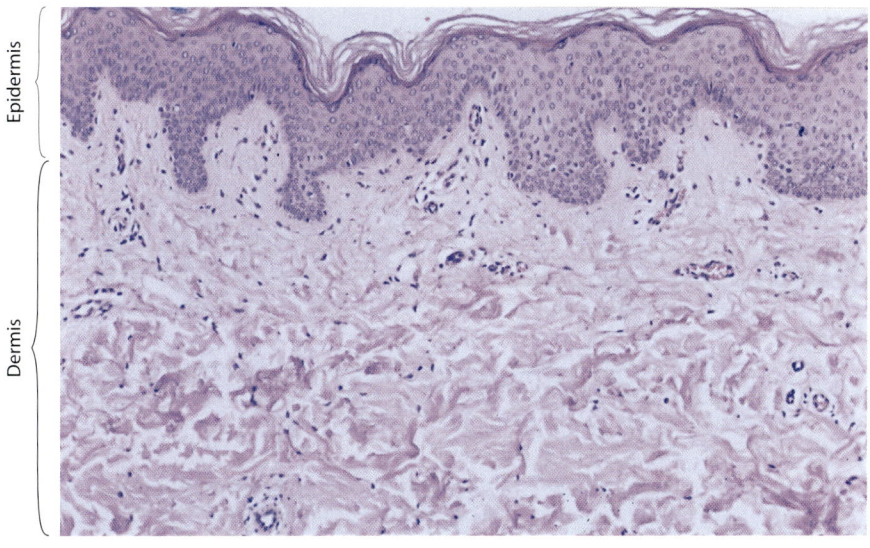

Transverse section through the skin.

Skin structure viewed through a microscope lens.

There is also variability in the thickness of the subcutis skin layer, which tends to be thicker in the thigh and abdominal areas, and particularly thin in the face.

FUNCTIONS OF THE SKIN

The skin

- acts as a protective layer,
- transmits sensations,
- helps to regulate the body's temperature,
- produces vitamin D, and
- plays a role in social interactions.

Protective Layer

The outermost layer of the skin is made of a tough keratin that serves as a covering that protects the body from mechanical damage such as that caused by friction, different levels of pressure and various kinds of impact, chemical toxins, ultraviolet rays from the sun, and infectious agents such as bacteria and fungi. The skin is continuously exposed to bacteria, but the tightly packed structure of the cells in the keratin layer renders it relatively impermeable and thereby prevents bacteria from penetrating the skin.

The skin serves not only to protect the body from the external environment but also to prevent loss of water from the body. If it were not for this important property, the body would lose substantial amounts of water to an extent that would threaten life. The importance of this function can be seen in patients whose skin has been damaged, for example, by widespread burns. These patients suffer enormous fluid losses, and initial resuscitation must always include the provision of large volumes of fluids.

Bacteria and Fungi

Many bacteria reside on the skin surface, but these usually cause no harm. Provided the skin is normal and healthy, and the keratin layer is intact, these bacteria cannot penetrate and enter the skin. As a rule, most bacteria found in the human body are not pathogenic, that is, they do not cause disease. However, any damage to the skin, be it a burn, a wound, or any other damage, can result in bacteria invading the skin and causing infection.

In contrast to bacteria, certain types of fungi can invade the keratin and damage its integrity; this explains why fungal skin infections are more common than bacterial infections. Furthermore, once the fungi have damaged the skin's integrity, it is easier for bacteria to invade the skin, so it is common for bacterial infections to occur in skin already infected by a fungus.

Transmission of Sensations

The dermis is richly supplied with nerves, which transmit sensations of touch, pressure, pain, and temperature from the skin.

Temperature Regulation

As water, such as perspiration, on the surface of the skin evaporates, it has a cooling effect. The amount of sweat released from the skin varies depending on the body temperature and the environmental conditions, and may reach several liters per day.

The body temperature is regulated by alterations in the amount of blood flowing to the skin, and in the evaporation of water.

Production of Vitamin D

Sunlight stimulates the production of vitamin D in the skin. The vitamin then passes from the skin into the blood, and reaches the various tissues of the body where it exerts its effects. Vitamin D is essential for the regulation of calcium levels in the body, and for the structure and growth of bones. Recent studies have also suggested that an appropriate amount of vitamin D may assist in preventing certain kinds of malignancies, diabetes, and certain disorders of the immune system.

Social Interaction

The skin—through its color, texture, and smell—"transmits" sexual and social messages. Thus, blushing, resulting from the dilatation of blood vessels in the skin, reflects embarrassment. Facial expressions reflect various emotions.

THE OUTER LAYER: EPIDERMIS

Epidermis: Keratinocytes

The epidermis is the outermost layer of the skin, made up of approximately 15 to 20 tightly packed layers of cells. Most of the cells in this layer are **keratinocytes**, or **squamous cells** (Latin: *squama* = scale). Each cell is a few thousandths of a millimeter in size.

As seen in the figure below, the lowermost layer of the epidermis is the **basal layer**, obviously called such because the cells that comprise it form the base of the epidermis.

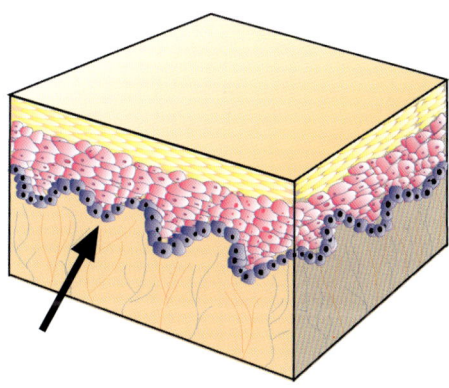

The basal layer of the epidermis.

In the basal layer, new epidermal cells are formed by cell division. The skin cells formed in the basal layer are pushed upward by younger cells until they are ultimately shed from the surface of the skin. This is a continuous process. Every moment, without our being aware of it, our skin is renewing itself as millions of cells slowly move outward.

As the cells move upward, their shape becomes flatter and flatter. As they move, they start to degenerate, and gradually lose their vitality. They lose water content, dry out, and flatten. By the time they reach the outermost layers, the cells are dead.

The outermost layer of the skin is the **keratinous (horny) layer** (Greek: *keras* = horn). There the cells are dead, flattened, and lie closely packed on each other like roof tiles. The cells of the outer layers contain large quantities of a protein called **keratin.** It takes approximately 28 days from the time a new cell forms in the basal layer until it is shed from the surface of the skin. This means that most cells of the skin are replaced by new ones every 28 days.

The keratinous layer is made of tightly packed dead cells, which gives the skin the protective capabilities listed above.

Increased Turnover of Cells in the Epidermis

In various diseases, such as psoriasis or seborrheic dermatitis, there is an increase in the turnover of cells in the skin, so keratin accumulates abnormally on the skin's surface. This takes the form of thick scales or flakes.

Other Epidermal Cells: Langerhans Cells, Melanocytes

In addition to the keratinocytes, there are also other types of cells contained in the epidermis: *Langerhans cells* and *melanocytes*.

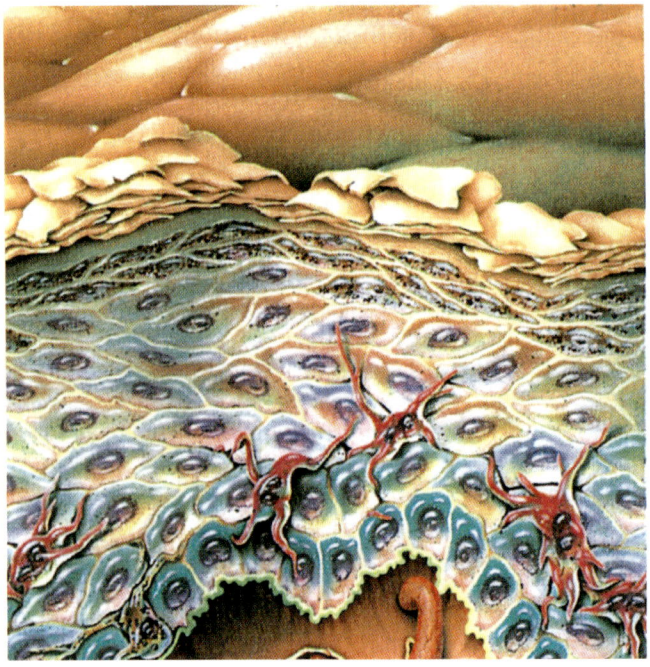

Melanocytes (shown in red) scattered throughout the cells of the epidermis.

Langerhans Cells

Langerhans cells are involved in the body's immune system.

Melanocytes

Melanocytes produce a pigment called **melanin**, which gives the skin its dark color. The melanin produced by melanocytes is passed on to the keratinocytes. Approximately 1 in 10 cells in the basal layer of the epidermis is a melanocyte.

The differences in skin color between individuals and races are determined genetically by the amount of melanin produced by the melanocytes and its distribution throughout the skin. In fact, differences in skin shade and color are determined not by the number and density of the melanocytes, which are basically identical in all humans of any race, but by their degree of activity.

Sunlight exposure stimulates the production of melanin.

DERMIS

The dermis lies beneath the epidermis. Its upper level has projections that extend into corresponding depressions in the epidermis.

The dermis is mainly composed of an amorphous (i.e., without shape or structure) intercellular substance that acts as a sort of "cement" for all the components of the dermis. Within this amorphic substance are

- cells of the dermis,
- collagen and elastin fibers,
- blood vessels,
- nerves and sensory organs,
- sebaceous glands,
- hairs, and
- sweat glands.

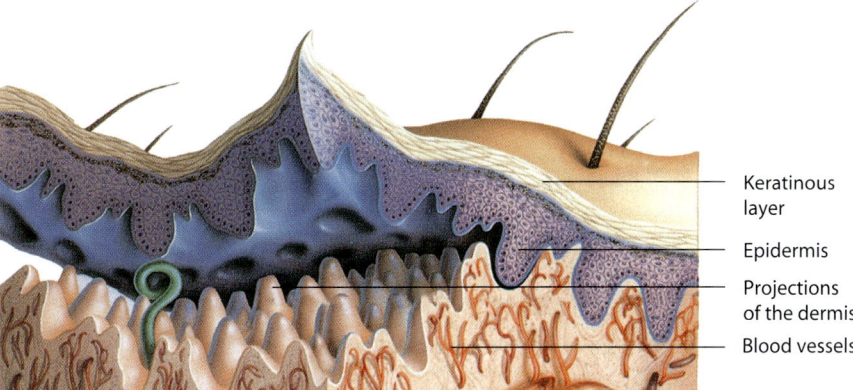

Schematic representation of the wave-like junction between the epidermis and the dermis, with corresponding projections and depressions.

Dermal Cells

The main cell of the dermis is the **fibroblast**. This cell produces the intercellular substance as well as collagen fibers.

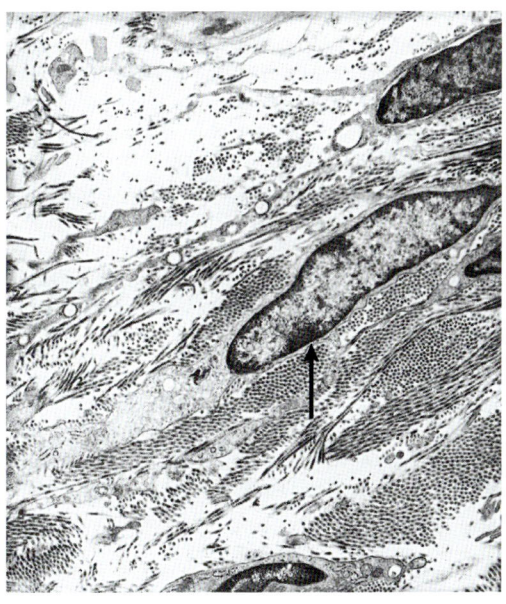

Fibroblast (indicated by the arrow) as seen under the electron microscope; the round-shaped bodies seen in this picture are collagen fibers in transverse section.

Other cells within the dermis include **white blood cells** (**leukocytes**), which are involved in the defense against infections. Under normal circumstances, their number in the dermis is negligible. The number of leukocytes increases when there is inflammation or infection in the skin.

Collagen and Elastin Fibers

Collagen and **elastin** are proteins in the form of fibers. The fibers are intertwined throughout the intercellular substance, and provide the dermis with its strength and elasticity. The collagen fibers give the skin its strength. Elastin fibers are thinner than collagen fibers; they are responsible for the skin's elasticity—its ability to "spring back" to its original form after being stretched. If these fibers are damaged as a result of aging, or from excessive, cumulative exposure to the sun, the skin becomes loose, does not return to its original state when stretched, and looks thin and wrinkled.

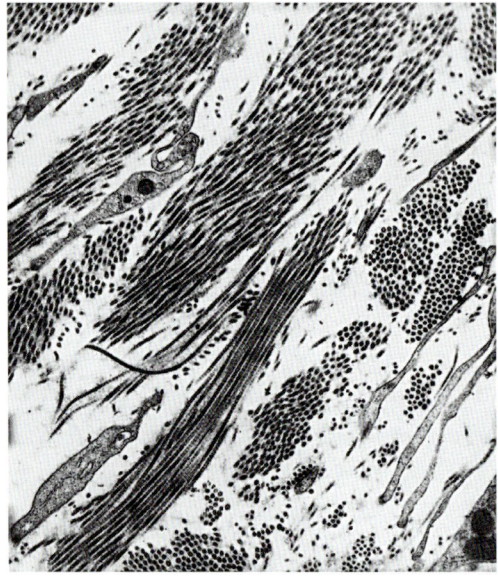
Collagen fibers as seen under the electron microscope.

Blood Vessels in the Dermis

The major function of the blood is to transport nutrients and oxygen to every organ in the body, including the skin, and to remove waste products and carbon dioxide produced in the various cells of the body. Note that there are no blood vessels in the epidermis. The epidermis receives its nutrients and oxygen directly from the dermis, which is richly endowed with blood vessels.

In the dermis, the blood vessels (which are continuations of larger vessels deeper in the body) branch out into smaller and smaller vessels that cover the entire area of the skin. Widening and narrowing (dilatation and constriction) of the blood vessels occurs in response to changes in temperature, and form one of the most important mechanisms for controlling the body's temperature. Dilatation of the blood vessels results in the skin becoming pinker, or even red—as seen in blushing or when the temperature rises.

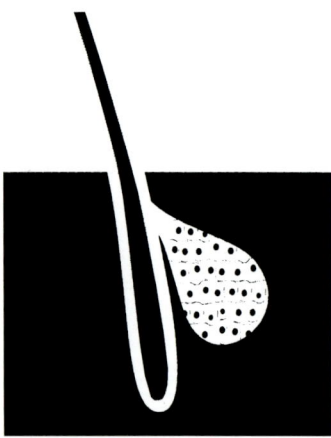
A hair follicle with its sebaceous gland.

Sebaceous Glands

These glands are attached to the hair follicles, and their contents are secreted into the follicle through a tiny duct. The glands secrete **sebum**—a fatty substance that emerges from the opening of the hair follicle onto the skin surface and coats the skin with an oily layer.

Hair

Hair is present on every area of the body except for the palms and soles, the red areas of the lips, the skin over the knuckles, and the genital organs. Hair grows out of an elongated tubular structure in the skin called a **hair follicle**, as shown in the diagrams on page 11.

Each hair has an elongated section, which grows from the dermis and protrudes above the surface of the skin, known as the **shaft** (or **body**) of the hair. At the lower end of the hair follicle, there is a swelling, where the **hair root cells** are found. These cells have a striking capacity for replication. As they divide, the new cells so formed at the root of the hair are aligned vertically and move upward; thus the hair grows longer and longer. As the cells move upward, they die off—in the same way as do the skin cells in the epidermis (the keratinocytes) as they move up to the surface of the skin.

The upper part of the hair that protrudes above the skin surface is therefore composed of keratinous "dead" matter. The main substance in the hair cells that died as they moved upward is a special form of the protein keratin. The keratin in hair is hard and is therefore called **hard keratin**, which differs in its chemical composition from the keratin of the horny layer of the skin.

The shaft of the hair is made up of a large number of thin, delicate, intertwined fibers. The main component of these fibers is, as noted above, keratin.

Attached to the hairs are tiny muscles (**arrectores pilorum muscles**). When these muscles contract, the hair stands up. These muscles have nothing to do with the secretion of sebum. In some animals, the contraction of these muscles causes the fur to stand up—in response to danger, etc.; in the human, the sudden contraction of these muscles in a given area causes "goose bumps." The structure and life cycle of hair is dealt with in more detail in chapter 30.

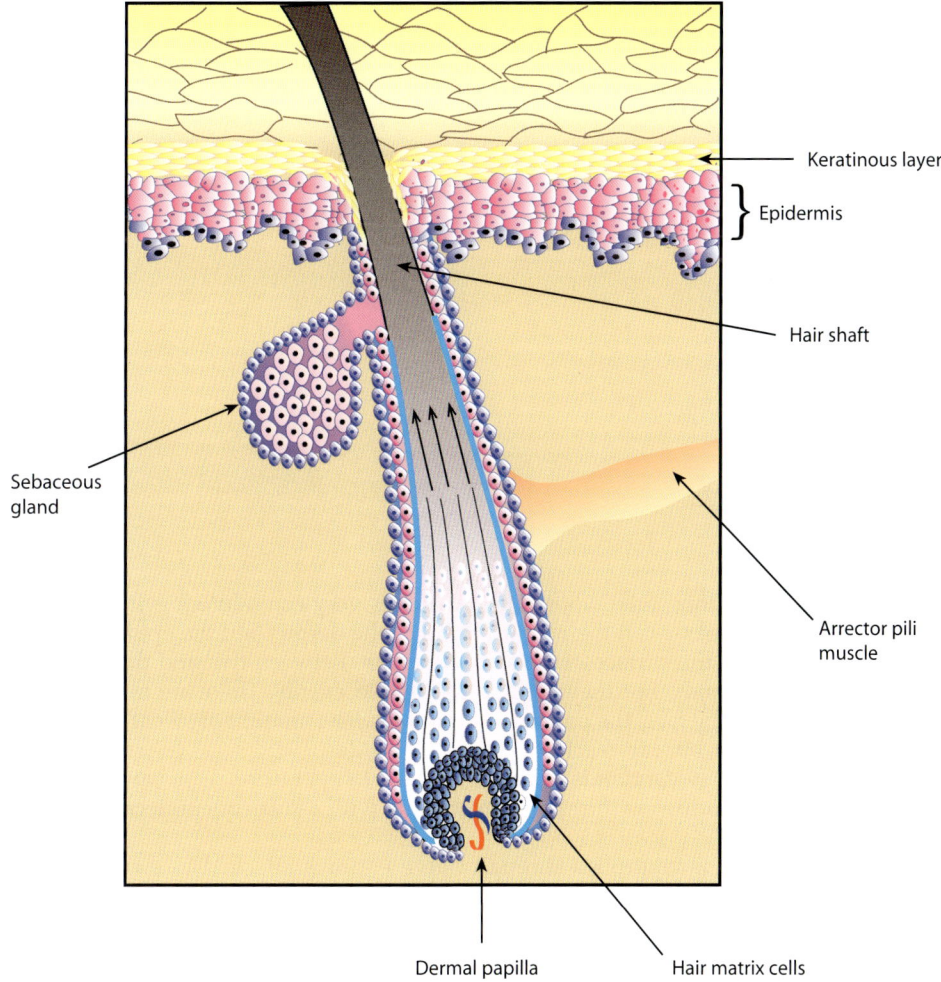

Structure of hair.

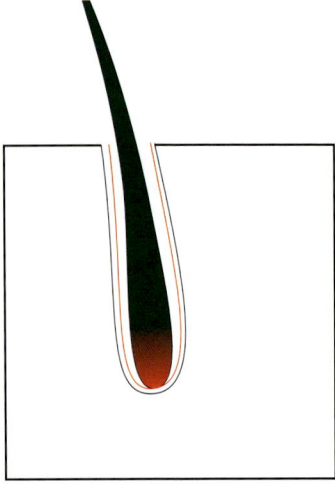
Schematic representation of a hair follicle (shown in red).

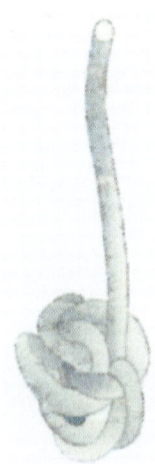
Eccrine sweat gland.

Eccrine Sweat Glands

An **eccrine sweat gland** is a long tube whose base, which is very convoluted, is in the lower part of the dermis. The tube passes all the way up through the dermis and the epidermis, and ends as a tiny sweat pore on the surface of the skin. There are between two and three million eccrine sweat glands in the body, but they are not distributed evenly. There are more eccrine sweat glands in the areas of the face, the palms, and the soles. The amount of sweat also varies considerably from day to day, but can reach several liters in a day.

The main function of the sweat glands is to regulate body temperature. As sweat evaporates from the surface of the skin, it lowers the skin temperature, with a subsequent decrease in the body's temperature.

The secretion of sweat is controlled through nerve endings attached to sweat glands. Physical effort, warm weather, fever, or emotional stress stimulate the sweat glands, which secrete sweat. Sweat is largely water, with small amounts of salts. Usually, the sweat secreted by eccrine sweat glands does not cause body odor.

> ### Apocrine Sweat Glands
>
> These glands, unlike the eccrine sweat glands, are not distributed on most of the skin surface. They are larger and more convoluted than the eccrine sweat glands and are found mainly:
>
> - in the armpits,
> - in the genital area, and
> - around the nipples.
>
> Similar glands are present in the external ear canals and the eyelids. These sweat glands are present at birth, but only develop and start to secrete during adolescence. They have no obvious physiological function in humans. In other mammals, the apocrine glands produce an odor involved in sexual attraction.
>
> The secretion from the apocrine glands is relatively thick and has a "milky" consistency. This secretion is responsible for the formation of body odor. When secreted, it has no smell. As the organic compounds in it are broken down by bacteria, the by-products of this process give off an unpleasant odor.

SUBCUTIS: THE LAYER OF FAT BENEATH THE DERMIS

This layer of fat beneath the dermis acts as a cushioning layer to protect vital inner organs from mechanical trauma, and also as an insulating layer to protect against cold. In addition, the fat is an important energy store for the body.

The amount and distribution of the fat depends largely on hereditary factors, on diet, and on physical activity.

Groups of fat cells are separated by rigid partitions made up mainly of collagen fibers, as illustrated in the figure below.

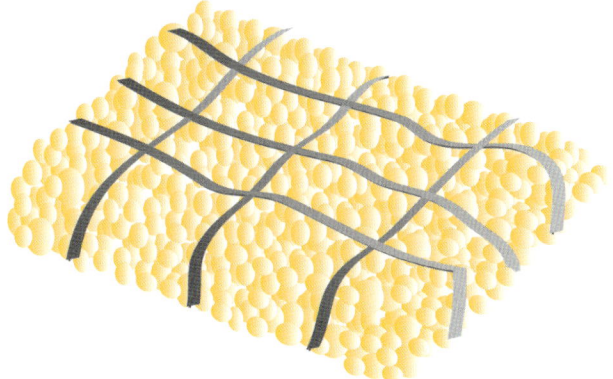

Groups of fat cells separated by collagen partitions.

3 | Principles in the Preparation of Medical and Cosmetic Products

Sima Halevy and Avi Shai

Contents Overview • Bases in cosmetic and medical products: fatty bases • Bases in cosmetic and medical products: aqueous solutions • Bases in cosmetic and medical products: powders • Combinations of bases • Combining a fatty base with water • Types of creams • Combining powder with water: suspensions • Combining powder with a fatty base: pastes • Other combinations • Gels • Preservatives • Organic cosmetic preparations • Summary

OVERVIEW

This chapter reviews the principles used in the preparation of medical and cosmetic products. The same principles are applied in the preparation of medical and cosmetic compounds for the skin, except that the former incorporates a medication or medications to treat a particular skin abnormality. Both medical and cosmetic preparations for application to the skin are called **preparations for external use**. A preparation for external use consists of the following three components:

- an active ingredient,
- a base (or vehicle), and
- an additional/auxiliary substance

In neither medical nor cosmetic use is the active ingredient meant to be applied to the skin in its pure chemical form. The active ingredient is combined with a base and with other substances to create the effective preparation. This combination ensures that the active ingredient penetrates the skin.

Active Ingredient
The active ingredient might be, for example:

- an antibiotic medication, used for the treatment of acne or a bacterial skin infection,
- an antifungal medication to treat a skin infection caused by a fungus,
- a substance intended to inhibit aging of the skin (e.g., retinoic acid or an alpha-hydroxy acid), or
- a substance that lightens dark lesions on the skin (e.g., hydroquinone).

The active ingredient is the main component of the preparation for external use, whose action produces the main effect. However, as stated above, the active ingredient does not appear on its own. It must be incorporated into the base of the preparation.

Base (Vehicle)
This is the material that "carries" the active ingredient into the skin. It is called the "base" or the "vehicle", in the sense of transporting something, since it "conveys" the active ingredient to the skin. The base must ensure that the active ingredient remains chemically stable, can penetrate the skin, and can be released effectively within the skin. The three elemental bases are:

- fatty bases,
- aqueous (water) solutions, and
- powders.

By using one of the above, or a combination of them, the wide array of bases used in dermatology and in the cosmetics industry can be produced: ointments, creams, emulsions, solutions, powders, pastes, suspensions, or lotions.

The role of the base in a medical or cosmetic preparation is not merely a wrapping for a medicine or an active ingredient in the preparation, or a vehicle that transports the active ingredient into the skin. In many cases, the base itself may have specific effects on the skin, such as increasing the moisture level, soothing, or cooling, as will be described further on.

A considerable portion of the cosmetics industry is devoted to these bases alone, without the addition of any active ingredients.

Additional/Auxiliary Substances

Medicinal or cosmetic preparations usually also contain other substances. Common additives are:

- fragrances and perfumes,
- dyes, and
- preservatives.

BASES IN COSMETIC AND MEDICAL PRODUCTS: FATTY BASES

The main uses of fatty bases in dermatology and cosmetics are as follows:

- Fatty bases may enable medicines incorporated within them to better penetrate the skin.
- Fatty bases increase the skin's moisture level by creating an oily film on its surface, thus reducing the amount of water evaporating from the skin.

Fatty bases may be derived from animal sources, plant sources, or mineral sources (the most common mineral source is crude oil, from which various oils can be derived after refining). In general, fatty bases from any of those sources can be in liquid, semisolid, or solid form. The terminology commonly used is as follows:

- A fatty base that appears in liquid form (at room temperature) is called an **oil**.
- A fatty base that appears in semisolid form is called a **fat**.
- A fatty base that appears in solid form is called a **wax**.

> Widely Used Terminology Regarding Fatty Bases and their Chemical Definitions
>
> The above definitions are those in everyday use but are not strictly accurate in terms of the chemical definitions of oils, fats, and waxes. Furthermore, it should be remembered that the chemical and cosmetics industries can alter the physical properties of fatty substances and mix them with other substances. Thus, for example, a substance that was originally a liquid (oil) can appear in a semisolid state as part of a particular compound.

Animal-Derived Fatty Bases

Lanolin
This complex compound, derived from sheep's wool, is made from the oily substance secreted by the sheep's sebaceous glands, and is a basic ingredient in many moisturizing compounds. In its original, pure form, lanolin is a yellowish-gray, sticky substance with a characteristic smell. By chemical and physical processes, numerous substances with different properties can be derived from lanolin, substances that are less sticky, odorless, of different shades, etc.

Since lanolin is fairly similar in composition to sebum, which is secreted by human sebaceous glands, it rarely causes irritation when applied to the skin. Nevertheless, skin sensitivity can occasionally occur due to lanolin or lanolin-based products.

Wool Alcohols
These substances are also derived from sheep's wool. Chemically, wool alcohols contain more alcoholic oily compounds than does lanolin—a quality that enables these substances to contain more water in their composition.

Spermaceti
This is an oily substance produced by whales. Its use is prohibited in the United States. In view of the source of this oil, consumers who have reservations about the killing of whales may prefer not to use moisturizing preparations that contain this substance, and should check the details on the package of any moisturizer to ensure that it does not contain spermaceti. Synthetic spermaceti, on the other hand, is a chemically synthesized wax that can be used as a replacement for natural spermaceti.

Note: The way in which all these animal-derived oils act on the skin is identical. There is no significant difference in the cosmetic or medicinal value of the different substances. They have no effect in preventing skin aging. There is no advantage in using oils derived from rarer animals, and their use is only an uncalled-for commercial gimmick. Mink oil, for example, produced from the skin of minks, or whale-derived oil has no advantage over lanolin in terms of their cosmetic or medicinal effects.

Plant-Derived Fatty Bases: Plant Oils
Oils derived from plants include, for example, olive oil, sesame oil, peanut oil, corn oil, sunflower oil, soy oil, and cocoa butter. The chemical composition of plant oils or animal-derived oils and the presence of saturated fatty acids or unsaturated fatty acids are significant in regard to diet and nutrition. However, it is of no relevance in regard to the external use of these oils. In terms of their cosmetic and dermatological effects, the efficacy of plant oils is similar to those that are animal-derived, and the ratio of polyunsaturated to saturated oils in their composition is irrelevant.

Fatty Bases Derived from Minerals
Fatty bases derived from minerals include the paraffin oils, which are products of the refining of crude oil. Substances derived from paraffin can be in a liquid, semisolid, or solid state:

- liquid paraffin (liquid petroleum),
- semisolid paraffin, white soft paraffin (petroleum jelly, semisolid petrolatum), or
- solid paraffin (wax).

The natural color of paraffin is yellow, but it usually undergoes chemical bleaching processes. Paraffin is an efficient occlusive and thus can inhibit water evaporation from the skin. Being inert, it very rarely causes skin irritation and sensitivity. However, it is not convenient for day-to-day use, since it produces an unpleasant greasy feeling on the skin.

In general, different fatty bases can be mixed together to achieve the desired properties. For further details on the cosmetic preparations that contain animal-, plant-, or mineral-derived fatty bases, see chapter 4 on skin moisture and moisturizers.

What Is an Ointment?
An **ointment** describes a preparation (medical or cosmetic) that is meant to be applied to the skin and whose base is composed of fatty substances; the fatty bases of the ointment produce the typical semisolid consistency.

The fatty base may allow better skin penetration of the active ingredients incorporated within the ointment. Thus, various medications can be incorporated into an ointment producing, for example, antibiotic ointments or corticosteroid ointments.

The "classic" ointments, such as petroleum jelly, are based on fatty substances derived from minerals. Petroleum jelly is an inert, water-repelling substance that creates an occlusive layer on the skin. Fatty preparations derived from minerals (as compared with other types of skin preparations) are better occlusives, which protect the skin more effectively, and also tend not to rinse off the skin so readily.

Products based on fatty substances such as lanolin or eucerin can contain water. The addition of water to the oil makes the product more aesthetically pleasing; it is less sticky, more pleasant to the touch, and easier to use.

As described below, when a small amount of water is added to a fatty base that is in a semisolid state, it is still called an ointment. However, above a certain amount of water, the preparation becomes a **cream**.

BASES IN COSMETIC AND MEDICAL PRODUCTS: AQUEOUS SOLUTIONS

The most common liquid used in cosmetic preparations is water. Usually, in dermatology, water is not used on its own, but with a medication or some other active ingredient dissolved in it (the same way as sugar or salt can be dissolved in water), producing a solution. In solution, molecules of the dissolved substance spread equally and are evenly distributed in the water. Therefore, a solution has a clear and uniform appearance.

Water can be combined with various forms of cosmetic substances. As discussed below, it can also be mixed with oils or powders.

Water has additional effects on the cooling and drying of the skin. Since water evaporates from the skin's surface, it has a cooling effect. As the water evaporates, it "drags" with it additional water found in the outer layers of the skin—so wetting the skin frequently with water actually has a drying effect! Consequently, in dermatology, when we want to dry out inflamed, weeping areas of skin, we do so by repeatedly wetting those areas.

Tinctures

Alcohol can also be used in cosmetic preparations. Since alcohol evaporates faster than water, it has an even stronger cooling effect. Alcohol is also effective, to some extent, in killing bacteria. However, the higher the concentration of the alcohol, the more it tends to irritate the skin. An alcohol-based solution is called a **tincture**.

BASES IN COSMETIC AND MEDICAL PRODUCTS: POWDERS

In both the cosmetics industry and dermatology, use is made of fine powders that do not contain coarse particles. Powders are made of one or more solid ingredients. They are intended for application to healthy skin. The main purposes of powders are to prevent friction and to absorb excess moisture.

Powders are usually used in skin creases (such as the groin), since those are the areas where moisture tends to accumulate, and where friction occurs. In addition, in cosmetics, powders are used in many types of makeup preparations to cover and conceal certain areas of the skin.

Substances Commonly Used in Powders

Among the substances used in powders are the following:

- **zinc oxide**, which has covering and protecting properties;
- **titanium dioxide**, which has protective properties against ultraviolet rays and is a significant component of sunscreens;
- **talc**, which is actually the commercial name for **magnesium polysilicate.** (Commercial preparations usually contain small amounts of other substances, such as zinc oxide or aluminium silicate. Talc is an inert substance that is effective in preventing friction);
- **calamine**, a mixture of zinc oxide with a small amount of iron oxide. It has a soothing effect on the skin and can decrease itching to some extent; and
- **starch**, which absorbs liquids effectively and is therefore used in the treatment of excessively moist skin.

In general, it is not advisable to use pure powders on babies, since, as the powder is being applied to the skin, the fine particles disperse into the air, and may be inhaled.

COMBINATIONS OF BASES

So far, we have discussed the three elemental bases—fatty bases, water and aqueous solutions, and powders.

A combination of various bases in different preparations creates the extensive range of cosmetic and medicinal substances intended for application to the skin. This is usually illustrated using a colored triangle, which shows how different combinations of the various bases can create a wide variety of preparations:

- Combining a **fatty base** and **water** produces a **liquid emulsion** or **cream.**
- Combining **powder and water** produces a **suspension.**
- Combining a **fatty base** and **powder** produces a **paste**.

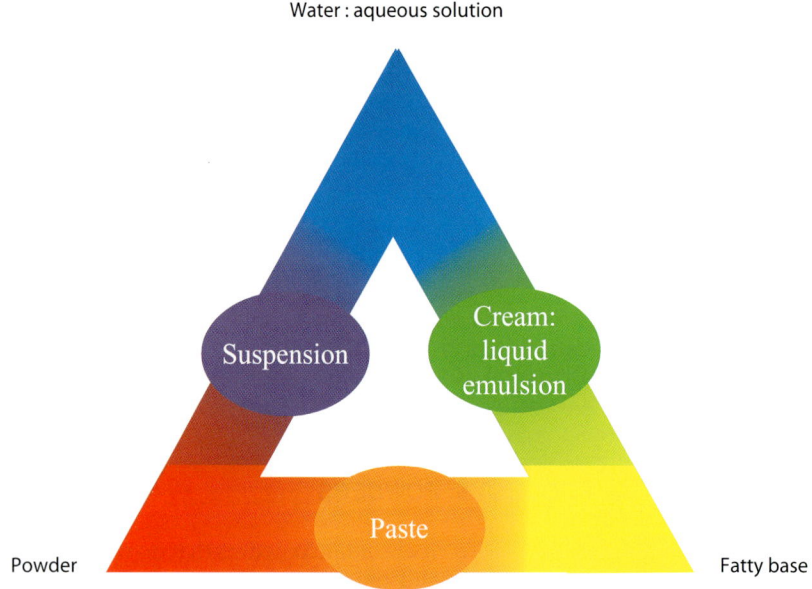

Triangle illustrating the various possibilities in combining bases.

COMBINING A FATTY BASE WITH WATER

Mixing Water and Oil

What happens when water and oil are poured together into the same vessel? Since oil does not dissolve in water, the answer is simple: the oil floats on top of the water, since its specific gravity is less than that of water.

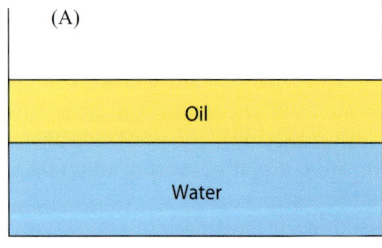
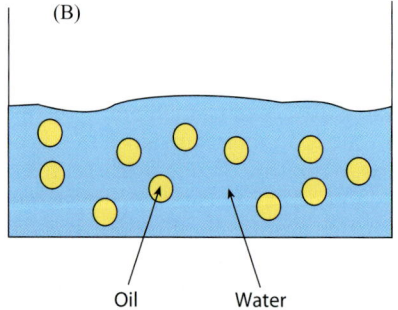

(A) Vessel containing oil and water.   *(B) After mixing the oil and water.*

When oil and water are mixed together, there is a brief moment when there will be a uniform mixture of oil and water, with drops of oil equally dispersed in the water.

Note that we are not talking here about dissolving oil in water (and creating a solution)—that is impossible, since oil is not soluble in water. We are referring to the even dispersion of oil droplets in the water. A mixture of oil and water is called an **emulsion**. When the mixing ceases, the oil will once again float to the top of the water.

To maintain the situation with the oil and water remaining uniformly mixed, we use a substance called an **emulsifier**. An emulsifier stabilizes the emulsion—the mixture of oil dispersed in water or water in oil—so that the oil and water remain "mixed" for a long time. There are two kinds of emulsions:

- When there is more water than oil, the oil is dispersed within the water.
- When there is more oil than water, the water is dispersed within the oil.

When the amount of water in the emulsion is relatively large, the end product is a liquid, and is called a **liquid emulsion**. If the end product of the emulsion is in a semisolid state, the product is a **cream**.

Creams are emulsions that appear in semisolid form, with varying degrees of viscosity. Both liquid emulsions and creams are based on a combination of a fatty base with water. The fatty content of these preparations provide moisture to the skin.

Liquid emulsions, creams, and ointments are themselves used as bases (vehicles) in dermatological preparations. Chapter 4 deals mainly with such preparations: liquid emulsions, creams, and ointments.

TYPES OF CREAM

There are many types of cream in cosmetics, each used for its specific purpose, and advertised under different names. Here, we shall review the main groups of creams:

- vanishing creams,
- night creams,
- cleansing creams,
- moisturizing creams,
- foundation creams,
- cold creams, and
- eye creams.

Vanishing Creams

These are creams with a relatively high water content. Because of their "watery" nature, they are easy to wash off. The water in the cream has a cooling effect. Since they do have some oil content, vanishing creams nevertheless have some moisturizing effect on the skin. However, they do not have a significant occlusive effect (compared to, for example, ointments, which have a much higher oil content). Since vanishing creams are easier to apply, and to wash and wipe off the skin, they are usually used as daytime creams. Usually other substances, such as sunscreens or various medications (e.g., antibiotics) or some other active ingredient (such as retinoic acid), are added to these creams.

The advantage of using a vanishing cream is that once it has been applied to the skin, it is almost transparent, and the thin film of cream on the skin surface is hardly noticeable.

Various medical and cosmetic preparations are promoted as vanishing creams to emphasize the fact that they are transparent, and invisible once they have been applied.

Night Creams

Night creams, because of their higher oil content, are greasier and more occlusive than vanishing creams but less oily and less occlusive than ointments. They are, therefore, used as moisturizers and are intended for use on dry skin. They have no cooling effect.

Night creams are also known as "nourishing" creams, since they are supposed to contain various substances that penetrate the skin. To enable these substances to penetrate better, the cream should remain on the skin for several hours. Hence, "nourishing" creams are applied at night, before going to bed. Because they are greasy, they tend to stay on the skin longer. The "nutritional" components of these creams comprise active ingredients that are supposed to have a beneficial effect on the skin once they have penetrated into the deeper skin layers. The topic of "skin nutrition" and the effects of various cosmetic substances on the skin are dealt with in chapter 16.

Cleansing Creams
Cleansing creams are basically mixtures composed of oil, water, and certain substances intended to cleanse the face. These creams are discussed in chapter 6 on creams and liquid emulsions for facial cleansing.

Moisturizing Creams
These creams, designed to increase the skin moisture content, are based on occlusives, which produce an impermeable barrier on the skin surface, and on humectants, which absorb water. This topic is dealt with in detail in chapter 4 on skin moisture and moisturizers.

Foundation Creams
Foundation creams are basically moisturizing creams. They usually contain coloring agents as well. Many of them also contain a sunscreen. As well as keeping the skin moist and protecting it from the sun, foundation creams provide a smooth, even color to the face and are used to conceal skin blemishes. These creams are available in a range of shades, so that every woman can find the appropriate color for her skin.

Cold Creams
Cold creams have a cooling effect. The cooling occurs because these creams are "pseudo" emulsions, rather than true emulsions. A cold cream is a simple mixture of oil and water. It does not contain an emulsifier, and so is not a stable product. Hence, when applied to the skin, the water separates from the oily component, and quickly evaporates from the skin, thus creating a cooling effect (hence the name "cold cream").

Cold cream was developed about 2000 years ago. In its original form, it contained olive oil, water, beeswax, and rose petals, creating its characteristic aroma.

The oily component provides a cleansing effect if the cream is wiped off the skin, since the oil removes the natural oily layer of the skin surface, in which the grime particles are embedded. Cold cream can serve as a moisturizer as well because of its oily component.

Over the years, many variations on the cold cream have been developed, but the original basic composition of oil, water, and wax still exists. Cosmetics companies still produce cold creams, some of which are marketed as moisturizing preparations, and some as cleansers.

Eye Creams
Preparations that are meant to be applied to the delicate skin around the eyes are mainly hypoallergenic preparations. This means that they do not contain components such as certain perfumes and/or certain preservatives that are known from past experience to have a higher-than-average risk of causing skin irritation and allergies. Nevertheless, there is no doubt that even eye creams may result in allergic reactions in some people, albeit very rarely.

COMBINING A POWDER WITH WATER: SUSPENSIONS

Salt and sugar dissolve in water. The salt or sugar molecules are disseminated uniformly throughout the water, and the end product is called a **solution**—characterized by its clear, uniform appearance.

The substance in which the solid is dissolved, i.e., the solvent, is usually water, but other substances can also function as solvents, for example, alcohol (as already mentioned, a solution in alcohol is called a **tincture**). Not all substances are soluble in water. The particles in talc, for example, are too large to dissolve in water. When mixed with water, the resulting fluid is turbid.

By combining an insoluble powder with water, we obtain a **suspension**. A suspension has a cooling effect on the skin, because of the evaporation of the water. Once the water has evaporated, a layer of powder remains on the skin. It is important to shake a suspension well before applying it to the skin, so as to spread the particles of powder evenly throughout the liquid.

COMBINING A POWDER WITH A FATTY BASE: PASTES

A **paste** is the result of combining a powder with a fatty base. The fatty base is usually petrolatum (petroleum jelly). The powder usually comprises 20% to 50% of the preparation. A paste is less greasy than regular ointment, but it still has occlusive and protective properties because of its fatty content.

Because a paste contains powder, it has the ability, as opposed to an ointment, to absorb liquids to a certain extent. This gives pastes certain advantages over ointments: the main use of pastes is for protecting babies' skin from urine and stool in the diaper area. It is the contact between the infant's excretions and the skin that causes the inflammation known as **diaper rash**.

A paste may be "hard" or "soft." Soft paste has more fatty component and less powder, rendering it with skin-protective qualities. Hard paste, on the other hand, has more powder and less fatty component, rendering it with absorbent qualities. In general, pastes are not used for cosmetic purposes, but rather for dermatological uses. As stated above, the combination of their protective function together with their absorbent properties makes pastes eminently suitable for treating diaper rash in babies.

There are preparations for the treatment of diaper rash that are not pastes. Some are fatty preparations that contain substances such as allantoin or Peru balsam, which are reputed to have a "soothing" effect.

Note: It is important to emphasize that preparations designed for use for diaper rash are only meant for simple, mild skin inflammation. If the inflammation is severe, or if there is no improvement within a reasonable time, there may be an associated bacterial or fungal infection, and in this case, the infant should be examined by a physician.

OTHER COMBINATIONS

Lotions

While the commonly understood meaning of the term "lotion" covers all the liquid preparations—solutions, suspensions and emulsions—in dermatology, a lotion is sometimes regarded as a unique combination of a powder and a solution, with glycerine (glycerol) added to obtain the desired texture.

A typical and well-known example of a lotion is **calamine lotion**, widely used to treat itching. It is mainly made up of calamine (zinc oxide with a small amount of iron oxide), together with a little glycerine. As mentioned above, the glycerine contributes to an appropriate texture and prevents the lotion from feeling too chalky on the skin.

Powder, Water, and Oil

Certain liquid preparations may contain not only powder and water but oil as well. Adding oil to the preparation helps to prevent dryness of the skin. By the same token, there are pastes that, in addition to the fatty and powder components, also contain water.

Note: The above definitions are the accepted medical/scientific ones. However, certain cosmetic preparations do not adhere strictly to those definitions. For example, certain products may be marketed as emulsions, or "facial cleansing emulsions," when, in fact, in terms of their composition, they are actually lotions or solutions.

GELS

Similar to the bases discussed earlier, a **gel** may also function as a base for various cosmetic and medical skin preparations. A gel is a semisolid, nongreasy, colorless, transparent substance that tends to evaporate when in contact with warm skin.

Composition of Gels

In its basic form, a gel is a solution, in which the solvent may be water, acetone, alcohol, or propylene glycol. Another type of gel is one whose basic state is that of a liquid emulsion: in other words, an oil/water combination. However, whether we are speaking of a gel that is basically a solution or one that is basically a liquid emulsion, there is an additional modification: in gels, the original preparation undergoes a process of thickening by the addition of various substances, resulting in a more viscous and less watery product—the extent depending on the desired degree of viscosity. The higher level of viscosity enables a gel preparation to adhere better to the skin than do liquid preparations.

When Is a Gel Preferable to a Cream?

Since creams do not contain thickeners, they need to contain a higher amount of fatty base in order to achieve the same degree of viscosity and adherence as a gel. Gel products can contain up to 70% water, and very low oil content. Therefore, gels are usually designed for use on oily skin, on which we do not want to use an oily substance but prefer a more watery preparation. Similarly, preparations intended for the skin of the scalp are usually gel based, in order to avoid excess oiliness of the hair.

Note that certain active ingredients mix better in a cream (or ointment) while others mix better in a gel.

PRESERVATIVES

A cosmetic or medical skin product may contain various microorganisms (bacteria or fungi) that come from the raw materials used in its manufacture, from the equipment used, from the packaging, or from exposure to the workers in the factory. Preservatives are chemical substances intended to prevent the proliferation of such microorganisms and the subsequent decay of the product.

Common Preservatives Used in Cosmetics

Nowadays, there are several dozens of chemicals that are used as preservatives in the cosmetic industry. These preservatives, which may be listed on the package, include:

- benzoic acid,
- imidazolidinyl urea,
- benzyl alcohol,
- parabens,
- formaldehyde,
- quaternium 15, and
- kathon CG.

A preservative may contain one ingredient or a mixture of certain ingredients. For example, the preservative Euxyl 400 actually represents a combination of several ingredients.

In cases where an allergic reaction develops following the use of a certain cosmetic preparation, the source of the reaction is not necessarily the active ingredient, but may be induced by one of the preservatives contained in the preparation.

Vitamin A and C, being antioxidants, may also be used as preservatives in the cosmetics industry. They are considered to be gentler than other preservatives and seem to cause less irritation or allergic reactions. However, for prolonged and efficient protection, many products have to include other preservatives as well.

As long as the level of microorganisms is within the required standards set by the relevant authorities, there should be no complications. However, with time, these microorganisms can continue to multiply within the cosmetic preparation, which could affect the properties of the preparation and may have a deleterious effect on the skin.

The use of preservatives is a necessary evil. It is better to add a preservative to a cosmetic preparation, as required by the relevant standard, than to use a defective or moldy preparation that may contain bacteria or fungi. Bacteria tend to replicate within the watery phase of cosmetic preparations, so in products with a high water content there is a higher risk of bacterial or fungal contamination.

How Can Contaminated Products be Recognized?

A substance infected by bacteria develops an unpleasant smell. Generally, it loses its uniform texture, and there is a definite separation into its two phases: watery and oily. There may be various discolored areas on the surface of the product—these discolored patches are, in fact, colonies of bacteria or mold.

How to Avoid Contamination

The shelf life of a cosmetic or medical product depends on the storage conditions. The more appropriate the storage conditions, the more stable the product. After leaving the manufacturer, it should not be exposed to sunlight or high temperatures; most cosmetic and medical products should be stored in a cool, dark, and dry place. Only products displaying an expiry date should be used.

Avoid leaving bits of paper or cotton wool inside the container after using the product, since these are the main sources of bacterial contamination.

Cosmetic or medical preparations should not be transferred to empty jars. Similarly, remnants of an older product should not be mixed with a fresh product of the same type, since this may lead to contamination of the latter.

A cosmetic product whose color, texture, or smell has changed should not be used.

ORGANIC COSMETIC PREPARATIONS

In its accepted meaning, a cosmetic preparation presented as "organic" is not supposed to contain chemicals and artificial additives such as preservatives, synthetic coloring agents, or artificial fragrances. Organic cosmetic preparations are usually perceived by the public as healthy and safe. However, in practice, the manufacturing of a 100% organic product cannot always be implemented. This requires avoiding the use of preservatives, which leads to a short shelf life of the product.

In some countries, the definition of "organic" is subject to manufacturers' arbitrary decisions. In other countries, there are organizations that closely supervise the manufacturing of what are claimed to be organic products.

SUMMARY

- The base of any cosmetic or medical product for use on the skin is either a fatty base, water, powder, or various combinations thereof.
- By using these bases or various combinations of them, different types of cosmetic and medical products are produced: powders, aqueous solutions, ointments, creams, emulsions, suspensions, pastes, and lotions.
- An active ingredient and other supplementary substances (where necessary) are added to the base to produce the final product.

4 | Skin Moisture and Moisturizers

Avi Shai, Howard I. Maibach, and Robert Baran

Contents Overview • What causes dry skin? • Significance of skin moisture: characteristics of dry skin • The beneficial effects of moisturizers • Natural factors that prevent skin dryness • Wetting the skin • Moisturizers: occlusives and humectants • How to select a moisturizer • Guidelines for use of moisturizers • The difference between moisturizers for the face and those for the body • Moisturizers for the hands • Summary

OVERVIEW

The water content in the skin (dermis and epidermis) is approximately 80%. The outer skin layer, the keratinous layer, is made up of dead skin cells, and has a lower water content of approximately 10% to 30%.

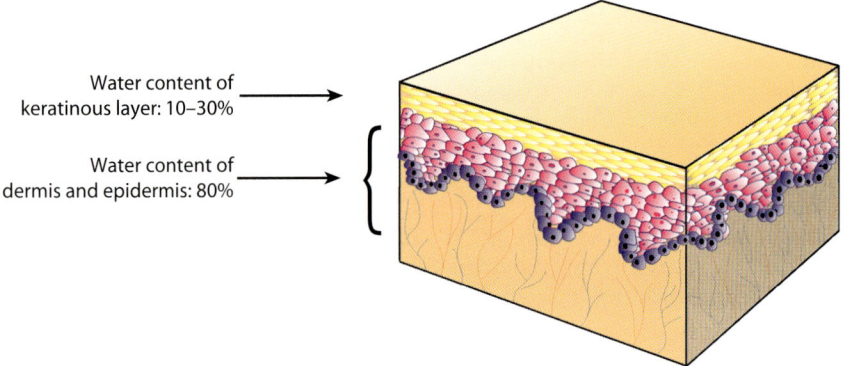

Water content of the skin.

The water content of the keratinous layer allows for a certain amount of suppleness. When the water content of the skin is normal, it appears soft, smooth, supple, and glowing. The skin is slightly filled out with water, which tends to smoothen the fine wrinkles.

In normal skin, there is a continuous movement of water from the deep layers to the superficial layers. Eventually, the water evaporates from the surface.

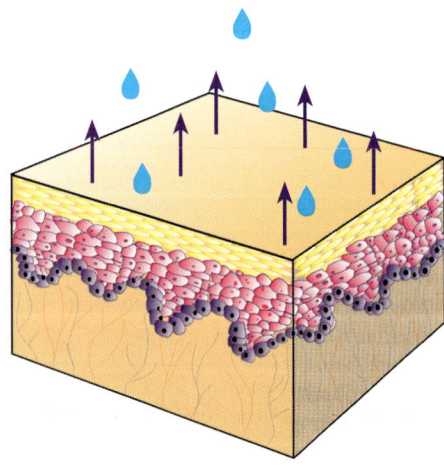

Evaporation of water from the skin surface.

WHAT CAUSES DRY SKIN?

Dry skin is relatively common: most people experience skin dryness, to some extent, from time to time. Dry skin can result either from external causes or from the skin's inability to retain its moisture.

External Causes

The major external causes of dry skin are exposure to dry environments and wind. Artificial indoor heating lowers the relative humidity, which dries out the skin even further. Therefore, the skin tends to be dryer in the winter. Air-conditioning, with cold, dry air being blown into the room, can cause the skin to become dry as well. Other external factors that influence the moisture level of the skin are:

- washing, and
- exposure to certain substances.

Washing
Frequent washing repeatedly removes the oily layer that protects the skin and actually serves to hold in the moisture. Certain types of soaps have a particularly drying effect.

Exposure to Certain Substances
Various occupations are characterized by exposure to substances that remove the natural oily layer from the skin surface, such as those occupations involving frequent exposure to detergents or solvents. Similarly, certain medical treatments (such as some for acne) cause dryness of the skin.

The Skin's Ability to Retain Moisture

Aging is associated with physiological processes whereby the skin loses its ability to retain moisture. Furthermore, there are diseases in which the skin fails to retain body water normally, and significant amounts of water are lost. This occurs, for example, in **atopic dermatitis**, and in certain skin disorders resulting from dietary deficiencies.

SIGNIFICANCE OF SKIN MOISTURE: CHARACTERISTICS OF DRY SKIN

Skin with a low water content appears dry, fissured, and rough. It has a delicate layer of scales on its surface. Fine lines are more apparent. The individual perceives a feeling of dryness, which may be accompanied by itching.

Dry skin is more prone to skin infections, both bacterial, and fungal. The common dermatological term for extremely dry skin is **xerosis**.

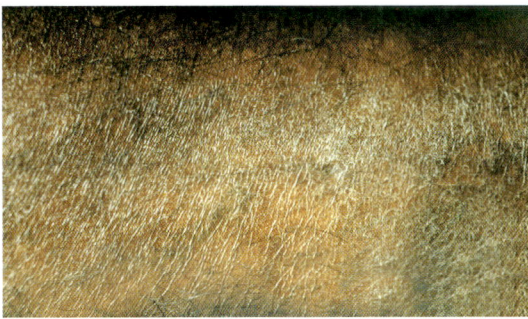

Dry skin.

Dry Skin

The skin loses its suppleness if its moisture content drops. Skin with a normal moisture content will slough off dead cells naturally. In dry skin, the superficial layers do not peel off easily and remain attached. The accumulated keratinous cells remain on the surface of the skin as scales.

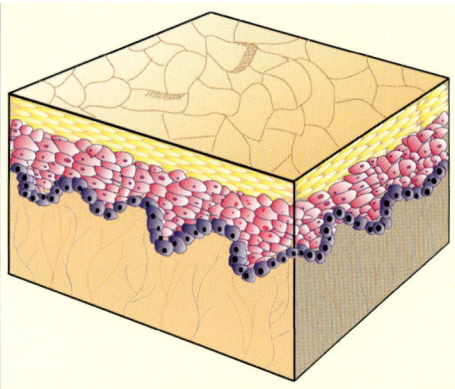
Microscopic structure of dry skin.

Dry skin seems rough and may be covered with a fine whitish scaling. It may also be itchy. In addition, extremely dry skin, which is tough and less pliable, tends to fissure. These fissures damage the integrity and continuity of the skin and interfere with its function as a protective layer. Subsequently, there is increased water loss, the skin becomes dryer, more fissures appear, and so the process is aggravated.

THE BENEFICIAL EFFECTS OF MOISTURIZERS

In stark contrast to advertisements concerning the "antiaging" or "age-reversing" qualities of certain moisturizing products, it has never been proven that standard moisturizers can prevent the aging process caused by advanced age or sun exposure. However, use of moisturizers may benefit the skin in several other ways by:

- **Preventing damage caused by dryness**: Protecting the skin from environmental factors and damage caused by dryness will help prevent deterioration in the appearance and quality of facial skin and will help maintain its texture.
- **Providing protection**: The thin oily layer on the skin surface can protect it from exposure to environmental factors such as soot particles, dirt, and dust.
- **Improving skin's appearance**: As previously stated, when the skin is well moisturized, it appears *temporarily* smoother and more refreshed. Since it is slightly swollen, there is flattening and virtual obliteration of fine wrinkles. The pores also appear somewhat smaller, since the skin surrounding them is slightly swollen. This temporary improvement may be exploited by advertisers claiming an "antiaging" effect in marketing various moisturizing products.

Note: Not everyone requires moisturizers, and individuals with oily skin usually have no use for them. However, during exposure to certain environmental conditions, such as dry air and cold wind, they may be needed. Older people, whose skin is usually dryer, may require such products more frequently.

NATURAL FACTORS THAT PREVENT SKIN DRYNESS

The skin is protected naturally from dryness by an oily layer and a natural moisturizing factor:

- **An oily layer on the skin—the lipid film**
- **Natural moisturizing factor**

The Lipid Film
The lipid film decreases water evaporation. It serves as a relatively occlusive layer above the keratinous layer. This layer is a combination of oily products on the skin surface, and includes mainly the sebum secreted by the sebaceous glands, and various lipid degradation products

that are formed during the process of skin maturation. As the epidermal cells traverse upward, chemical changes occur in them. Eventually, cell death occurs, and various degradation products, partly lipid, are formed.

Natural Moisturizing Factor

The "natural moisturizing factor" is the name given to a combination of several compounds created in the skin, comprising approximately 20% to 25% of the keratinous layer. These compounds serve to retain the water content of the keratinous layer.

> Natural Moisturizing Factor
>
> Among the compounds that compose the natural moisturizing factor are
>
> - urea,
> - lactic acid,
> - glycolic acid,
> - phospholipids,
> - malic acid,
> - pyruvic acid, and
> - salts of pyrrolidone carboxylic acid.
>
> We mention these compounds, since some may appear in various moisturizers and may be listed on the packaging.

WETTING THE SKIN

Wetting of the skin can be achieved in two ways:

- Soaking
- Repeated washing or repeated application of a damp cloth

Prolonged Soaking

When the skin is soaked in water, for example, when putting/immersing one's hand into a bucket/container full of water, the water penetrates the skin. If the soaking is prolonged, the water may cause damage. At first, the keratinous layer appears swollen and pale. At a later stage, maceration of the skin appears and the damage is more pronounced. An increase of the moisture to such a level causes a predisposition to infections, both bacterial and fungal, in the skin of the hands.

Repeated Washing or Repeated Placing of a Damp Cloth on Skin

When we allow the water that we have added (by washing or repeatedly placing a damp cloth on skin) to evaporate, a different situation arises. Here, the added water evaporates, and with it, water previously located in the outer layers of the skin. Thus, the quantity of water evaporated is *greater* than that which was applied. Subsequently, the skin's water content is less than it was at the beginning of the washing process. Although there is no conclusive scientific explanation to this phenomenon, frequent washing of the skin with water does have a drying effect. In dermatology, physicians apply this principle for drying inflamed and secreting skin areas by repeated washing, for a few minutes several times a day. Hence, water is not useful for retaining sufficient skin moisture. In order to preserve skin moisture one must apply moisturizers.

MOISTURIZERS: OCCLUSIVES AND HUMECTANTS

There are two principal preparations intended for preserving the moisture of the skin:

- occlusives
- humectants

Occlusives

Occlusives produce an oily layer on the skin, enriching the skin's natural lipid film, which prevents water evaporation. The keratinous layer dampens, becoming more fully saturated with water.

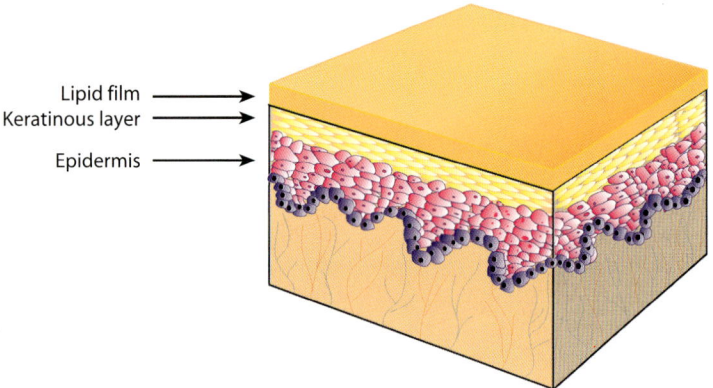

Lipid film over the keratinous layer.

These products are more effective if applied directly after washing, trapping a layer of water beneath them. Substances such as the following can be used:

- Mineral-derived fatty compounds such as paraffin or petroleum jelly (the most common mineral source is crude oil, from which various oils can be derived after refining). Cetomacrogol is another occlusive, mineral-derived compound that can be found in various moisturizers. Moisturizers based mainly on minerals are highly effective, but they are sticky and greasy. They are intended for people with very dry skin or for those having certain skin medical problems.
- Substances derived from animal fat, such as lanolin and its derivatives (derived from sheep's wool).
- Vegetable oils such as olive oil, oat oil, peanut oil, sesame seed oil, and many others.

Vegetable oils are less occlusive than animal-derived oils or mineral oil, yet allow sufficient occlusion.

Note: Oily products all function in the same way, preventing water evaporation from the superficial layers of the skin. There is no significant difference among the various fatty products derived from animals. None have any proven age-reversing abilities. Oils derived from rare animals are not superior, and their use is only an uncalled-for commercial gimmick.

Some moisturizing products contain a substance called **spermaceti**, which is produced from whales. The use of these products is prohibited in the United States. Those consumers who have reservations about the killing of whales should avoid using products containing this substance. One can read the label of contents on the product to ensure that it does not contain spermaceti.

Remember that occlusive products tend to be sticky and oily, so consumers will generally refrain from using products that appear in an oilier form (such as an ointment). Therefore, these products are generally combined as creams or lotions (which have a greater water content). These are easier to apply and are preferred by most consumers. After water evaporation, the occlusive components that remain will protect the skin and fulfill their function.

Humectants

Humectants absorb water. This group includes numerous substances, some of which are able to penetrate the keratinous layer and increase its water content.

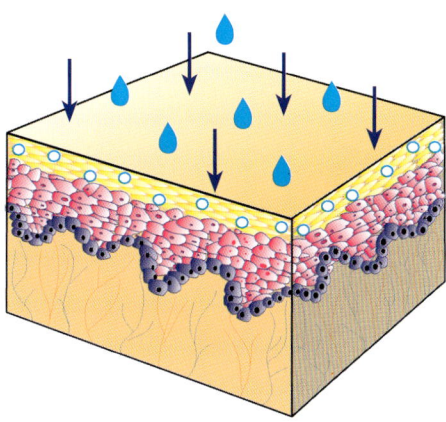

Water-absorbing substances (shown as clear circles) in the keratinous layer.

Other products from this group have large molecules that do not penetrate the keratinous layer, but form a hygroscopic (water-absorbing) layer on the skin. The effectiveness of several of these products is debatable. In a relatively arid environment, they may actually absorb water from the skin (rather than the environment), causing increased dryness. On the other hand, in a humid environment, they are clearly efficient. In conclusion, their efficacy is not as great as occlusive products in a cold, dry environment. Therefore, an efficient moisturizer suited to cold, dry weather, should contain a combination of occlusives and humectants.

In daily usage, moisturizing cosmetics made only from water-absorbing substances are called **nonoily moisturizers**.

From a practical point of view, the various approaches to skin moisturizing are not distinctly segregated. Most moisturizers have a number of components from each group. They usually contain occlusive, oily products along with humectants. In addition, a number of the components have a combined effect: lanolin and its derivatives, for example, are occlusives but they have a certain degree of absorptive capacity as well.

Humectants

The subtypes of humectants in use are as follows:

Products composed of relatively small molecules with efficient absorbing capabilities:

- glycerine (glycerol)
- sorbitol
- propylene glycol

Macromolecules
Products composed of larger molecules that are not able to penetrate the keratinous layer form a hygroscopic, water-absorbing layer on the skin. These include:

- glycosaminoglycans (such as hyaluronic acid),
- elastin, collagen, and other proteins.

Components of the natural moisturizing factor
The humectant group includes other products with absorbing capabilities. Since the natural moisturizing factor was identified, it was only logical to use its components in order to increase skin moisture. These components include

- sodium salts of pyrrolidone carboxylic acid,
- urea (in 10% to 20% concentrations),
- lactic acid, and
- phospholipids.

> Note that lactic acid belongs to the group of α-hydroxy acids. These have been introduced for cosmetic and dermatological use in recent years and are notable for their ability to increase the water content of the skin.
>
> The liposomes found in various cosmetic products are made up of phospholipids. Products containing liposomes also have a certain ability to increase the skin's moisture level (in addition to other advantages of the liposomes).
>
> Detailed descriptions of α-hydroxy acids and liposomes appear in chapters 18 and 23, respectively.
>
> In order to identify which moisturizers contain humectants, one can read the label of contents on the package and refer to the above list.

HOW TO SELECT A MOISTURIZER

Hundreds of moisturizers are available. They may contain substances previously mentioned. They may contain occlusive products, water-absorbing products, or a combination of these. They are sold in various formulations:

- Liquid emulsions
- Ointments
- Creams

The water content and lipid components differ in each formula type. Products rich in water are cool to the touch, and appear matte; products with a higher oil content cause a warm sensation, and the skin appears smooth and glossy. How does one determine the preferred moisturizer?

Skin Type
The foremost factor in selecting a moisturizer is the skin's lipid content.

Dry Skin
Dry skin lacks sheen. The pores are hardly noticeable. These individuals usually have lighter-toned skin. In extreme cases, as previously detailed, the skin will be scaly and fissured.

Oily Skin
Oily skin is glossy, especially on the forehead, nose, and chin. The skin is oily to the touch. Large pores are apparent. Individuals with this type of skin tend to suffer from acne as adolescents.

Normal Skin
This is somewhere between dry and oily skin. The skin is neither glossy nor oily to the touch, yet appears smooth and well moisturized. The pores are not large.

Combination Skin
This skin type is almost identical to the normal skin type. The T-zone, which includes the forehead, nasal bridge, nose, and center of the chin, has an increased level of sebaceous gland activity. The skin tends to be oily in these areas.

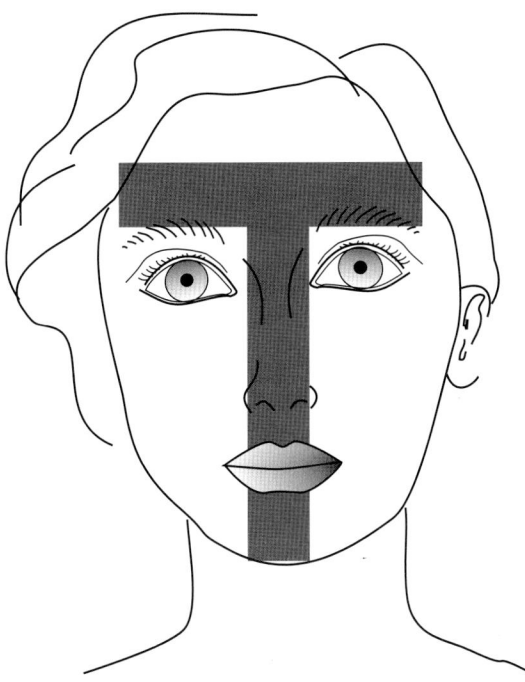

The T-zone: forehead, nasal bridge, nose, and center of the chin.

Note: Skin type must be determined on a "clean" face. No conclusions should be drawn concerning the quality of skin when a moisturizer has recently been applied, or the skin has recently been washed with a drying soap.

Which Moisturizers Should Be Used for which Types of Skin?

For an individual with **dry facial skin**, using moisturizers containing only humectants will not be enough. Oily moisturizers containing occlusive components are required. If the skin is fairly "normal" and not dry, one should use a preparation that has both occlusives and humectants.

An individual with **oily skin or a tendency toward oily skin** does not need moisturizers (except at those times when the face becomes drier, e.g., following exposure to a cold wind). Similarly, one should avoid applying moisturizers on *acne-affected skin*.

For skin that is **normal or near normal**, one should use a moisturizing preparation that incorporates less of the oily, occlusive substances. In this case, preparations containing humectants are recommended.

If the skin type is **combination**, one should avoid applying moisturizing preparations in the T-zone. On the rest of the face, one should use nonoily products (containing humectants).

Note: Remember that the skin tends to dry with age. An individual who did not require moisturizers in the past may require them later in life. If one moves to a more arid environment, moisturizers will be required as well. Certain seasons, such as in winter, may cause one to feel a need for extra moisturizing.

In addition to the skin type, other variables may influence the choice of a moisturizer:

- **Consistency**: The product's texture and consistency is a significant factor. Certainly a product that is not pleasant to the touch, such as one that feels sticky or oily, should not be selected. The flood of products on the market enables the consumer to select a moisturizer perfectly suited to one's aesthetic needs.
- **Additives**: Fragrances and preservatives may irritate and sensitize. For some individuals, it is necessary to avoid using products containing these components which may cause skin irritation, and are not necessarily required. Cosmetic companies are currently manufacturing hypoallergenic products, which contain fewer potentially allergenic compounds. These may be preferred for sensitized individuals. However, even cosmetic products labeled as "hypoallergenic" may contain various preservatives and fragrances as well, with the potential (albeit reduced as compared to standard preparations) to induce allergic reactions.

Note: The skin surrounding the eyes is particularly sensitive. Products marketed as eye creams should contain as little potential irritants, such as fragrances and preservatives, as possible.

- **Sunscreens**: There is no justification for using a moisturizer containing sunscreens if it is planned for evening or night use. However, it may be recommended to use a moisturizing lotion that contains an efficient sunscreen, if applied in areas exposed to the sun during daytime.
- **"Exotic" ingredients**: Exotic ingredients such as allantoin, gelatin, vitamins, proteins, and royal bee jelly are not superior to conventional compounds in retaining skin moisture. There is no scientific evidence that they have additional benefits, such as age-reversing qualities.

Various preparations, including exotic ingredients in cosmetic products, are detailed in chapter 16 on active ingredients in cosmetic preparations.

GUIDELINES FOR THE USE OF MOISTURIZERS

As a rule, individuals with dry skin should avoid frequent washing of the face with soap; they should also avoid exposure to harsh environmental factors such as cold wind and dry weather.

The application of moisturizers after skin cleansing is recommended. The product should be applied after washing when the skin is still slightly damp. Application should be gentle. The frequency of application should be determined according to skin type. Dry skin will require a more frequent application of moisturizers. Extremely dry skin requires several daily applications, depending on the product used. The moisturizer should be applied to the face and neck. If the T-zone (forehead, nasal bridge, nose, and chin) is oily, one should avoid moisturizing this area unnecessarily.

Note: Moisturizers that contain relatively large amounts of water (i.e., liquid emulsions or creams) should not be applied just before exposure to cold weather. In this case, the wet skin is exposed to the drying effect of the cold wind. As water on the skin's surface evaporates, it has a cooling effect. Cold, dry conditions may harm facial skin. One should consider the following:

- Apply the moisturizer 20 to 30 minutes prior to exposure to a cold, dry, or windy environment.
- Under these conditions, oily moisturizers may be preferable.

THE DIFFERENCE BETWEEN MOISTURIZERS FOR THE FACE AND THOSE FOR THE REST OF THE BODY

In principle, there is no significant difference between moisturizers designed for the face and those for the rest of the body. Any moisturizer that increases the moisture of the face will also be effective in increasing the moisture elsewhere. Nevertheless, since applying moisturizer to the body involves much larger areas, manufacturers generally make body moisturizers in the form of liquid emulsions (rather than creams or ointments), to make them easier to apply. This is not a rigid rule. There are some facial moisturizers that appear in a liquid form, and there are many body moisturizers in the form of creams or ointments.

Most people will take more care to apply moisturizer to the face and neck than elsewhere, because of the aesthetic importance of the skin in these regions, and also because those areas are more exposed to the elements, such as sun and wind.

Some body moisturizers are meant to be used in the bath or shower, for people with particularly dry skin. The advantage is that while bathing, a layer of water is trapped between the skin and the moisturizer, which further increases the moisture content of the skin. Each preparation comes with detailed instructions as to how much to add to the bathwater, for both infants and adults. There is no need to use most of these preparations in the bath. One can simply apply them in a thin layer on the skin areas after having a shower provided they do not contain any cleaning agents.

MOISTURIZERS FOR THE HANDS

Moisturizers designed for the hands are based on the same principles as other moisturizers. They contain occlusives or humectants, or a combination of both. However, there is another aspect to hand moisturizers: the skin of the hands is subjected to repeated washing with soap and water. Therefore, moisturizers for the hands contain oils that may be water resistant, which create an impermeable, occlusive layer on the skin that does not wash off easily.

Furthermore, hand creams often contain an additional ingredient: **oil-based silicone**. This substance is water repellent. Owing to the presence of this water-repellent silicone layer, the natural lipid film on the skin is not washed away, and the skin remains moist.

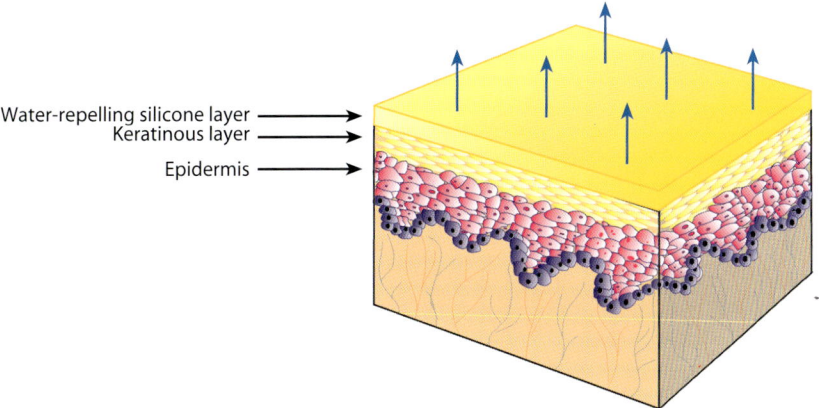

A water-repellent layer of silicone over the keratinous layer.

For people engaged in manual work involving exposing their hands to various harsh substances, silicone-containing moisturizers may provide a layer protecting the skin from toxic substances, allergens (substances producing allergic reactions), and irritants. The degree of moisture achievable with these substances is, in general, less than that achieved by using occlusive or water-absorbent substances. However, as stated earlier, the presence of a water-repellent layer on the skin may be a possible advantage.

SUMMARY

- Moisturizers consist of occlusive substances, water-absorbent substances (humectants), or a combination of the two.
- The use of a moisturizer must be adjusted to the type of skin.
- For dry skin, one needs an oily moisturizer that contains a relatively higher concentration of occlusive compounds.
- For normal or near-normal skin, it is advisable to use a moisturizer that combines an occlusive substance with a water-absorbent substance. The skin type also determines the frequency of application of a moisturizer. The drier the skin, the more often it should be used.
- Moisturizers should be applied gently, after cleaning the skin and washing it with water.

5 | Skin Cleansing

Avi Shai and Howard I. Maibach

Contents Overview • Soap and its mode of action • Possible disadvantages of regular soap • What is pH? • Synthetic soaps (soapless soap) • What does soap contain other than the active ingredient? • "Mild"/hypoallergenic soaps • Soaps for use in acne • Washing the face

SKIN CLEANSING: OVERVIEW

Skin cleansing is a basic to maintaining its health and contributing to its aesthetic appearance. What is the dirt that has to be removed? It consists of:

- dust,
- soot (from the air),
- sweat,
- breakdown products of sebum,
- residues of cosmetics and makeup previously applied to the skin, and
- other substances carried in the air which vary depending on the geographical location and immediate environment.

All the above substances stick to the thin, oily layer on the skin's surface. Since the dirt is embedded in the oily layer, washing with water is not effective enough to cleanse the skin. Water is repelled by the oil, and therefore is not able to remove the oily layer of the skin surface containing the dirt particles. Anyone who has ever tried to wash oil or fat off one's hands will know that water alone cannot remove it. Thus, to effectively remove the dirt embedded in the fine oily layer on the skin's surface, one has to use soap.

SOAP AND ITS MODE OF ACTION

The active ingredients in soaps consist of salts of various fatty acids.

Fatty Acids Commonly Used in Soaps

Stearic acid
Palmitic acid
Oleic acid
Myristic acid
Lauric acid

In terms of its basic chemical composition, regular, classic soap, known as **hard soap** or **toilet soap**, comprises the sodium salts of fatty acids. These fatty acids are derived from either animal or vegetable sources.

Because of soap's particular molecular structure, the soap particles "coat" the fat droplets in which the dirt is embedded, and allow them to be washed off the skin with water. These soap structures, called micelles, coat the fat (and dirt) particles, allowing them to be removed from the skin. The soap molecules arrange themselves in the form of micelles because of the electric charge they carry. The soap micelles surround the fat droplet, and thus enable its removal from the skin.

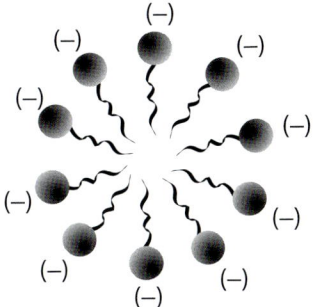

A soap micelle.

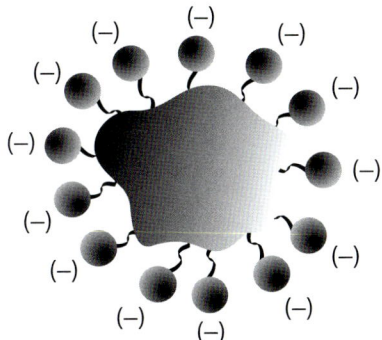

A micelle coating a fat droplet.

POSSIBLE DISADVANTAGES OF REGULAR SOAP

Normal tap water contains calcium and magnesium. When ordinary soap is used with tap water, calcium and magnesium salts of fatty acids are formed. These are "sticky," not readily soluble salts. The salts remain on the skin surface and may lead to skin irritation.

Another reason regular soap may cause skin irritation is that it has a high pH. The pH of regular soap lies between 9 and 10 (and sometimes higher than 10)—much higher than the normal skin pH (which is between 4 and 6.5). Consequently, it raises the skin's pH (see below for an explanation of the concept of pH). However, healthy skin has mechanisms for adjusting its pH, so that shortly after it has been exposed to regular soap, its level of acidity returns to normal. (The pH returns to normal any time from half an hour to two hours after soap has been used.) Nevertheless, in some people, abrupt changes in pH can cause significant skin irritation. Therefore, the current trend in the cosmetics industry is to adapt the pH of cleansing agents and other cosmetic preparations to that of normal skin.

> **Skin Acidity Protects Against Infections**
>
> The acidity of the skin is a protective mechanism of the body against bacterial and fungal infections. The natural pH of the skin acts as a protective acid mantle.

WHAT IS pH?

The "pH factor" is a numerical value that expresses the level of acidity or alkalinity of a solution. The acidity of a solution is determined by the concentration of hydrogen ions in it. pH values range from 0 to 14. The actual value of the pH of a solution is derived from a logarithmic calculation based on the concentration of hydrogen ions in the solution.

- A very strong **acid**, such as hydrochloric acid, has a high concentration of hydrogen ions, and a pH close to 0.
- A very strong **base** (or **alkali**), such as sodium hydroxide, has a low concentration of hydrogen ions, and a pH close to 14.
- The pH of pure water, which is **neutral**, is 7.
- The pH of blood is 7.4.
- The pH of milk varies from 6 to 7.
- The pH of lemon juice is between 2 and 3.
- The normal skin pH ranges from 4 to 6.5.

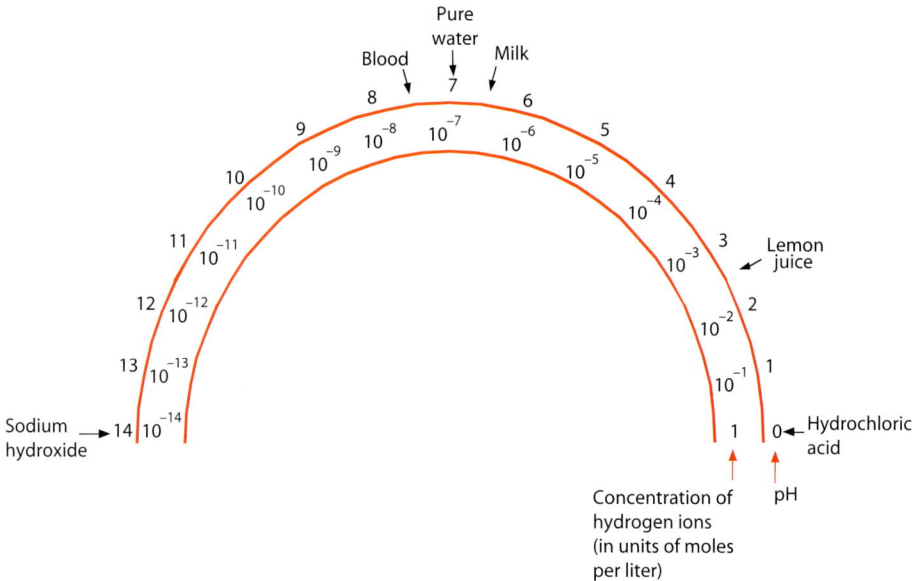

The pH scale.

SYNTHETIC SOAPS ("SOAPLESS SOAP")

The disadvantages of regular soap created the need for new kinds of soaps. As early as the 1940s, cosmetic companies started manufacturing synthetic soaps, largely derived from by-products of crude oil refining.

Surfactants, or **surface-active agents**, are water-soluble compounds that make up the major components of soaps and shampoos. The surface-active agents in these soaps act in exactly the same way as in regular soaps. Because of their electric charge, they form micelles. Small particles of oil are trapped inside the micelles. In this way, the oil and particles of dirt embedded within them can be washed off with water. All the other cleansing agents made of surface-active agents are called:

- artificial soaps,
- soapless soaps,
- nonsoaps, or
- synthetic soaps,

and they may be in the form of solids or liquids.

> Surfactants
>
> There are four groups of surfactants such as:
>
> - anionics,
> - cationics,
> - nonionics, and
> - amphoterics.
>
>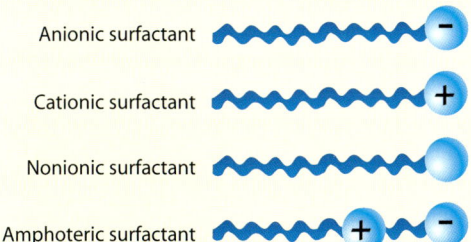
>
> The nature of each group is determined by its chemical charge. Each surfactant group has different chemical properties that affect the way it cleans.

Clarification of the Term "Detergent"

Some people include any cleaning agent under the definition "detergent." However, the term "detergent" actually refers to a "soapless soap." In general, manufacturers avoid using the term "detergent" in relation to skin cleansing agents or shampoos; they prefer to use the terms "soapless soap" or "surfactant." This is because the average person tends to associate the word "detergent" with those strong detergents used for cleaning dishes, etc. In fact, all detergents accomplish their cleaning action by the same principle described in this chapter.

Possible Advantages of Synthetic Soaps

Synthetic soaps usually cause less skin irritation than regular soaps do. The pH of synthetic soaps can be adjusted to that of the normal skin by the addition of substances such as lactic acid or citric acid.

"INTERMEDIATE" GROUP OF SOAPS

Some of the soaps on the market are a combination between regular soaps and synthetic soaps. Hence, they are actually made up of regular soaps, composed of sodium salts of fatty acids, to which surfactants have been added. The resulting pH lies somewhere between the two types of soaps, according to the amount of surfactants added.

> Are Surfactants in Soaps and Shampoos Hazardous to Health?
>
> Sodium lauryl sulfate and sodium laureth sulfate are surfactants contained in a wide range of cosmetic products, mainly liquid soaps and shampoos.
>
> Since the 1990s, an increasing number of publications has started to appear in the Internet, warning of the risk of exposure to these substances. Consequently, the Cosmetic Ingredient review Expert Panel, the U.S. cosmetic industry's independent body of experts for the safety of cosmetic ingredients, has examined this issue. The panel concluded that these substances are safe for use in low concentrations, intended for cleaning skin and hair, and when washed out shortly after being applied.
>
> However, similar to the effect of other surfactants, these substances may irritate the skin and eyes of some people. The severity of irritation increases with the amount of surfactant in the preparation. Irritation is fairly common when dealing with concentrations of over 2%.

> On the basis of current knowledge, there is no substantial evidence that preparations containing sodium lauryl sulfate and/or sodium laureth sulfate are not safe, when used in the commonly accepted concentrations for cleaning skin and hair. However, it is not recommended to let them get into the eyes and mouth, especially when washing babies. They should always be rinsed off as soon as possible after they have been applied.

WHAT DO SOAPS CONTAIN APART FROM THE ACTIVE INGREDIENTS?

As already stated, the active ingredients in all cleansing agents and soaps are surface-active agents (surfactants). Nevertheless, apart from surface-active agents, soaps contain other ingredients such as:

- moisturizers,
- preservatives,
- coloring agents,
- fragrances and perfumes,
- antibacterial substances,
- substances that alter the pH, and
- other ingredients.

Moisturizers

All regular and synthetic soaps tend to remove the oily layer on the skin surface. However, it is not only the oil containing the dirt particles that is removed but the soap also removes the natural oily layer on the skin, which is important for skin protection. Hence, the use of soap, with the subsequent removal of the natural oily layer, dries out the skin. Loss of the oily protective layer also increases the likelihood of irritation. For this reason, most soaps contain moisturizing agents, such as lanolin, glycerine, and various vegetable fats. These substances leave a thin protective layer on the skin to counteract the drying effect of the soap. However, both the action of the soap itself (in removing oily substances) and the rinsing with water remove moisturizers from the skin. Thus, significant amounts of moisturizers will not be left on the skin surface following the use of soap. Therefore, anyone who has a tendency to dry skin should apply moisturizing agents in the form of creams or ointments, instead of relying on the use of soaps containing moisturizers. Moisturizing agents are dealt with further in chapter 4.

Soaps Meant for Use on Oily Skin

These soaps contain minimal amounts, if any, of moisturizing agents. In addition, they contain surfactants that are particularly effective in removing the oily layer from the skin. In general, the use of moisturizing agents should be tailored to the type of skin: someone with dry skin needs a soap that contains moisturizing agents. On the other hand, there is no need (and indeed it is unwise) for someone with oily skin, or someone with acne, to use moisturizing soap.

Some dermatologists claim that liquid soaps tend, more than bar soaps, to dry out the skin. Therefore, it would be desirable, for those suffering from dry skin, to minimize their use.

Transparent Soap

Transparent soap represents another type of soap which contains moisturizers. These soaps usually contain a higher than usual concentration of glycerine or various sugars. The high glycerine content gives the soap its transparent appearance. Some dermatologists maintain that glycerine tends to absorb water contained in the skin, causing these soaps to have a drying effect in certain cases. For this reason, some transparent soaps contain additional moisturizing agents; hence each transparent soap can be tailored specifically for dry, normal, or oily skin. In general, transparent soaps are considered to be relatively mild.

Preservatives and Coloring Agents

The same preservatives used in various cosmetic preparations may be used in soaps as well. However, irritation as a result of preservatives used in soaps is less likely to occur than those contained in cosmetic preparations, because of the fact that the soap is usually washed off shortly after application, as opposed to cosmetic preparations. Preservatives are dealt with in detail in chapter 3.

Coloring agents, as in other cosmetic preparations, are mainly synthetic and are intended to contribute to the marketing appeal of the product. Some dyes have been blamed for being potentially hazardous to health. There is, however, no concrete scientific evidence to support this claim. Note that white soaps do not necessarily have a remarkable advantage over colored soaps. Most white soaps contain synthetic bleaching agents in order to impart the impression of purity and "cleanness."

Some manufacturers use natural dyes which are, sometimes, by-products of substances contained anyway in the soap and are not suspected of being harmful. Thus, for example, extracts of mint may impart a green color to the soap, while carrot extracts will enrich it with an orange hue. In general, natural dyes give to soaps hues which are less striking than synthetic dyes. A label that clarifies which types of colors are included may be found in some products and may assist the consumer.

Fragrances and Perfumes

It is common practice in most cosmetic preparations, including soap, to add scents of various types to hide the odors of the raw ingredients used. Sometimes these substances can cause allergic reactions.

Antibacterial Substances

"Antibacterial" soaps usually contain triclocarban and triclosan. Residues of these substances remain on the skin surface after washing, thereby inhibiting the growth of bacteria.

Soaps that contain antibacterial substances are used mainly to prevent unpleasant body odors. They are also used for several types of superficial skin infections such as folliculitis (infection of the hair follicles), or acne, as well as following exposure to dirt or any other potential source of contamination.

Unpleasant Body Odor

Unpleasant body odor results from the breakdown of organic substances present in the secretions of certain types of sweat glands, called **apocrine glands**, found in the armpits and groin. These substances are broken down by bacteria. Hence, using antibacterial soaps that inhibit the growth of bacteria prevents, to a certain extent, the formation of unpleasant body odor.

The antibacterial effect of these soaps depends on how often they are used during the day. Since there are no apocrine sweat glands on the face, and if the purpose of these soaps is to prevent body odor, their use should be confined to washing the body.

Unpleasant body odor derived from the apocrine glands in the armpits and groin develops after puberty. Therefore, there is no justification using these soaps in children for this purpose.

Are Antibacterial Soaps Beneficial?

The beneficial effect of antibacterial soaps containing materials such as triclosan remains controversial. Some warn that the use of these substances in an uncontrolled manner may lead to a selection of resistant bacteria to these antibacterial agents and, perhaps, similar antibacterial agents, that share similar biochemical structure. In any case, there is no substantial evidence as to the advantage of "antibacterial" soaps over usual soaps on the market. Some researchers claim that it is reasonable to assume that most of the removal of bacteria from the skin by soaps, in general, is due to washing them from the skin, and not to any specific antibacterial effect.

There are other soaps with antibacterial properties:

- Some soaps contain benzoyl peroxide. This substance is an antimicrobial agent and is used in the treatment of acne.

- Soaps containing a high concentration of lactic acid have a pH of about 3.5. These soaps are said to have some antibacterial action.
- Soaps containing povidone iodine—an iodine-based antibacterial compound—have marked antibacterial properties but can cause skin irritation. They should therefore be used only after consulting a physician, who will advise whether there is a medical problem that justifies their use. Gynecologists sometimes recommend these soaps for vaginal douching.

Substances that Alter Skin pH

Substances that alter skin pH are usually acids, such as lactic acid and citric acid. The aim is to adjust the pH of the substance to the normal pH of healthy skin (the normal value being between 4 and 6.5). Certain soaps are designed to deliberately lower the skin pH, since lowering the skin pH is supposed to produce some antibacterial effect.

Other Ingredients

Certain soaps contain other ingredients, such as vitamins, various medical preparations, and a variety of exotic "natural" ingredients (usually derived from fruits, other plants, etc.). In most cases, these additives are of no documented medical value. Soap is in contact with the skin for a brief period only, and, in any case, if the soap performs as it is supposed to, these substances would quickly be washed off the skin.

The effect of any additive on the skin must be considered. If a certain ingredient really does benefit the skin, it would be preferable to use some other cosmetic preparation (such as a cream or an emulsion) containing the required ingredient. That way, by applying the preparation to the skin, the substance in it would be in contact with the skin for a longer period and may truly have some beneficial effect on the skin.

"MILD" OR HYPOALLERGENIC SOAPS

"Mild" or "hypoallergenic" soaps have had certain ingredients, such as fragrances and coloring agents, removed. The substances excluded are those that, statistically, have a higher chance of causing skin irritation or allergic reactions. Another feature of these soaps is that they may contain substances from the betaine group, which are amphoteric surfactants. These are known to be relatively mild, and do not tend to cause stinging of the skin or eyes. Nevertheless, even "mild" and hypoallergenic soaps can cause skin irritation and allergic reactions—although the likelihood of this happening is theoretically less than with regular soaps. Hypoallergenic soaps are designed for use by people with delicate skin and for infants.

SOAPS FOR USE IN ACNE

As noted above, some of the soaps intended for use in acne contain antibacterial substances such as benzoyl peroxide. Benzoyl peroxide is a strong oxidizing agent that penetrates the hair follicle and acts on the bacteria that are involved in the development of acne.

The other soaps intended for use in acne are mainly those designed for use on oily skin, which have very potent cleansing properties. Reducing the oiliness of the skin may help in the treatment of acne. Note, however, that most of the medical preparations used nowadays in the treatment of acne may dry out the skin. This, in addition to excessive use of soaps that also tend to dry out the skin, can lead to extremely dry skin.

WASHING THE BODY AND FACE

- A mild soap, suited to the skin type, should be used. For dry skin, soap with moisturizer should be used.
- Excessive scrubbing of the face while washing is unnecessary. There is no advantage in using an abrasive substance or device to remove dead cells. They will fall off anyway.
- When drying the skin, vigorous rubbing, which may irritate the skin, should be avoided. The face can be wiped by gently dabbing with a soft towel.
- For the skin of the face, lukewarm water should be used.

6 | Creams and Liquid Emulsions for Facial Cleansing

Avi Shai, Howard I. Maibach, and Robert Baran

Contents Overview • Creams and liquid emulsions for facial cleansing vs. soap • Abrasive cleansers • Summary

OVERVIEW

Creams and liquid emulsions for cleansing the face are basically mixtures of oil and water. The difference between a cream and a liquid emulsion lies in their degree of viscosity. When the preparation is thin and fluid, we speak of a **liquid emulsion**; if the preparation contains more fatty components, so that it is semisolid, we speak of a **cream**. Both creams and liquid emulsions intended for facial cleansing are composed of oils, water, and cleansing substances (usually the same substances as are found in the mild soaps), with the proportions between the various components differing from product to product.

When the skin is washed with a soap, the soap, with the addition of water, disperses the oil along with the dirt particles embedded in it. Water is then used to rinse off this mixture of soap and oil from the skin.

In contrast to soaps, cleansing creams and emulsions already contain water and they disperse the oily dirt particles from the skin, without the addition of tap water. These preparations should be applied to the skin with the fingertips and left on the skin briefly. When they are removed from the skin with a tissue or a wet facecloth, or by rinsing off with water (preferred!), the fatty layer with the dissolved dirt is removed with them.

As with other cosmetic preparations, the cosmetics industry adds various auxiliary substances to cleansing creams and emulsions: **emulsifiers** to stabilize the product, **antiseptics** (to act against bacteria), various solvents, and moisturizers.

CREAMS AND LIQUID EMULSIONS FOR FACIAL CLEANSING VS. SOAP

Makeup preparations, especially those based on heavy oils, are removed from the skin more easily using cleansing creams or emulsions, which have a relatively high fat content compared with normal soap. Cleansing creams and emulsions dissolve the fatty substances (which contain the makeup pigments), making removal of makeup easier. These substances are more effective at removing sebum from the skin than soap and water.

Since cleansing creams and emulsions contain oils, a thin layer of oil may still remain on the skin after rinsing them off. For this reason, these preparations are generally more effective for people with dry skin and are not usually recommended for people with oily skin or acne. Nevertheless, many cleansing creams and preparations are manufactured in a range of variations, as subgroups of the original product, designated specifically for use with dry, normal, or oily skin—depending on the customer's requirements.

Cleansing creams and emulsions are usually made of relatively delicate cleansing agents (compared with the wide variety of soaps and "soapless" soaps). If they are rinsed off with water after use (not just wiped off), their cleansing effect is gentler and usually does not cause skin irritation.

> **Cleansing Cream Should not be Used as Moisturizing Cream**
>
> Since cleansing creams and emulsions contain cleansing agents, they should be removed from the skin as soon as possible, since they are liable to cause irritation if left in contact with the skin for too long. Leaving a cleansing cream on the skin, as one does with a moisturizing cream, is the same as leaving soap on the skin—not a good idea! Furthermore, for this reason, it is definitely preferable to wash cleansing creams and emulsions off with water and not merely to wipe them off the skin with a tissue paper or cloth.

ABRASIVE CLEANSERS

Abrasive cleansers are creams or emulsions designed for cleaning the face. In addition to the standard ingredients described above, the "abrasive effect" is achieved by the presence of tiny, fine granules—some natural and some made of synthetic compounds. These preparations are supposed to remove the keratin layer of the skin that normally peels off. This is achieved by mechanical means, by the abrasive effect of the granules on the skin. Removing the outermost layers of keratin may help produce a uniform, smooth surface on the skin and improve its appearance.

Even though these preparations are effective in removing the peeling skin layers, there is no proof that they offer any additional benefit in cleaning the skin, or caring for it, than soaps or other facial cleansing creams or emulsions. In general, healthy, normal skin does not require such treatment. The outermost layers of skin are normally constantly peeling off and do not need any assistance in doing so! Furthermore, several dermatologists have pointed out the possibility of damage to the epidermis if this abrasive cleaning is carried out too vigorously and roughly.

For those who nevertheless decide to use these preparations, this type of cleansing should not be carried out more than once weekly, since the defensive properties of the skin may be affected if the outer layers are removed. Massaging and rubbing these preparations onto the skin must be done with the utmost care and gentleness, and in strict accordance with the manufacturer's instructions.

SUMMARY

Cleansing creams and emulsions offer another means of cleaning the face, but hold no significant advantage over soap and water, except to remove waterproof makeups, or to be used by people with delicate skin, since the cleansing substances they contain are relatively mild compared to other types of soaps. Cleansing creams and emulsions must not be used as moisturizers, should not be left on the face for long, and should be rinsed off with water, not just wiped off with a tissue paper or cloth.

7 | Facial Cleansing Masks
Avi Shai, Howard I. Maibach, and Robert Baran

Contents Overview • Functions of a facial mask • Masks that rinse off and masks that peel off • "Absorbent" masks that rinse off • Masks that peel off • Exotic facial masks • Possible undesirable effects from facial cleansing masks

OVERVIEW

Facial masks represent a unique approach to cleaning the face and skin care: the preparation is applied to the skin as a relatively thick layer and then removed some time later, usually 15–30 minutes. The facial mask does not represent an essential technique of skin care. The effects achieved by facial masks can all be achieved by simpler means, such as washing the face with soap and water, applying moisturizing creams or using astringent preparations. Nevertheless, facial masks have certain advantages.

FUNCTIONS OF A FACIAL MASK

Facial masks are used for:

- **Effective cleansing of the skin**, while removing the outer parts of the keratinous layer. This type of thorough cleansing, in fact, has a certain "peeling" effect, but it is extremely superficial and the degree of peeling is negligible compared to the medical procedure of skin peeling as carried out by an experienced physician (see chapter 24 on chemical peeling).
- **Moisturizing the skin**, giving it a smooth, moist appearance—provided that the mask contains moisturizers. After using a facial mask, the skin becomes slightly swollen, which has the effect of temporarily smoothing out fine wrinkles. This effect of skin moisturization is achieved by virtue of the occlusive effect of the facial mask, which becomes more effective the more moisturizing substances the mask contains.
- **Treatment of acne**—provided the mask is designed for that purpose and contains the appropriate ingredients.
- **Improvement in the overall feeling of well-being**: through the perception that the facial skin is being coddled and the feeling of calmness and tranquillity while the mask is on the face. In addition, removal of the mask is followed by a pleasant, fresh, and clean feeling; and usually there is a sensory effect of tautness, resulting from the drying out of the mask on the face, which is even more pronounced if the mask contains astringents.

Note: A facial mask does not nourish the skin. It cannot smooth out wrinkles (other than the temporary smoothing due to skin moisturization). As part of the vigorous marketing and advertising of these products, claims are made to the effect that a facial mask can, for example, stimulate the blood flow to the skin. In fact, simple physical or sporting activities will stimulate blood flow in the body and skin much more effectively than will a facial mask—not to mention all the other advantages of physical exercise.

MASKS THAT RINSE OFF AND MASKS THAT PEEL OFF

Masks That Are Rinsed off

Masks that rinse off are removed from the skin by lukewarm or warm water. They consist of absorbent masks, which are based on insoluble powders, natural clay and mud, or gel masks, which contain ingredients such as tragacanth. In addition, some of the masks that are rinsed off are not actually masks, but rather a mixture of moisturizing agents or cleansing agents (or a combination of both) that are marketed, for commercial reasons, as facial masks.

Masks That Are Peeled off

Masks that are peeled off are made of rubbery substances, such as polyvinyl alcohol or rubber-based substances such as latex or other natural rubber compounds. As these masks dry on the skin, they harden and form a thin, flexible, usually transparent sheet on the skin. In this case, the mask is not removed by rinsing with water but is peeled off the face.

With both masks that are rinsed off and those that are peeled off, it is important that the time for which they remain on the face is in accordance with the manufacturer's instructions. The mask is usually removed 15 to 30 minutes after application.

In spite of the division into masks that are rinsed off and those that are peeled off, this distinction is not necessarily clear-cut. Masks can be made that contain a mixture of ingredients, such as clay (used in masks that are rinsed off) with rubber components (used in masks that are peeled off). Hydrocolloid substances (such as carboxymethyl cellulose) may be added to any type of mask. The final composition of the mask determines whether it can be rinsed off or peeled off.

"ABSORBENT" MASKS THAT RINSE OFF

The basic ingredient of rinse-off masks is powder, which is made up of inorganic substances such as zinc oxide, titanium dioxide, kaolin, calamine, and others. Other masks in this group are based on processed clay and natural mud. Before the mask is applied to the face, the powder is mixed in accordance with the manufacturer's instructions, with water, milk, various fruit or vegetable juices, other extracts, or any liquid specified in the instructions. These masks are also available in the form of a paste, in which the powder has already been mixed by the manufacturer. Usually, some liquid such as propylene glycol, with a small amount of soap, has to be added, to make it easier to remove the mask from the face. These masks usually absorb fats from the skin and are recommended for people with oily skin.

The material is gently applied to the face and left in place in accordance with the manufacturer's instructions, for some 15 to 30 minutes. It is then rinsed off with soap and water.

MASKS THAT PEEL OFF

These masks do not absorb fats from the skin, as do powder- or clay-based masks. The major effect of these masks is to prevent the evaporation of water from the skin's surface. As a result, the amount of moisture in the skin increases, as long as the mask is on the face. These masks are recommended for women with relatively dry facial skin.

When these masks are used in a cosmetics salon, a thin layer of gauze can be placed under the mask. This allows the ingredients of the mask to coat the client's skin (since they pass through the gaps in the gauze material), while at the same time allowing the mask to be removed quickly and efficiently in one piece as shown in the illustrations.

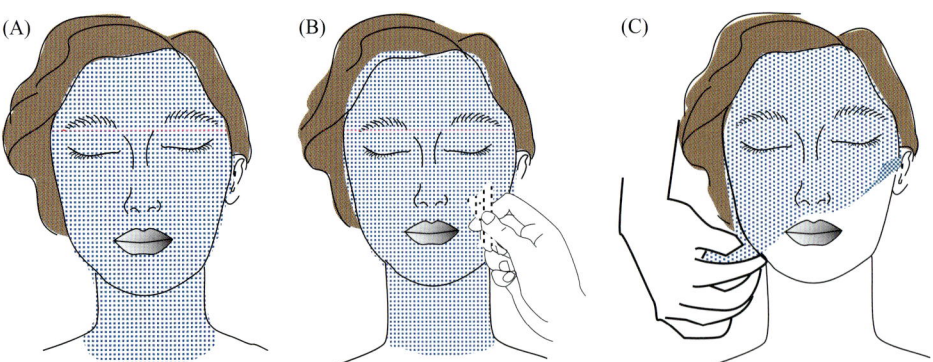

(A) A piece of gauze soaked in water is placed over the face. (B) The mask is applied to the face on top of the gauze. (C) After the required treatment time, the gauze is lifted and rolled up off the face, taking the mask with it.

EXOTIC FACIAL MASKS

In addition to the types of masks already discussed, other sorts of masks are used in various health resorts and cosmetic clinics, each place having its own "speciality." The masks used are, for example, mud masks (depending on the soil composition of the region) and masks containing beeswax, seaweed extracts, or extracts of a wide variety of plants. In general, a wide range of cosmetic ingredients can be added to any type of mask. There is no scientific proof that any of the components of these "exotic" masks have any advantage in terms of skin care. Furthermore, facial masks may not be very useful in helping cosmetic or other ingredients penetrate into the skin, since they are only on the skin for a relatively short time.

Facial Masks for Acne

Another type of facial mask is that used in the treatment of acne. These masks are based on:

- substances that absorb oil from the skin, and
- the incorporation of active ingredients that are used for treating acne, such as sulfur or benzoyl peroxide.

These masks may well be an effective adjunct to other acne treatments.

POSSIBLE UNDESIRABLE EFFECTS FROM FACIAL CLEANSING MASKS

Facial cleansing masks may cause:

- skin irritation, which is usually because of an allergic reaction to one or more components of the mask, and
- skin infection.

These complications are more likely to occur from the use of masks of dubious origin. The risks of such problems are much fewer when using masks from a reputable cosmetics manufacturer. In general, before using any mask, one should establish that the client is not allergic to any of its ingredients.

Note: Following the use of a mask, and after it has been rinsed off, moisturizing cream should be applied to the face. This is because a facial mask tends to cause slight superficial peeling of the outermost layers of the skin. Hence, it is important to avoid exposure to wind, sun, or polluted air after removing a facial cleansing mask.

8 | Skin Aging and Its Management

Avi Shai, Howard I. Maibach, and Robert Baran

Contents Overview • Skin and age: chronological aging • Photoaging: aging of the skin due to sun exposure • Major characteristics of skin aging • How to control skin aging • A comment regarding hormone replacement therapy for postmenopausal women

OVERVIEW

We are all too familiar with the aging process. Young individuals with soft, smooth, and supple skin become aware, with the passage of time, of signs of aging: the development and deepening of wrinkles, the appearance of age spots, and loosening of the skin. These changes occur in all layers of the skin. They can be classified as follows:

1. Changes due to the natural aging process: **chronological aging**. Skin aging is the natural expression of an individual's age. Yet, people of identical chronological age may appear to have younger- or older-looking skin. Genetic factors have a great impact on determining skin quality over time. Genetics determines the rate at which the skin ages by controlling certain factors such as:
   ○ skin durability,
   ○ hormonal mechanisms, and
   ○ skin thickness (thicker skin tends to wrinkle less).
2. Changes due to **environmental factors**: the leading factor here is **solar radiation**. These changes appear, of course, in areas of the body exposed to the sun. Prolonged exposure to cold, wind, and environmental pollutants such as smog may also cause cumulative damage to skin.

The desire to preserve a youthful appearance has led to the development of a myriad of cosmetic products, marketed with labels such as "prevents skin aging" and "removes wrinkles." Not all of these products are based on biological reasoning that supports the advertising claims. Most "before and after" photographs reflect the photographer's technical skill rather than the product's effectiveness.

This chapter reviews the skin-aging process, possible preventive measures, and corrective methods that have proven to be effective.

SKIN AND AGE: CHRONOLOGICAL AGING

The following changes occur with the natural passage of time. They appear in all areas of the body, regardless of exposure to the sun. They include:

- degeneration of elastin fibers,
- degeneration of collagen fibers, and
- thinning of the skin.

Elastin Fibers
Thin, functioning elastin fibers of the skin undergo a degenerative process, gradually becoming lumps of fibers of poor quality. The changes in the elastin fibers are the major cause of the development of wrinkles and the loss of skin elasticity.

Collagen Fibers
In addition to the degeneration of elastin fibers, there is a gradual degeneration and reduction in the amount of collagen fibers. This causes a decline in skin strength, with subsequent loosening.

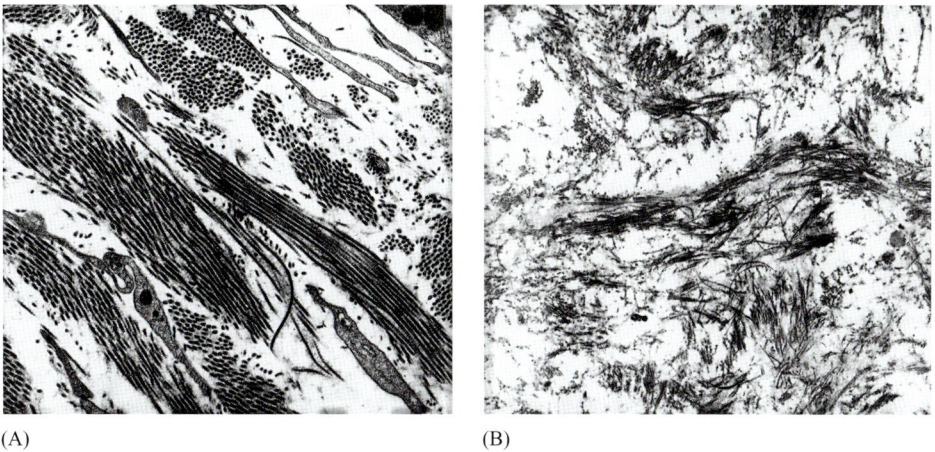

(A) Collagen fibers in the dermis of young skin. (B) Collagen fibers in the dermis of old skin.

Thinning of the Skin

In general, starting at approximately 45 years of age, there is a gradual thinning of all skin layers, including the epidermis, dermis, and the subcutis. This process is more pronounced in women than in men. There is also a gradual flattening of the wavy attachment between the epidermis and dermis.

The subcutaneous fatty layer becomes thinner. Loss of the fatty layer is more prominent in certain areas: face, hands, and calves. This process of degeneration and waning of tissue is called **atrophy**.

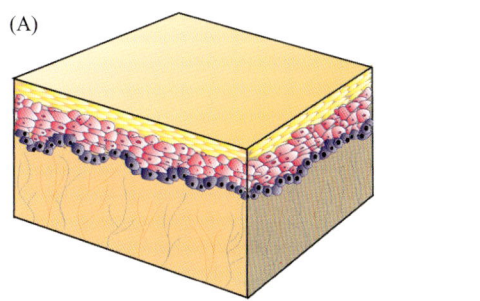 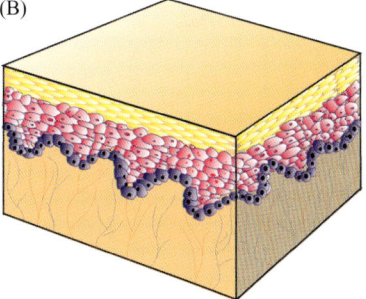

Flattening of the attachment between epidermis and dermis in older skin (A), compared with the wavy attachment in younger skin (B).

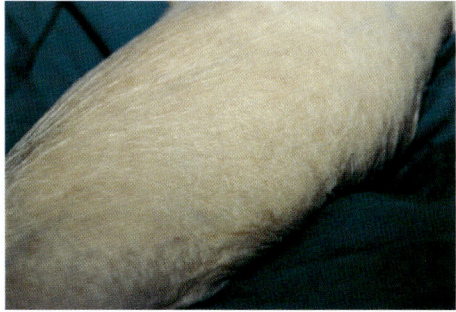

Extremely thin atrophic skin.

All of the above changes cause the appearance of wrinkles and loss of skin elasticity. The loss of strength and thickness in the skin, and the layers beneath it, causes it to become more vulnerable. With advancing age, there is a tendency to develop local hemorrhages as a result of minimal trauma: this is termed "easy bruisability." It occurs as a result of the poor quality of the skin, as well as the increased fragility of the blood vessels.

Additional Changes that Appear with Age

With increasing age, significant changes occur in the skin that affect:

- moisture content,
- rate and location of hair growth,
- pigmentation, and
- the size of the sebaceous glands.

Moisture Content

With increasing age, the skin becomes drier. Dry skin partially results from a gradual decline in the activity of the sebaceous glands. This decline is apparent after menopause in women, and at a later age in men. The sebum produced by sebaceous glands forms a fine lipid layer over the skin surface. This lipid layer serves as a barrier preventing evaporation of water from the skin. A decrease in the production of sebum will therefore cause the skin to become drier.

There is also a decrease in the ability of skin to retain its water content.

Extremely dry skin in older individuals may become a nuisance and may cause severe itching. The medical term for extreme dryness is **xerosis**.

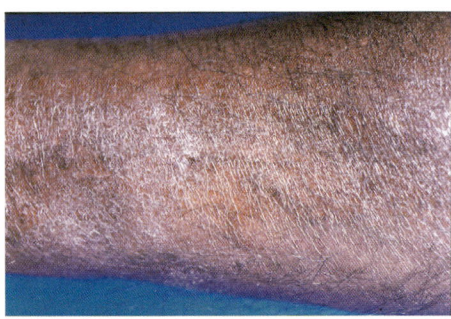

Dry, cracked, and xerotic skin.

Changes in Hair Growth

Thinning of hair appears in most areas of the body. As an individual ages, the quantity of hair decreases, as well as its thickness. However, the reverse process occurs in certain areas, such as the ears and eyebrows in men: hair that was previously unnoticeable in these areas becomes thicker and darker, posing a significant aesthetic problem.

Changes in Pigmentation

With increasing age, there is a decline in the number of melanocytes (melanin-producing cells) in the skin, which results in a decrease in the production of melanin. The skin tone, in general, becomes lighter. The decrease in melanin means that the skin's function as a barrier against the sun's radiation is less effective.

On the other hand, in areas of the skin that are exposed to the sun, there may be a proliferation of melanocytes. This will be manifested by the appearance of darker spots on the skin.

Enlargement of Sebaceous Glands

In certain areas, despite a decrease in the amount of sebum produced by the skin, the sebaceous glands increase in size. As a result, the skin's pores may widen. The glands enlarge and may appear to the naked eye as flat yellowish blemishes, up to 3 mm wide, upon the skin's surface. Because of the high density of sebaceous glands on the nose, this process causes gradual thickening, enlargement, and a general change in the appearance of the nose.

PHOTOAGING: AGING OF THE SKIN DUE TO SUN EXPOSURE

Exposure to the sun is the primary environmental cause of skin damage, along with other external factors such as prolonged exposure to cold and wind. As previously stated, the major factor in the formation of wrinkles and loss of skin firmness is the destruction of elastin fibers. Degeneration of these fibers, which occurs naturally in gradually aging skin, is intensified by prolonged exposure to the sun. The elastin degenerates as exposure to the sun continues.

Chronological aging, which occurs naturally with the passage of time, differs in its presentation compared to photoaging. For example, in photoaging, more cells are formed in the epidermis, which thickens in an irregular pattern. This is in stark contrast to the thinning of the epidermis, which occurs during normal aging in skin not exposed to the sun. Additional characteristics of photoaging are:

- uneven pigmentation,
- the appearance of "age spots," the medical term for which is **solar lentigines**,
- the possible development of skin tumors, typical of photoaging, and
- the appearance of dilated blood vessels in the skin, the medical term for which is **telangiectases**.

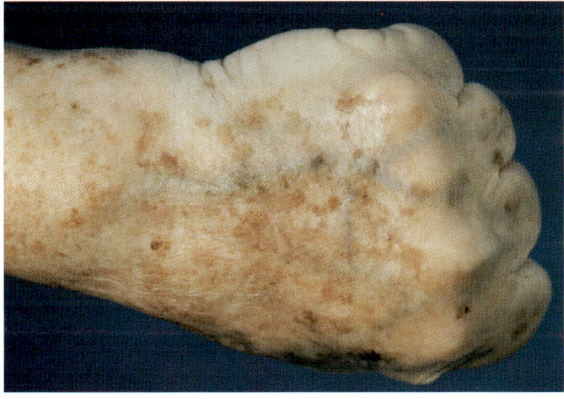

Solar lentigines ("age spots").

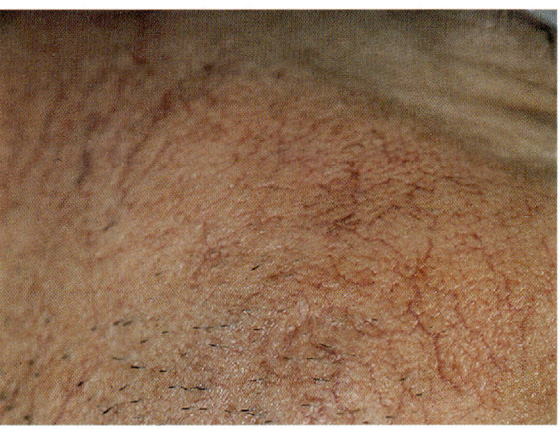

Telangiectases in facial skin.

Chronological Aging	Photoaging
Thin, atrophic skin	An irregular pattern of thicker skin; an increase in the number of epidermal cells
Degeneration of collagen and elastin fibers	Accelerated degeneration of collagen and elastin fibers
Possible development of skin tumors	Possible development of skin tumors, which are typical of photoaging
Lighter skin due to decline in melanin production	Uneven pigmentation: appearance of "age spots" (solar lentigines)
Additional features such as: • drier skin, • changes in hair growth, and • enlargement of sebaceous glands.	• Telangiectases (dilated blood vessels in the skin)

Differences between chronological aging and photoaging.

How to Differentiate Between Chronological Aging and Photoaging

Compare, in a middle-aged individual, the skin on the inner part of the upper arm—skin that is not exposed to the sun—with that on the back of the hand—which is constantly exposed:

- The skin on the inner arm is smooth and looks younger.
- The elasticity of the skin on the outer hand is significantly reduced. The skin is wrinkled and characterized by irregular pigmentation.

Older people may show the first signs of skin lesions and tumors, depending on their personal history of sun exposure.

MAJOR CHARACTERISTICS OF SKIN AGING

Degeneration of elastin and collagen fibers occurs, as previously discussed, both in chronological skin aging and in photoaging. These changes lead to the appearance of:

- fine wrinkles,
- pronounced lines of expression, and
- skin sagging.

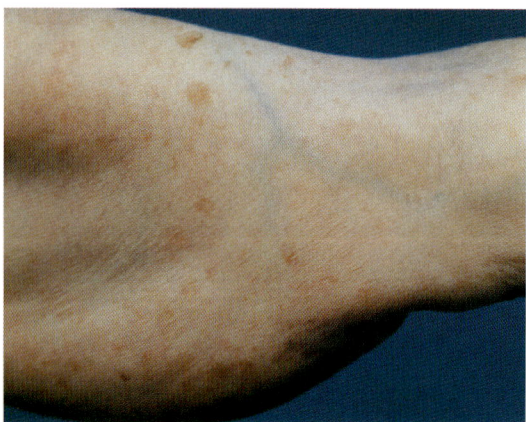

Inner arm.

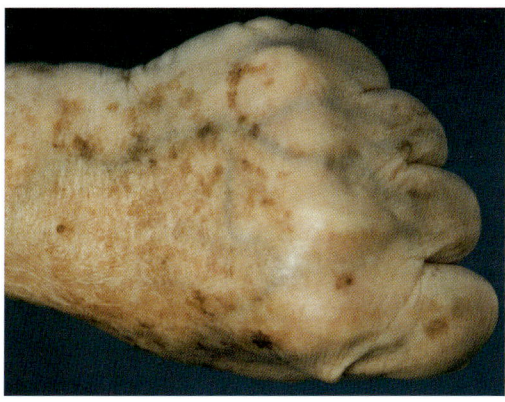

Outer hand of the same person after prolonged exposure to the sun.

Fine Wrinkles

With the decline in quantity and quality of the elastin fibers, the skin loosens. It loses its elasticity and its ability to return to its original state after stretching. When the elastin fibers degenerate, the skin gradually acquires a large number of fine wrinkles. Everyone older than 75 years has wrinkling over the skin's surface.

Pronounced Lines of Expression

The facial muscles are attached directly to the skin. The facial region is relatively poor in its subcutaneous fat content. Thus every facial expression causes folding of the skin, because muscles can contract, but skin cannot.

In the young, facial expressions disappear when the muscles are relaxed because elastin fibers function properly in the skin. But when the muscles contract beneath degenerated elastic tissue, fine wrinkles appear. They remain even when the face is passive and devoid of all expression.

These wrinkles are formed uniquely in each person. Expressive habits are formed late in childhood, and remain habitually throughout life. Eventually, they form an individual pattern of facial expressions. With time, these facial lines become permanent and may lead to a misinterpretation of moods or feelings. These lines may impart an expression of fatigue, anger, or depression that in itself does not necessarily represent the individual's actual mood.

In observing people's expressions, it is easy to understand the formation of wrinkles. For example, when the eyebrows are raised, horizontal expression lines are formed on the forehead.

Expressions also affect the formation of fine wrinkles. One can observe the wrinkling of the fine skin of the eyelids when squinting or raising the eyebrows.

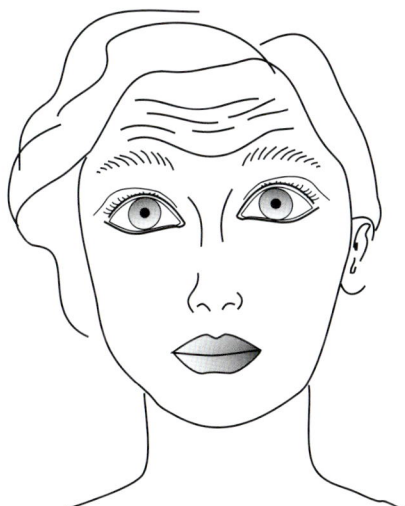

Raising eyebrows form horizontal expression lines on the forehead.

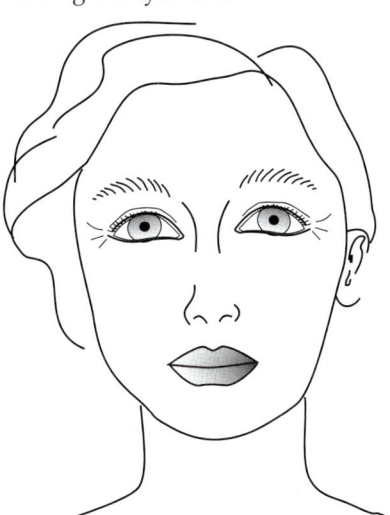

Squinting may contribute to development of lines, termed "crow's feet," at the outer edges of the eyes.

Skin Sagging

A combination of decreased skin thickness and strength, as well as a decrease in the thickness of the subcutaneous fatty layer, causes loosening and sagging of the skin. Gravity pulls the slack skin even further. In addition, bone loss begins at an age of approximately 60 years. Resorption of the lower jawbone and cheekbones, as well as a loss of muscle tension (muscle hypotonia), further contributes to the appearance of loose facial skin.

HOW TO CONTROL SKIN AGING

The process of skin aging is not fully understood. Currently, there is no definitive way to prevent this process. However, there are practical measures that can be taken to minimize the effects:

- Avoid excess sun exposure.
- Don't smoke.
- Prevent unnecessary stretching of the skin.
- Change facial expressive habits, if necessary.
- Use certain topical products.
- Lead a healthier emotional and physical lifestyle.

Sun Exposure

Excess exposure to the sun causes:

- damage to the elastin fibers in the skin,
- the development of tumors, both benign and malignant, and
- changes in skin pigmentation.

Excessive exposure to solar radiation must be avoided. Moderate periods of time spent outdoors and the use of hats and sunscreens are recommended.

Note: Sunglasses prevent damage caused by the penetration of ultraviolet rays to the eyes. In addition, they prevent the inevitable response of squinting that occurs in sunlight. Such prolonged, repeated squinting may accelerate the appearance of "crow's feet" type wrinkles, so the use of sunglasses is highly recommended. Photoaging is discussed in detail in chapter 10 on sun and the skin.

Smoking

Smoking affects the health of the skin, not to mention the damage it does to the blood vessels and heart, lungs, brain and other organs.

The characteristics of a smoker's face are well recognized. Chronic smokers have pale, yellowish-gray skin. Deep lines typically appear radially from the upper and lower lips, and laterally from the eyes. The skin between these wrinkles is somewhat thicker than in nonsmokers.

In 1992, the *American Journal of Epidemiology* published an article entitled: "Does cigarette smoking make you ugly and old?" The answer, in short, was yes! Since then, many other research studies have been published confirming further the detrimental effects of smoking on the skin.

Causes of Skin Damage Due to Smoking

- Nicotine causes vascular constriction that decreases the normal nourishment of the skin by the blood.
- Additional toxic products in the smoke causes damage to external layers of the skin (through direct contact).
- Absorption of these toxic products and their introduction to the skin through the circulation damages the collagen and elastic fibers.
- Smoke also causes dryness and irritation. If prolonged, this will damage the skin.
- Exposure to smoke is irritating to the eyes. This causes repeated squinting, which results in the appearance of "crow's feet" type wrinkles.

- Staining of fingers and teeth.
- After plastic surgery (such as a face lift or peeling procedures), the healing is delayed and is not as effective as it is in nonsmokers. This is probably because of damage to blood vessels.

Stretching of the Skin

Gradual stretching of the abdominal skin during pregnancy results in an increase in surface area. Excess skin is formed by its gradual expansion. After delivery, the skin may appear more slack and loose. In younger women, the skin is more supple; therefore, the actual effect of pregnancy on the skin is minimal.

The cosmetic significance is that any stretching of the skin, whether gradual or repeated, causes the skin surface to expand. When this process is not intended for medical purposes, the skin is not utilized for covering adjacent surfaces. This skin remains loose, slack, and wrinkled. The cosmetic implications are clear: **unnecessary stretching of the skin should be avoided**.

Unnecessary facial expressions, as detailed later in the text, cause repeated stretching of the skin, and should be avoided. Training and exercising of the facial muscles can cause unnecessary stretching of the skin. It is a myth that these exercises are beneficial to facial skin. As previously explained, such exercises may actually accelerate the process of wrinkling. Even when one is applying facial cosmetic products, this should be done gently to avoid stretching of the skin.

The same principle holds for **abrupt changes in weight**. Extreme weight gain accompanied by an increase in the amount of subcutaneous fat causes stretching of the skin above the thickened fatty layer. With weight loss, skin that was previously stretched becomes slack, and the excess skin becomes wrinkled and loose. So a balanced diet should be followed, in order to avoid repeated weight gain and loss.

And one more comment . . . It has been suggested that sleeping on one side causes stretching of the face in certain directions due to gravity, so diagonal wrinkles are formed on the cheeks and forehead. Therefore, sleeping in a supine position may be recommended. There is some degree of biological logic in this argument, but it is difficult to substantiate. No medical studies on this issue have been conducted. Because of the complexities involved, and the long periods of follow-up required, it is unlikely that such studies will take place.

Tissue Expanders—What Does Stretching of the Skin Result in?

The use of tissue expanders in plastic surgery also illustrates this concept. A tissue expander is a bag or balloon made of inert materials and is filled with water.

This procedure is utilized in regions where there is an absence of skin. It is performed in various medical conditions, including traumatic injury, burns, and certain diseases. The surgeon requires supplementary skin to cover areas devoid of skin. In order to obtain additional skin, the expander is transplanted below the patient's skin, adjacent to the deficient area. This results in expansion of the healthy skin, which is later used to cover skinless areas.

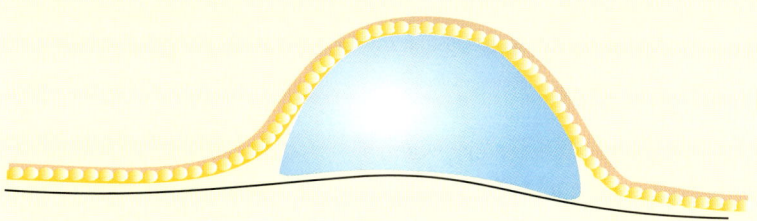

A transplanted expander.

Over a period of several weeks, additional water is injected into the transplanted expander, increasing its volume. As a result, the overlying skin is stretched, and its surface gradually expands.

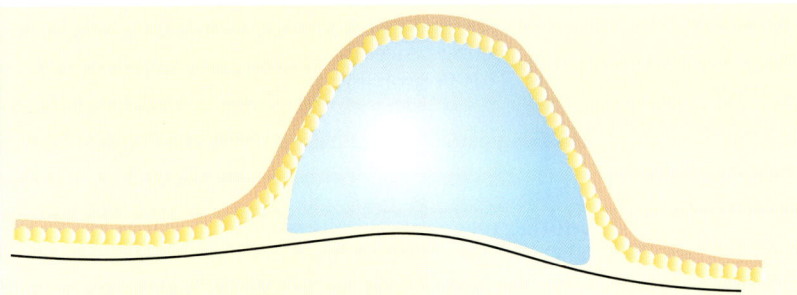

Volume increase of the expander, with subsequent expansion of the skin surface above.

The expander is then removed from the patient's body. After removal, the excess skin remains loose and can be stretched to cover adjacent areas, as necessary.

This is the main idea in using tissue expanders: a gradual stretching of the skin causes an increase in the skin's surface area, with the production of excess skin.

Facial Expressions

As previously described, when observing people during animated conversation, it is easy to see why expressive lines are formed. What can be done? Certainly, the object is not to develop a "poker face," nor is the intent to achieve total lack of facial movement. Normal expressions and expressive lines impart unique facial characteristics. One's personality, characteristics, and history are defined in the expressions and lines of one's face. Some suggest, however, that excessively exaggerated facial expressions be avoided during normal conversation in order to prevent the formation of unnecessary expressive lines over time.

Injection of botulinum toxin is a unique form of therapy that demonstrates the connection between facial expressions and wrinkles (detailed in chapter 27). Following injections of botulinum toxin, the targeted muscle becomes temporarily inactive. Subsequently, the formation of expression wrinkles is prevented to some extent. This form of treatment should only be carried out by an experienced professional in order to avoid the appearance of a "masked" face devoid of natural expression.

Facial Expressions and Wrinkles: Unilateral Paralysis

There is additional proof that facial expressions can cause wrinkles. In people with unilateral paralysis, after a number of years, the paralyzed side of the face appears younger. In contrast, the side of the face with normal movement and expression gains lines with time.

Use of Certain Topical Products

Skin aging, whether chronological or sun-induced, was previously considered to be irreversible. In the past few years, a number of new products that can affect the aging process have been developed, revolutionizing cosmetic dermatology. These include:

- retinoic acid, and
- α-hydroxy acids

These products are discussed in detail in chapters 17 and 18, respectively. The scientific literature does not provide clear data as to the effectiveness of other products, such as herbal extracts and preparations containing topical vitamins. Some of these products are detailed in chapter 16 on active ingredients in cosmetic preparations.

Until recently, products advertised as effective against wrinkles were simply based on increasing skin moisture. Moisturizers increase the water content of the skin. They give the skin a healthier, swollen appearance, blurring and diminishing the appearance of fine wrinkles—although only temporarily.

Do Moisturizers Prevent Skin Aging?
Certain moisturizing products are marketed as having "age-reversing" and "antiaging" qualities. However, moisturizers have never been established in the prevention of the skin aging process—whether caused by advanced age or by sun exposure. Nevertheless, the use of moisturizing products does have benefits.

- It can prevent skin damage caused by excessive dryness.
- An oily layer on the skin surface can protect it from exposure to various environmental factors such as soot particles, dirt, and dust.
- As previously stated, when skin is well moisturized, it appears temporarily smoother and more refreshed. Since it is slightly swollen, there is flattening and virtual fading of fine wrinkles. The pores appear somewhat smaller because the skin surrounding them is distended. This temporary improvement is exploited by advertisers, who claim that various moisturizing products have "antiaging" qualities.

Protecting the skin from environmental factors and preventing damage caused by dryness are highly significant, and without a doubt minimize deterioration in the appearance and quality of facial skin. Moisturizers are recommended for dry and normal skin, but not for oily skin. Details are given in chapter 4.

Leading a Physically and Emotionally Healthy Lifestyle
A healthy lifestyle will significantly improve one's general health. This includes the skin, a unique organ of the human body. The term "healthy lifestyle" includes:

- physical activity,
- regular sleeping hours,
- a healthy, balanced diet, and
- a healthy mental and emotional state.

All these will affect the body as a whole, and the skin specifically.

Physical Activity
As a rule, physical activity bestows well-being. During physical activity, there is an increase of blood flow to the skin, creating a rosy color. In the long run, this may also improve the skin's texture.

Sleep
After a sleepless night, red eyes and dark shadows around them are a familiar sight. Sleepless nights should be minimized. It is reasonable to assume that, in the long run, sleeplessness may cause cumulative damage to the skin texture.

Growth hormone is essential for appropriate growth during childhood and adolescence. After the period of active growth, it also plays a significant role in maintaining the quality of tissues, including muscles and skin. Inappropriate sleep may hinder the secretion of growth hormone that, in any case, tends to decrease after 40 years.

A Healthy, Balanced Diet
The significance of remaining at a steady weight was stated previously. One should avoid fluctuations in weight. In addition, various nutritional deficiencies are closely linked to dermatological diseases.

For example, severe vitamin C deficiency causes **scurvy**. This disease is manifested by the appearance of hemorrhages in the skin; the gums swell and bleed, with eventual loss of teeth; the body's ability to heal wounds is also adversely affected. Another example is **pellagra**, a disease caused by vitamin B3 deficiency. The appearance of inflamed rashes in areas exposed to the sun is typical of this disease.

Other nutritional deficiencies may manifest themselves by various skin lesions. These include lack of other vitamins, proteins, fatty acids, and trace elements such as iron or zinc. Although these diseases will only manifest themselves with extreme deficiencies, it is reasonable to assume that persistent minimal deficiencies may result in accumulative damage and should be avoided. So a balanced diet, composed of all the food groups and vitamin requirements, is highly recommended.

In the last decade, much attention has been devoted to vitamins functioning as **antioxidants**. These include:

- vitamin C,
- β-carotene, and
- vitamin E (α-tocopherol).

The assumption is that these products entrap the **oxygen free radicals** that cause damage to the body tissues.

Vitamin E, vitamin C, and β-carotene are able to entrap oxygen free radicals. Studies have been conducted in order to establish whether dietary supplements of these vitamins can decrease the incidence of malignancies and cardiovascular disease. Despite publications defending this statement, it remains a controversial issue. Whether or not supplementary vitamins improve the skin's quality and delay the aging process has not been established, either.

> What Are Oxygen Free Radicals?
>
> Oxygen free radicals are by-products formed by the chemical changes that the oxygen molecule undergoes. They are produced naturally and regularly in the body's tissues. The production of these free radicals in the body is much higher in response to several situations, for example, exposure to sunlight, X-rays, smoking, and environmental pollutants.
>
> Free radicals damage cell membranes and DNA and alter various biochemical compounds within the cells. It seems that they play a significant role in the development of heart and blood vessel diseases and the induction of malignancies.
>
> Scientists believe that oxygen free radicals accelerate the process of aging in various body systems.

A Healthy Mental and Emotional State

The relationship between mental health and skin health has been well documented for thousands of years. A person's mental and emotional state may be externalized, expressed on the skin—going pale or blushing, for example. Emotions, such as rage, anxiety, or fear, cause a drop in the temperature of the fingertips. A prolonged state of anxiety may therefore cause damage to the skin texture and its health.

Many diseases, including various skin diseases, are linked to mental stress, and may be exacerbated following a deterioration in the patient's mental health. Diseases whose association to emotional state have been vastly documented are, for example, acne, atopic dermatitis, and psoriasis. Expressive worry lines, anger, and depressed facial expressions are established and etched gradually, over years, on the face.

We shall not elaborate on this subject; ample literature has been published regarding this issue. In brief, it may be helpful to lead a happy lifestyle—it certainly cannot hurt.

A COMMENT REGARDING HORMONE REPLACEMENT THERAPY FOR POSTMENOPAUSAL WOMEN

During the reproductive years in women, **estrogen** is released from the ovaries. This hormone significantly contributes to the young, fresh, soft appearance of the skin. With the approach of the menopause, there is a decrease in the level of oestrogen released from the ovaries. Therefore, as well as the general effects of the menopause, there is also a progressive damage to the appearance of the skin and its function.

Hormone replacement therapy (HRT) is prescribed, in most countries, by gynaecologists. The replacement therapy can be taken orally, as tablets, or as hormone-containing patches that adhere to the skin. The advantages of this therapy include prevention of hot flushes, prevention of dryness of the vagina, and a decrease in symptoms of depression and fatigue, as well as slowing the detrimental processes of osteoporosis.

Several studies have documented the effects on the skin of HRT with oestrogen. This treatment has been reported to prevent, to a certain extent, the decrease of collagen content in the skin that appears after menopause. In addition, HRT may delay the undesirable accumulation of subcutaneous fat in various areas of the body that accompanies the aging process.

However, in 2002, the results of a large-scale American research study were published, indicating that HRT may increase the risk of developing cardiovascular diseases and may be associated with malignant diseases—mainly breast cancer. However, on thorough analysis of the results of this study, together with the results of subsequent research studies, the data showed that factors such as the timing of therapy and the age group of women treated had a crucial impact on the HRT medical effect. It seems that women that start HRT rather early may even have a reduced risk of cardiovascular diseases. HRT seems to have undesirable effects on the heart and blood vessels if started several years after menopause.

Other research studies suggested that HRT may increase the risk of developing breast cancer. The accurate extent of association between breast cancer and HRT still has to be assessed and future studies are required to clarify this issue.

In addition to age, certain other factors may influence the therapeutic ramifications: form of administration (tablets vs. patches), dosage, and identity of hormones included in the preparation and combination. Thus, the use of hormone preparations must be tailored to suit each woman according to her specific medical profile, and a physician should be consulted in all cases.

Note that several topical cosmetic products contain hormones and therefore are advertised as having "antiaging" qualities. These products contain oestrogens in very low concentrations. Because of the minimal amount of hormones they contain, these products remain categorized as cosmetics and are not labeled as drugs. It has not been confirmed scientifically that these hormone-containing products have any beneficial effect on the skin. Most dermatologists do not recommend them.

9 | Acne
Alex Zvulunov

Contents Overview • Acne lesions • The basis for the appearance of acne lesions • Diet and acne • Facial cleansing • Sun and acne • Drugs, chemicals and acne. • Cosmetics and make-up • Treatment by a cosmetician • Treatment by a dermatologist • Tailoring treatment • Final comment

OVERVIEW

Acne is an inflammatory disease of the hair follicles and their associated sebaceous glands. It is related primarily to hormonal changes that occur during adolescence. Acne is very common, affecting approximately 85% of adolescents. In most cases, acne first appears at 12 to 14 years of age. As sexual development begins earlier in girls than in boys, acne appears earlier in girls. However, in view of the effect of testosterone on sebaceous glands, boys, in most cases, tend to present more severe forms of acne as opposed to girls. Acne may become quite severe after a number of years—between the ages of 15 and 19, following which there is a gradual improvement and disappearance of the acne lesions, usually in the mid-20s. Acne can persist into the 40s in a minority of patients. The afflicted person should be aware of the fact that the problem may last for more than 10 years, and treatment may be necessary from time to time during this period.

ACNE LESIONS

Acne is characterized by the appearance of:

- **open comedones (blackheads)**
- **closed comedones (whiteheads)**

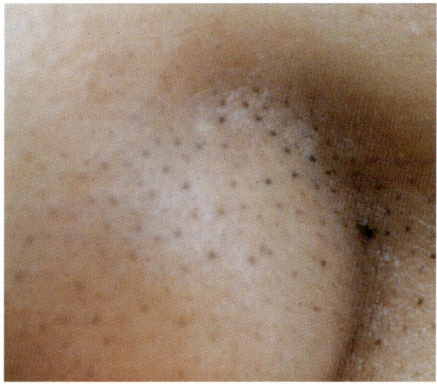

Open comedones (blackheads).

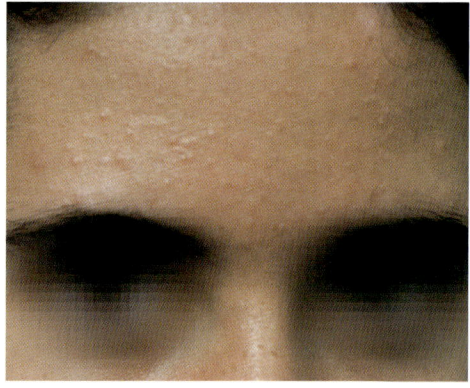

Closed comedones (whiteheads).

The correct medical term is "comedo" (plural "comedones"). The term "comedone" is commonly used as well—and we shall do so here.

The comedone is the basic, primary lesion of acne. Other lesions that appear in acne represent various degrees of inflammation and include the following:

- **Papules**, which are small, raised lesions, up to 0.5 cm in diameter, usually pink/red in color.
- **Pustules**, which are lesions containing pus.

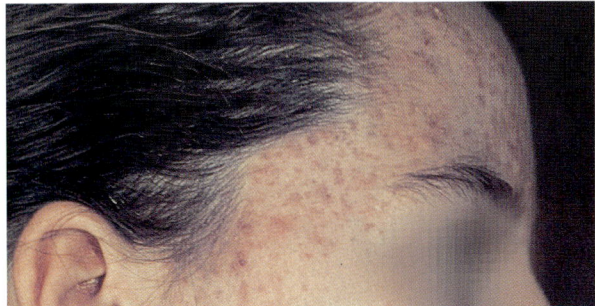
Papules.

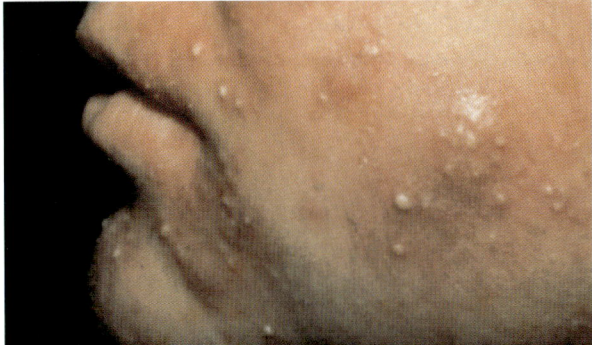
Pustules.

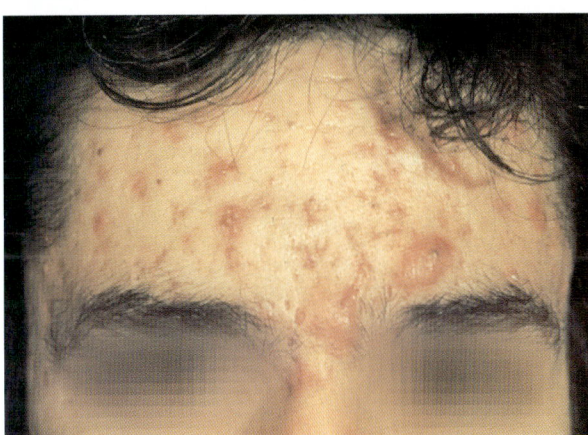
Nodules.

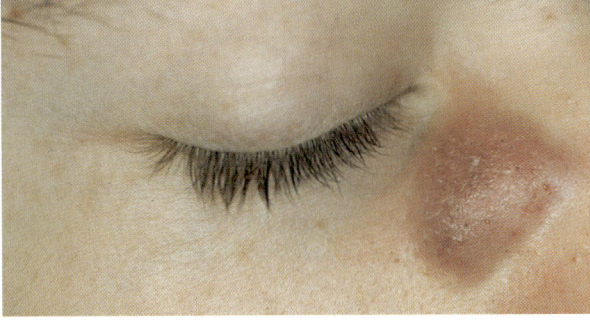
Cyst.

- **Nodules**, which are inflammatory swellings that, in comparison to papules, are located deeper under the skin. When large, a nodule may change the contour of the skin, thus creating a bulge.
- **Cysts**, which are closed spaces under the skin's surface, containing liquid or semisolid material.

THE BASIS FOR THE APPEARANCE OF ACNE LESIONS

Structure of the Hair Follicle and the Sebaceous Gland

To understand why acne lesions appear and the reason for their development, one should be familiar with the microscopic structure of the skin, the hair follicle, and the sebaceous gland.

A **hair follicle** is an elongated tube–like structure, out of which the hair grows—as shown in the diagram. Each hair follicle has at least one **sebaceous gland** attached to it. The sebaceous glands secrete **sebum**, an oily substance that coats the skin and hair. Sebum is not secreted directly onto the surface of the skin, but into the hair follicle from where it reaches the skin's surface. The length and width of each hair are not necessarily correlated with the size of the sebaceous gland whose contents drain to the same hair follicle. For example, on the skin of a woman's face, or on the nose, sebaceous glands are relatively large, while hairs in this area are barely discernible. When the hair is small, and the opening of the hair follicle is wide and gaping, it looks as though there is a tiny pore on the skin's surface.

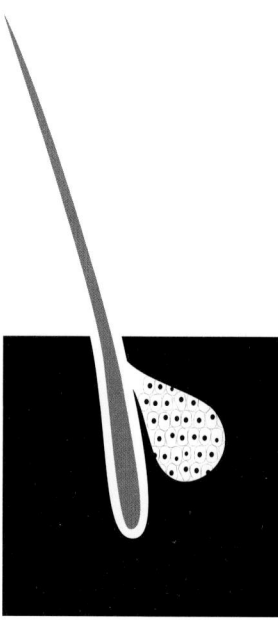

Hair follicle with a hair growing out of it, and the sebaceous gland attached to it.

Sebaceous glands are distributed throughout the skin of the whole body, except for the palms and soles. They are deeper and more numerous on the face, upper chest, and upper back. These areas are indeed more prone to acne.

Primary Lesions in Acne: Closed Comedones and Open Comedones

There are two main reasons for the appearance of the primary acne lesions (the closed comedone and the open comedone):

- An increase in the number of cells in the hair follicle, which results in an increase of the horny substance (keratin) found in the hair follicle.
- An increase in sebum production by the sebaceous glands.

Normally, cells in the hair follicle replicate steadily and continuously, as do other cells on the skin surface. Similarly, there is a constant, steady secretion of sebum by the sebaceous glands. Under normal circumstances, cells that are shed within the follicle are swept out of the follicle onto the surface of the skin along with the secreted sebum.

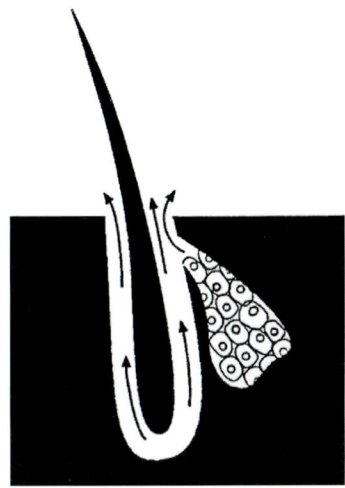

Normally the contents of the skin follicle are swept onto the skin surface.

However, in acne, the replication of cells within the hair follicle is excessive. Within the follicle, there are increasing amounts of oily substances and keratinous material (originating from the secreted sebum and the accumulation of dead cells) that cannot drain easily from the follicle to the surface of the skin. With time, these keratinous and oily substances block the tiny ducts through which the sebum drains to the surface of the skin. In the next stage, the draining duct widens and the sebaceous gland grows larger and wider due to the accumulated material. This process is shown in the following four illustrations.

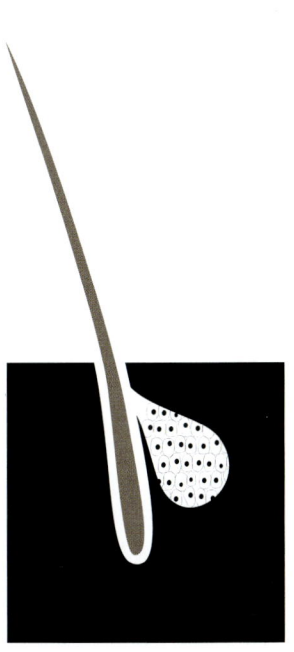

(**A**) Cross-section of a hair follicle: normal sebaceous gland.

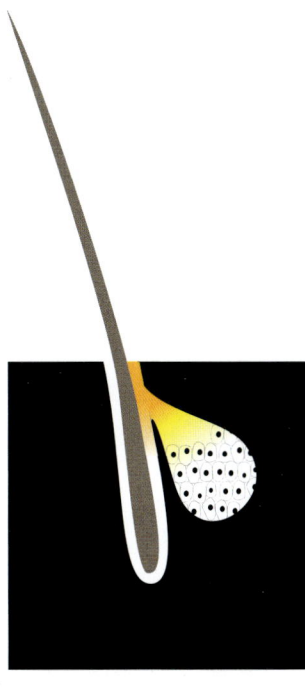

(**B**) The duct leading from the sebaceous gland is blocked by sebum and keratin.

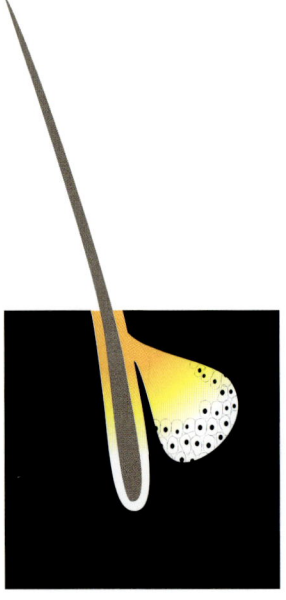

(C) The sebum, produced in the sebaceous gland, accumulates behind the area of blockage.

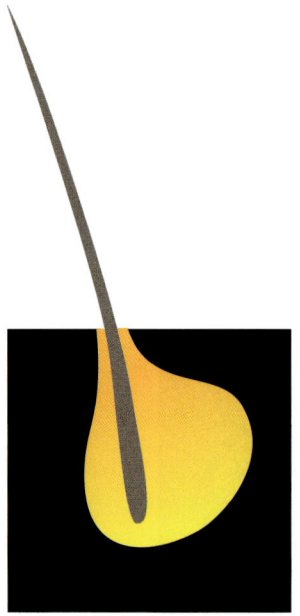

(D) The accumulated sebum distends the sebaceous gland and its duct.

As a result of this process, the two basic lesions of acne appear. At this point these lesions are not yet inflamed.

Open Comedones (Blackheads)

These are caused by a widening of the follicle opening owing to the accumulation of dense keratinous material and sebum. The black color seen in the pore comes from the presence of pigment, which is also found among the substances that plug the opening of the follicle.

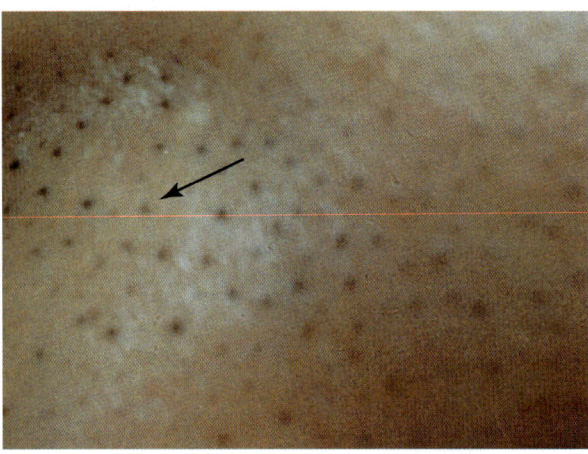
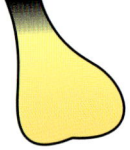

An open comedone (blackhead).

Closed Comedones (Whiteheads)

These occur when the follicle's opening remains closed. Underneath the opening of the follicle, the dense keratinous material and sebum accumulate. A closed comedone, in itself, is not an inflammatory lesion, but it is the initial lesion from which the various inflammatory lesions in acne may develop.

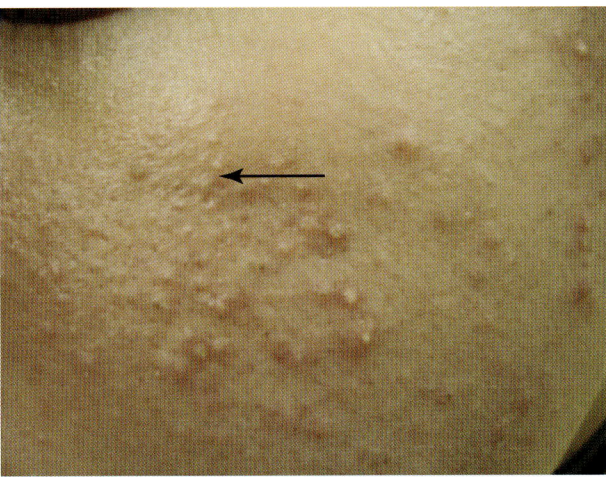
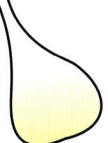

A closed comedone (whitehead).

Inflammatory Lesions of Acne

As already pointed out, the inflammatory lesions of acne develop from the closed comedone (whitehead), which is a closed space filled with sebum, fatty substances, compressed keratinous material, and remnants of dead cells. These conditions permit a proliferation of bacteria naturally found within the hair follicles and on the skin surface. However, within the closed comedone, bacteria in the depths of the follicle enjoy ideal conditions for proliferation—a nutritional environment rich in fats (sebum) and without oxygen, within the enclosed space. The bacteria replicate rapidly and excrete substances that induce an inflammatory reaction. This bacterial activity produces the inflammatory lesions in acne. These lesions were listed earlier in the chapter, and we now review them in detail, together with schematic illustrations.

Papules

These are the primary inflammatory lesions. A papule is a lesion that is usually smaller than 0.5 cm in diameter. It is raised above the skin's surface. As a result of the inflammatory process in acne, it acquires a pink to red color.

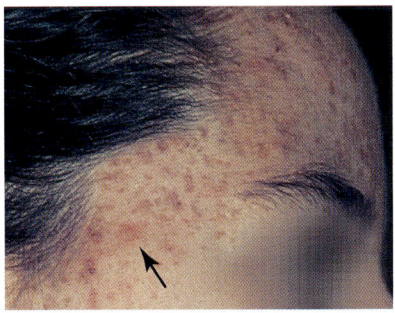
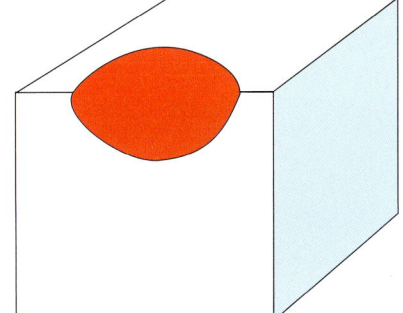

A papule.

Pustules

If the follicle's space becomes filled with pus, the result is a pustule. Pustules are tiny spaces containing pus. Their color ranges from white/yellow to orange/green. Puncturing a pustule releases its liquid pus content.

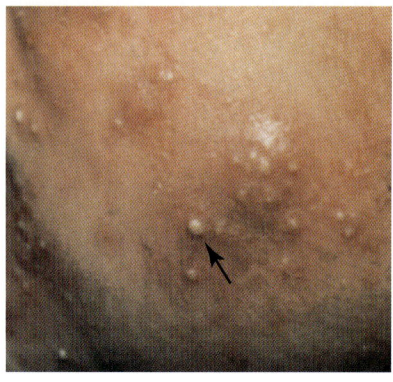
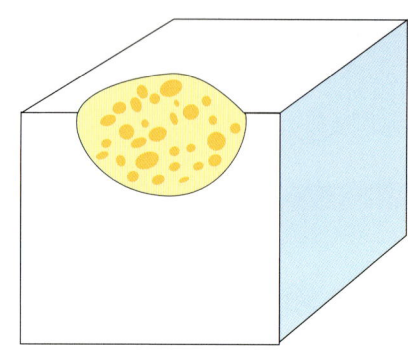

A pustule.

Nodules

When more and more keratinous remnants and sebum accumulate within the follicle, it becomes larger and deeper, resulting in a nodule. A nodule is an inflamed swelling located deeper in the skin than a papule. The distinction between a papule and a nodule can be made by feeling the lesion with the fingers.

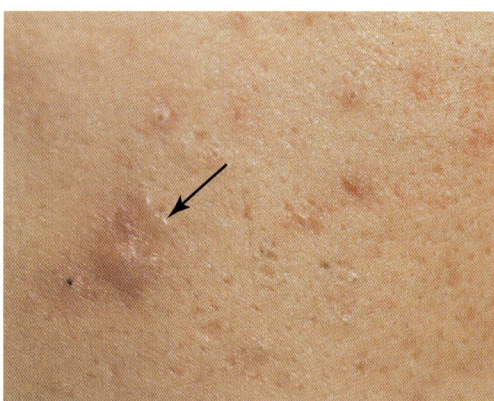
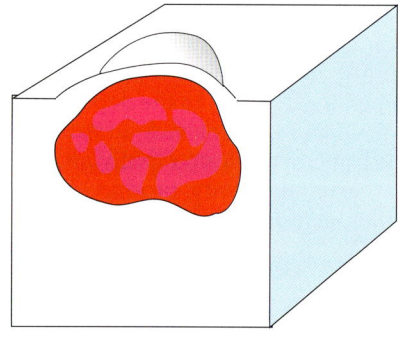

A nodule.

Cysts

When the hair follicle becomes filled with a liquid substance, the result is a cyst. A cyst is a fluid-containing space within the skin. By carefully feeling a cyst, one can feel the presence of the liquid substance contained within it.

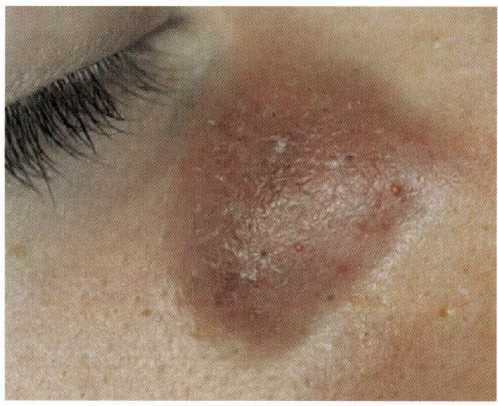
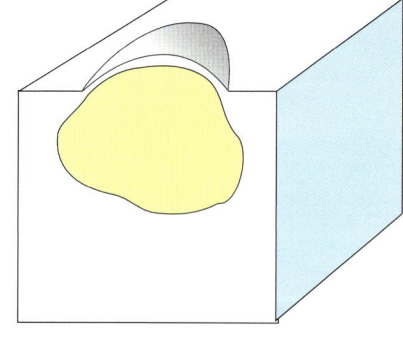

A cyst.

DIET AND ACNE

Traditionally, certain foods such as chocolate, peanuts, fatty foodstuffs, and dairy products have been blamed for causing or aggravating acne. Research studies, however, have failed to find any association between certain diets and acne. This conclusion is now widely accepted amongst dermatologists. However, a few dietary recommendations may be given for acne patients.

Sensitivity to Particular Foods

Although, for most patients, there is no association between dietary factors and acne, there are exceptional cases where a certain food does cause acne to appear within days of its ingestion. If there is an apparent correlation between consumption of that food and acne, the patient should avoid that specific food.

Milk Products and Acne

An acne patient being treated with antibiotics of the tetracycline group should avoid milk products while taking these drugs. After ingestion of milk products, one should wait at least two hours before taking these antibiotics. For acne patients who are not taking tetracyclines, there is no special reason to avoid milk products.

Alternative Medical Treatments Associated with Diet

In the standard medical literature, there is no proof that alternative therapies are effective in acne. Nevertheless, these forms of treatment are usually harmless. Therefore, if an acne sufferer is interested in alternative therapies (whether or not they involve dietary changes), they can be tried, provided there is no possibility that they will harm his/her health. In any case, these therapies should be used in conjunction with conventional medical acne treatment. Nowadays it is quite rare for acne not to improve with conventional medical treatment, taking into account the wide range of treatments currently available.

FACIAL CLEANSING

Acne is a process that does not originate from the skin's surface, but from the deeper layers—inside the follicles and the sebaceous glands. Therefore, merely cleaning and washing the face cannot solve the problem. People with clean skin can most definitely develop acne, just as those whose skin is less clean may escape the disease.

However, cleansing does remove sebum, sweat, dirt, and dead cells from the surface of the skin. Removing the oily layer and dirt from the skin's surface may, to some extent, reduce the blockages in the pores, allowing a more effective drainage of the contents of the hair follicles. By the same token, applying oil to an oily skin that is prone to acne tends to seal the pores and aggravate the acne. Furthermore, even though the cleansing process does not reach deep into the follicles and the sebaceous glands, it may possibly remove bacteria found on the skin's surface and prevent them from penetrating into the follicles. Surface cleansing of the skin is not supposed to cure a preexisting comedone—at most, it may limit the spreading of infection and may prevent the development of new lesions. Hence, acne sufferers are advised to wash the face gently in order to remove excess dirt, oily substances, bacteria, and dead cells from the skin's surface. Vigorous rubbing and scrubbing has no additional benefits, and indeed may worsen the acne by spreading the inflammation to new areas. A relatively mild soap should be used rather than a drying one, because most of the preparations used in the treatment of acne already contain substances that tend to dry the skin. If the skin becomes red, irritated, or scaly while using a certain soap, another more gentle type should be tried.

Soaps

The soaps recommended for acne patients are relatively mild. They do not tend to cause irritation. Another group of soaps used to treat acne contains antibacterial compounds. These soaps are detailed in chapter 5 on skin cleansing.

> **Benzoyl Peroxide in Acne Soaps**
>
> Benzoyl peroxide is a common antibacterial compound used in acne soaps. This peroxide is an oxidant that acts against the bacteria that cause acne. It is found in many acne preparations for application to the skin, and has been found to be effective in the treatment of acne (see later). However, benzoyl peroxide is less effective when in a soap or other cleansing preparation that is rinsed off shortly after being applied to the skin than when in a preparation that is left on the skin for several hours.

SUN AND ACNE

Upon sun exposure, the majority of acne patients will show some improvement. About one-fifth of patients will not respond, and in a minority of patients, aggravation of the skin lesions will occur. The improvement is related to a certain anti-inflammatory effect of the ultraviolet rays. In addition, tanning may conceal the acne lesions to some extent. However, exposure to the sun's rays may also cause an excess production of keratin and sebum, both on the skin's surface and in the pores, which may, in turn, cause a relative worsening of the acne. Some dermatologists therefore recommend that the face be gently cleansed after being moderately exposed to the sun. In summary:

- Exposure to the sun should be gradual and moderate.
- If patients notice an aggravation of acne after exposure to the sun, they should avoid it.
- Gentle cleansing of the skin after exposure to the sun may be recommended.
- A nonoily sunscreen that suits the patient's skin should be used. It should be remembered that the use of some oily moisturizers may aggravate the acne.

Note: The above discussion relates to noninflammatory lesions of acne. If **active inflammatory lesions** of acne are present, it is best to avoid sun exposure, because these lesions sometimes heal by the formation of scars. In general, sun exposure may permanently darken the final color of scars, including acne scars, thus making them more apparent.

DRUGS, CHEMICALS, AND ACNE

Certain medications may induce the development of acne. In cases where a specific medication is known to inflict acne, the most reasonable step would be to discontinue its use and, if necessary, replace it by an alternative medication. Numerous drugs have been reported to cause acne. The most common are steroids, androgenic hormones, certain anti-convulsives, anti-tuberculosis drugs, lithium, and others. In addition, exposure to certain oils (especially at work) may induce acne. Exposure to iodides, bromides, and chlorines has also been reported to cause acne.

COSMETICS AND MAKE-UP

Two types of cosmetics may cause acne:

- Certain cosmetic preparations may induce a **comedogenic** effect. These substances cause the appearance of comedones. In such cases, the acne usually appears after using the cosmetic for several months. Comedones begin to appear—both whiteheads and blackheads.
- Certain cosmetic preparations may induce an **acnegenic** effect. In these cases, the acne appears in the form of pustules within one to two weeks of using the formulation.

Usually, make-up preparations that are too oily may cause occlusion of the skin's pores, interfering with the normal drainage of sebum secretion, and therefore have comedogenic or acnegenic potential. In the cosmetics industry, emphasis has been put on the identification of certain ingredients that may reduce acne. Many cosmetics include a label specifying that they are either non-comedogenic or non-acnegenic. In general, cosmetics for women who suffer from acne are designed for use on oily skin. These preparations, as a rule, contain a relatively larger concentration of water and less oil, and may even contain oil-absorbing substances.

Similarly, there are creams intended for acne treatment in which the medical preparations are combined with coloring ingredients. These can be used simultaneously as make-up. The user

TREATMENT BY A COSMETICIAN

The main functions of a cosmetician in treating acne are:

- cleansing of the face,
- expressing the contents of the comedones, and
- instructing patients about how to clean and treat the skin.

Note: The part of the cosmetician's treatment described below, namely, opening and draining comedones, has no effect on the duration and the general course of the acne. The treatment is aimed at preventing the inflammation and infection of comedones, but new comedones will continue to appear. However, appropriate treatment by a cosmetician does produce an immediate cosmetic improvement, with all its psychological benefits.

The stages in treating comedones are:

1. softening the comedones,
2. cleaning and sterilizing the skin,
3. expressing the contents of the comedones, and
4. further cleansing of the affected area.

Softening the Comedones

It is preferable to soften the comedones before draining them. Ideally, this is achieved by the use of creams containing retinoic acid. The cream should be applied to the affected area, daily, for one month, before the cosmetician commences treatment. This preliminary treatment can only be prescribed by a physician. Alternative methods for softening and loosening the comedones are:

- steaming,
- applying hot, moist compresses 15 minutes before the treatment,
- the application of preparations with salicylic acid or sulfur salicylic acid before the treatment is given, and
- using alpha-hydroxy acid preparations.

Cleaning and Sterilizing the Skin

Cleaning and sterilizing the skin can be achieved by using alcohol (70% solution) or any other antiseptic solution.

Releasing the Contents of Comedones

There are two ways to release the contents of comedones:

- squeezing with the fingertips, or
- using a **comedone extractor** (often termed "comedo extractor").

Both methods are acceptable, and each has its advocates.

Squeezing the comedones with the fingertips, if not done correctly, may cause the contents of the comedones to burst into the surrounding tissue. This may cause inflammation in the area and result in scarring.

Nowadays, with the emergence of HIV and an increase in the incidence of hepatitis B infection, any contact with the blood or secretions of a patient requires the use of gloves. A cosmetician who squeezes comedones with the fingertips must also wear gloves, because the treatment may cause some localized bleeding. However, by wearing gloves, the cosmetician may lose the delicate feeling in the fingertips needed for the treatment, and the whole process becomes awkward and much less efficient.

On the other hand, many cosmeticians prefer the old method of squeezing the comedones with the fingertips. They maintain that in fact, the firm vertical pressure that the comedone extractor exerts on the follicle (downwards, towards the deeper layers of the skin) may

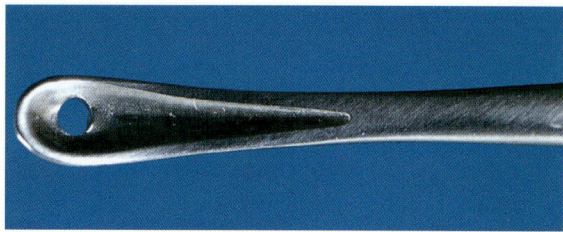

Comedone extractor.

actually cause the follicle to burst—which, they believe, does not happen when an experienced cosmetician uses the fingertips. Some proponents of this method recommend covering the fingers with a thin layer of cotton/wool soaked in a weak alcohol solution.

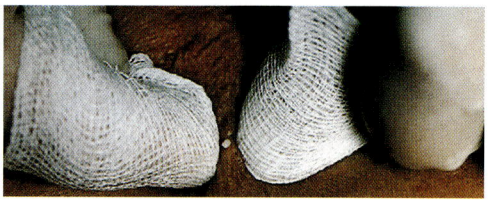

Expressing the contents of a comedone by squeezing with the fingertips.

Note: All the treatments described here must be performed under optimal conditions, with a bright light and a magnifying glass.

How to Release the Contents of Comedones?

- **Open comedone (blackhead)**: This is expressed by applying vertical pressure—gentle, yet steady—pressing downwards around the sides of the lesion. The pressure applied to a comedone ought to push the contents up and out, onto the surface of the skin. If nothing comes out, the fingers should be moved a little bit to a different location around the lesion and the procedure is repeated. If fatty material starts to ooze out of the comedone, one should press gently in a few places (using two opposing fingers) until all the contents have come out, or a little bleeding occurs. The extruded material should be wiped from the skin with cotton/wool (not gauze or tissue, which have a rougher consistency than cotton/wool), and the area is then wiped again with antiseptic.

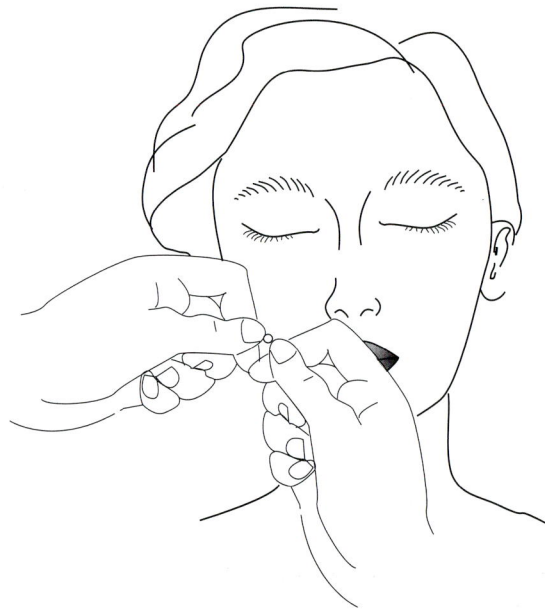

Expressing the contents of a comedone by finger pressure.

- **Closed comedone (whitehead)**: If the comedone does not open easily, it should be punctured gently in its center with a sterile needle. Following that, the contents of the comedone should be expressed by pressure as described above.

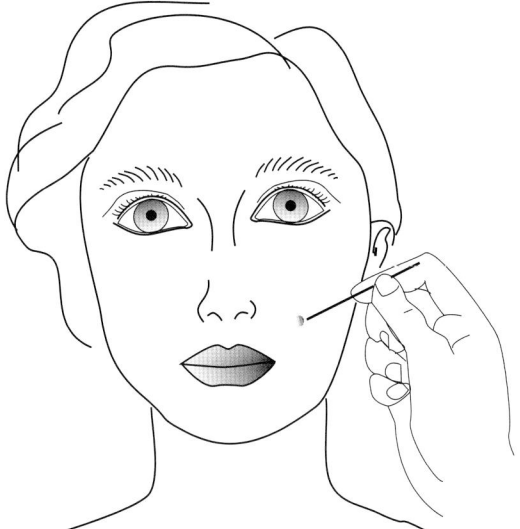
Puncturing a comedone.

Treating Other Acne Lesions
- The contents of **small pustules** (up to about 3 mm in diameter) may be drained by puncturing the center. Following the puncturing, the contents should be expressed with pressure as described above. For the treatment of **larger pustules**, the patient should be referred to a doctor. If there are more than four or five pustules, the patient might also be referred to a doctor.

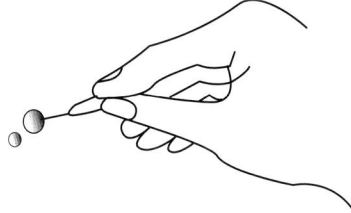
Puncturing a pustule.

- On the other hand, **nodules** or **cysts** should not be punctured or squeezed. These must be treated by a dermatologist.
- **Inflamed, red papules**: One must avoid any manipulation of inflamed lesions. They should not be touched, squeezed, or punctured. If punctured, they will just bleed without any drainage of the follicle's content. Fiddling with inflamed papules will only result in unnecessary tissue damage, which can later develop into a scar. No fatty or purulent (pussy) material can be obtained from such a lesion.

Further Cleansing
After treatment, the area should be cleansed again with alcohol or another antiseptic solution.

TREATMENT BY A DERMATOLOGIST

This section presents the treatment of acne by a dermatologist. Two types of treatment are performed by a dermatologist:

- by using preparations for external use, applying them to the skin, and
- by using oral medications (systemic treatment).

Note: This section is not meant to encourage cosmeticians to treat acne sufferers with medications. Its aim is to broaden cosmeticians' knowledge of the subject, and to let them know which medications are commonly used for acne. Obviously, medicinal treatment should only be prescribed by a physician.

Preparations for External Use (Application to the Skin)
Preparations for external use are designed to be applied to the skin in the areas affected by acne. They are usually in the form of creams or liquids (as emulsions, suspensions, aqueous solutions, or alcohol solutions). These preparations generally cause drying and scaling of the skin to a variable degree; this is particularly true for those preparations that cause a decrease in the amount of sebum secreted in the skin.

When starting to use a preparation for the first time, one should be cautious: First the substance should be applied over a small area of the skin that is out of sight, and only if no skin irritation occurs should it be applied over a wider affected area and over the face.

It is an acceptable practice to use a combination of different preparations, for example, one type of preparation in the morning and a different one for nighttime.

If a certain preparation causes skin irritation or aggravates the acne, even if it has been used for a certain period of time without any adverse effects, it should be discontinued and a physician consulted.

Preparations Containing Salicylic Acid, Sulfur, or Resorcinol
Preparations containing salicylic acid, sulfur, and/or resorcinol are the "traditional" preparations, which are less commonly used nowadays, because newer preparations have been found to be much more effective. These preparations are **keratolytic** substances, that is, they dissolve the keratinous substance in the skin. Dissolving the keratinous layer helps remove the material that is plugging up the opening of the hair follicle. However, the keratolytic action of salicylic acid, sulfur, and resorcinol is considered to be weak. These preparations have a drying effect and may irritate the skin. They have mild antibacterial properties.

Alpha-Hydroxy Acids
The main rationale for using alpha-hydroxy acids in acne is that these preparations, as chemical exfoliants, weaken the adhesion between the degenerating and dead cells of the outer layers of the skin, thereby preventing plugging up of hair follicles. Research has demonstrated the beneficial effect of alpha-hydroxy acids at low concentrations in mild and moderate acne, with subsequent reductions in the number of acne lesions. In low concentrations, they are intended for application once or twice a day. Alpha-Hydroxy acids are discussed in more detail in chapter 18.

Benzoyl Peroxide
This is an antimicrobial substance that acts by oxidizing the bacterial proteins. When applied to the skin, it penetrates the follicles and decreases the bacterial population of the follicle, which is responsible for the various phenomena of acne. In addition, it has a certain keratolytic effect. It is available in the following forms:

- cream
- gel
- lotion
- facial mask
- in some soaps used for acne

Benzoyl peroxide is usually used in concentrations of 2.5%, 5%, or 10%. Preparations containing benzoyl peroxide may cause drying and irritation. Hence, it is advisable to begin with a lower concentration and if there is no skin irritation, then move up to a higher concentration.

Antibiotic Preparations for External Application
Antibiotic preparations for external application contain one of the following antibiotics:

- erythromycin
- clindamycin
- tetracycline

These preparations act directly on the bacteria in the hair follicle. Their use could potentially result in allergic reactions, albeit in a minute percentage of patients.

Retinoic Acid

Retinoic acid is chemically related to vitamin A. Its main effect is to regulate the rate of reproduction of cells within the follicle. In that way, it ensures an effective turnover of cells within the follicle, with more effective disposal of dead cells. It prevents the formation of "plugs" that block the opening of the follicle, thus preventing the formation of comedones. Hence, it is particularly useful in noninflamed acne, which consists mainly of open and closed comedones. Retinoic acid is present in various preparations, be they in the form of a solution, cream, or gel.

The usual concentrations of retinoic acid are 0.025% and 0.05%. When it is first used, the skin may become red and scaly, but after a few weeks of use the irritation subsides. Sometimes, at the beginning of the treatment, there may be a transient worsening of the acne, but this resolves with time. Retinoic acid increases the skin's sensitivity to sunlight; therefore, it should be applied only at night. During the day, people using retinoic acid should avoid exposure to sunlight as much as possible, and should apply a sunscreen preparation. Retinoic acid is also used to prevent aging of the skin and for lightening dark spots (see chapter 17).

Retinoic acid should not be used in pregnancy and breast-feeding mothers.

Examples of Preparations Containing Retinoic Acid, in Various Countries:

Airol®
Avita®
Locacid®
Renova®
Retin-A®
Retisol-A®
Vesanoid®

Adapalene

The mechanism of action of adapalene, a drug used for topical treatment in acne, is similar to that of retinoic acid. Adapalene is incorporated in gel preparations, in a concentration of 0.1%. Research has demonstrated the beneficial effect of adapalene in mild-to-moderate acne. It has some anti-inflammatory activity.

The adverse effects of adapalene basically resemble those of retinoic acid. Skin irritation may occur, manifested by redness, dry skin, and a sensation of stinging, itching, or burning.

Adapalene preparations are applied as a thin film on the affected skin areas, once before bedtime, after washing the face.

Other Topical Retinoids

In recent years, other forms of retinoid compounds that are intended to be applied to the skin have been developed. Tazarotene and isotretinoin are typical examples of these preparations. These preparations are not approved in all countries. In some countries, they are intended for other indications apart from acne. In all these compounds, the mechanism of action in the treatment of acne is basically similar to that of retinoic acid.

Retinoids should not be used in pregnancy. In women with childbearing potential, they should only be used if precautionary measures are being undertaken to avoid pregnancy, according to the gynecologist's instructions.

Azelaic Acid

Azelaic acid is a substance made naturally in the body. It has been used in several relatively new preparations that have been found to be effective, to a certain degree, against acne. Azelaic acid has a combined therapeutic activity—it is both antibacterial and anti-inflammatory. In addition, azelaic acid regulates the cell turnover within the follicle, and in that way prevents blockage of the follicle by keratinous material, and hence the formation of comedones. Preparations containing azelaic acid are useful for both inflammatory and noninflammatory acne lesions.

Azelaic acid is also used for lightening dark, pigmented areas of skin (see chapter 20 on bleaching).

Orally Administered Medications (Systemic Treatment)

Antibiotics
Antibiotics are used in acne for inflamed and infected lesions. They are directed against the bacteria in the follicle that result in inflammatory acne lesions. The antibiotics generally used in acne are:

- tetracyclines
- erythromycin

Of the antibiotics that can be taken orally, tetracyclines are usually preferred. The most popular medication of this group is **minocycline**. It is given in a dosage of 50 mg twice daily for several weeks. Following that, the patient continues on a maintenance dose of one 50-mg tablet a day for a variable period. Minocycline focuses on those bacteria that are involved in the development of acne; however, it has a general effect against inflammatory processes as well. (**Doxycycline** is another medication of the tetracycline group that is commonly used in acne.)

Tetracyclines
As tetracyclines are common medications in the treatment of acne, note the following:

- While taking tetracyclines, exposure to sunlight should be minimized, because these drugs increase the skin's sensitivity to sunlight. People who are exposed to sunlight while taking tetracyclines may develop exaggerated sunburn.
- Tetracycline preparations may cause damage to mucosa after its ingestion. It is recommended to drink at least half a glass of water after taking the medication, while sitting or standing. Most doctors advise not to lie until 30 minutes after taking it to ensure the tablet/capsule does not stay in the upper parts of digestive system.
- Drinking milk or eating milk products, such as cheese, together with tetracyclines interferes with the absorption of the medication in the body, lessening its effect. At least two hours should elapse between taking a tetracycline and ingesting a milk product. Similarly, tetracyclines should not be taken together with antacid preparations, substances containing iron, or preparations containing vitamins.
- Tetracyclines, as with other types of antibiotics, may affect the efficacy of contraceptive pills. Women taking such pills should consult their physicians regarding the use of additional or alternative contraceptive precautions while taking tetracyclines.
- **Tetracyclines must not be taken during pregnancy or while breast-feeding!**
- Tetracyclines may cause a disturbance in the growth of bones and may stain the teeth of children (and embryos). They should not be given to children younger than 12 years in the United Kingdom. In other countries, the age threshold varies. Yet, in children, other optional treatments should always be considered prior to prescription of tetracyclines.
- The development of an unusual or severe headache or visual disturbances while taking the drug may be the clinical manifestation of increased intracranial pressure. In that case, the medication should immediately be discontinued.
- In case of any other medical problem while taking the drug, it should be discontinued and a physician consulted.

The above list is not complete. All patients should consult their physicians prior to taking the drug.

Hormonal Preparations
The commonly accepted hormonal preparations in the treatment of acne (for women only) contain an estrogen (ethinyloestradiol) and/or an anti-androgenic substance that counteracts the male hormones (cyproterone acetate). These preparations are usually used as birth control pills, prescribed by a gynecologist. Sometimes they are also used for the prevention of excessive hair growth in women.

Common commercial names of the medication in various countries are Diane®, Dianeal®, and Dianette®.

Isotretinoin

Isotretinoin is an orally administered medication from the retinoid group of compounds, that is, substances that are chemically similar to vitamin A. It has been used in the treatment of acne for more than 30 years, widely known as **Accutane®** or **Roaccutane®**. In recent years, other commercial products based on isotretinoin have been released to the market (only the original product has been approved by the FDA). Isotretinoin exerts its beneficial effect on acne by:

- reducing the size of sebaceous glands,
- decreasing the activity of sebaceous glands, thus decreasing sebum excretion,
- reducing the bacterial population within the follicles,
- reducing the level of inflammation in follicles, and
- restoring the keratin formation process and the return of cells (turnover) within the follicle to a normal state.

Isotretinoin is an effective drug that has been found to be highly beneficial in the treatment of acne that has not responded to previous modes of therapy. This medication is only ever taken after consulting a physician and after having a medical examination; it requires a doctor's prescription and monthly follow-ups.

Precautions for Patients Taking Isotretinoin

- In isolated cases, patients taking isotretinoin may experience headaches and visual disturbances due to increased intracranial pressure. In such cases, the drug should be discontinued and the treating physician should be consulted.
- Isotretinoin treatment may cause fluctuations in mood. In rare cases, the occurrence of depression may be severe. However, one should take into account that acne, as a disfiguring disease, may cause depression in itself, which is expected to abate following successful treatment. Patients taking isotretinoin should be aware as to the possible development of depression and consult the physician if any problems arise.
- **Isotretinoin may not be taken before puberty.**
- **Isotretinoin must not be taken during pregnancy!** If taken during pregnancy, it may cause fetal malformations, particularly in the heart and nervous system. The patient must not become pregnant for at least one month after discontinuation of isotretinoin. Women of childbearing age should consult a gynecologist for advice on a birth control regimen. In most countries, two different contraceptive methods are required, and pregnancy tests must be repeated every month, up to one month after isotretinoin treatment is terminated. In the United States, women of childbearing potential taking isotretinoin are required to participate in an approved program to ensure against becoming pregnant.
- Patients treated by isotretinoin should not undergo skin peeling or plastic surgical procedures (especially on the face), during therapy and one to two years thereafter. Similarly, one should avoid hair removal by laser, by wax, and using abrasive facial cleansers during treatment and for a certain period (to be considered by physician) thereafter.
- Avoid taking any other drugs without informing the treating physician.
- Update the treating physician if any unusual health problems or changes appear. The main problems to look out for are headaches, pain in the eyes or visual disturbances, and changes in mood.

What Are the Side Effects of Isotretinoin?

The following table presents common adverse effects of isotretinoin and suggestions on how to deal with them.

If any of the following adverse effects appear, or any not listed here, the treating physician should be consulted. Discontinuation of isotretinoin or reducing the dose for a certain period may be considered. (The severity of the adverse effects of isotretinoin is usually proportional to the amount of drug being taken.)

Side Effect	Therapeutic Approach
Dryness of the skin appears during the first few weeks of treatment. The skin may peel and become scaly.	In most cases, one may decrease the severity by appropriate use of moisturizers and emollients. The use of oily soaps is recommended. When drying, one should avoid vigorous rubbing. The skin should be wiped by gentle dabbing with a soft towel.
Dry eyes.	This can be moderated by frequent use of eye drops containing artificial tears. It is absolutely forbidden to wear contact lenses during the treatment period to avoid damage to the cornea. In case of eye irritation or visual difficulties, the drug should be discontinued and a physician/ophthalmologist consulted.
Dryness in the mouth and nose. A bleeding nose may also result from dryness and fragility of the nasal blood vessels.	Some doctors recommend applying small amounts of petroleum jelly to the nostrils before bedtime. The warmth of respiration liquefies the jelly, increasing the moisture level in the nasal mucous. If bleeding occurs, it is usually sufficient to press the affected side of the nose for several minutes.
Increased skin sensitivity to sunlight, ranging from mild redness to severe rashes.	In most cases, this is not a concrete reason to avoid using isotretinoin during the summer. Appropriate use of sunscreens should be carried out during the treatment period. It is not advisable to postpone acne therapy (especially not severe acne that may undergo scarring), but to initiate treatment as early as possible, while avoiding unnecessary sun exposure.
Dry, scaly lips.	This requires frequent application of lip balms. Note that repeated wetting of the lips may aggravate the dryness (see chapter 4). A possible way to moisturize the lips is to wet them and then apply an occlusive ointment, thus trapping in the layer of water. Evaporation is prevented, with subsequent increase in the moisture level.
Temporary hair loss.	Washing, drying, and brushing of the hair should be done as gently as possible. If the hair loss worsens, the medication may be discontinued or reduced for a certain period of time. In any case, other possible causes for hair loss should be ruled out by the treating physician.
Disturbance of liver function (usually temporary).	Liver function should be monitored in patients receiving isotretinoin by regular blood tests once a month.
An increase in blood triglycerides or cholesterol.	This can be reversed following dose reduction or discontinuation of therapy. Blood tests should be carried out every month, and dietary consultation if needed.
Muscle discomfort and pain following physical exercise.	In most cases, this is not an indication to avoid any kind of physical activity. However, during treatment, it would be advisable to avoid extreme sport/physical activity.

Common adverse effects of isotretinoin with their appropriate therapeutic approaches.

The Usual Course of Isotretinoin Therapy

Usually, in the first or second week, there is dryness of the skin and mucous membranes inside the mouth and nose. Within the first six weeks of treatment, there may actually be a mild worsening of the acne in a small percentage of patients, which may be prevented if therapy is initiated in low doses. However, in most cases, after several weeks of treatment, the severity of the acne lessens, and from that stage onwards there is gradual healing of most of the acne lesions.

Isotretinoin is highly effective and has been found to have significant beneficial effects in cases of acne that have not responded to previous treatments. The main advantage of taking isotretinoin is that the acne will disappear without recurring in most patients. However, if the acne does happen to reappear, it tends to be in a much less severe form. In such cases, one may repeat another course of isotretinoin treatment.

Even though the list of adverse effects seems to be long, isotretinoin is considered to be a relatively safe drug when administered according to the accepted guidelines.

The Recommended Dosage of Isotretinoin

To achieve a desirable clinical outcome, the recommended total cumulative dose of isotretinoin is around 120 mg/kg. For instance, a patient of 60 kg will require an overall quantity of 7200 mg. If the patient takes 40 mg/day (2 tablets), the treatment period will last six months. Some recommend administering even lower doses in cases of mild acne.

Treatment with Light

The common bacterium that is associated with acne is *Propionbacterion acne*. This type of bacteria contains certain compounds called porphyrins. Porphyrins are affected by light, if they are exposed to it in a particular wavelength and sufficient intensity. Hence, treatment by using blue light may cause the destruction of these bacteria. In about 80% of patients, one may expect a reasonable degree of improvement. This treatment is fairly safe, and no adverse effects have been observed thus far.

This mode of treatment usually requires one or two sessions per week, with each session lasting approximately 15 to 20 minutes. Considering the fact that nowadays the accepted treatments for acne are fairly effective, treatment with light may be of value only in certain cases. For example, if a patient prefers to avoid systemic treatment, or in cases when isotretinoin treatment is contraindicated, such as in pregnancy, severe acne in an unusually young age, or in cases of intolerance to isotretinoin.

Other similar modes of therapy exist, such as laser treatment (pulsed-dye laser) or photodynamic treatments.

TAILORING TREATMENT

Treatment should be adjusted to the clinical appearance of the acne.

Mild Acne

In mild acne, the aim is to rely on externally applied preparations, that is, preparations to be applied locally to the affected areas of skin. If the only lesions are comedones, preparations containing salicylic acid, sulfur, or resorcinol usually suffice. Alternatively, one can use preparations containing retinoic acid, or alpha-hydroxy acids. In acne, where there are **inflammatory lesions** (such as papules or pustules), one adds antibacterial treatment: benzoyl peroxide or antibiotics that are applied to the skin (such as erythromycin or clindamycin solutions). A combination of preparations can be used, such as one type in the morning and a different type at night.

The decision as to the type of preparation to be used is also determined according to the level of moisture in the skin. In oily skin, relatively drying preparations are preferred such as solutions or gels. In dry skin, it is advisable to use preparations that tend to increase the degree of moisture in the skin such as those containing α-hydroxy acids.

Severe Acne

In cases of severe acne, orally administered medications are usually necessary in addition to local treatment. The treatment is usually based on antibiotics (generally tetracyclines), special contraceptive pills for females, or isotretinoin. The general approach to treating acne lesions is demonstrated in the following illustration.

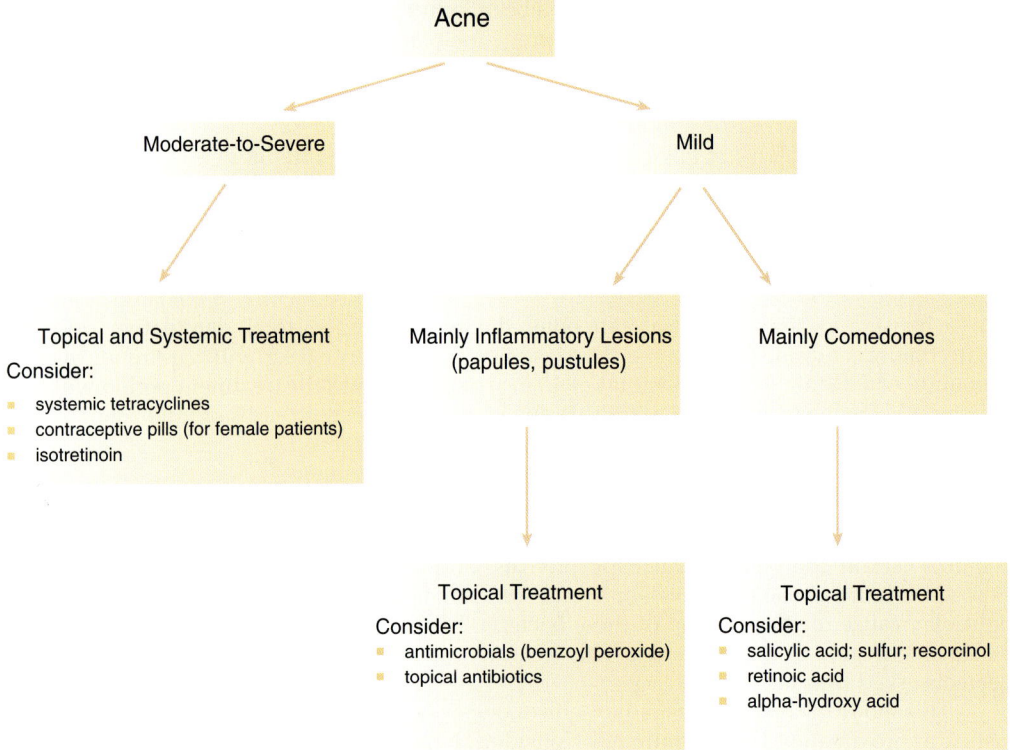

Tailoring treatment according to the clinical appearance of acne.

FINAL COMMENT

Both the physician and the cosmetician must make it clear to the patient that the standard medical treatment of acne is effective. Over 90% of acne sufferers will show significant improvement within months. Even patients who do not see any improvement within a few months should not despair. There is an extremely wide range of possibilities available for acne treatment, and it is more than likely that one of these treatments will help the patient.

10 | Sun and the Skin
Dafna Hallel-Halevy

Contents Overview • Solar radiation • Short-term effects of sun exposure • Long-term effects of sun exposure: solar damage • Types of skin • Protection from the sun • Artificial tanning and alteration of skin color

OVERVIEW

There is an increasing awareness of the damage caused to skin by cumulative sun exposure. Solar radiation is responsible for most of the deleterious skin conditions that are often erroneously attributed to aging, such as:

- the appearance of sun spots—those brown spots that tend to appear on areas of skin exposed to the sun,
- the appearance and accentuation of wrinkles and sagging skin,
- enlargement of blood capillaries on the face, and
- the development of various skin tumors.

This chapter discusses the detrimental effect of short-term and long-term exposure to the sun, as well as ways to protect against it.

SOLAR RADIATION

The sun's radiation ranges over a wide spectrum of wavelengths. Visible light, made up of the familiar colors of the rainbow, is in fact only a thin band of the wide total range of radiation, as shown in the illustration.

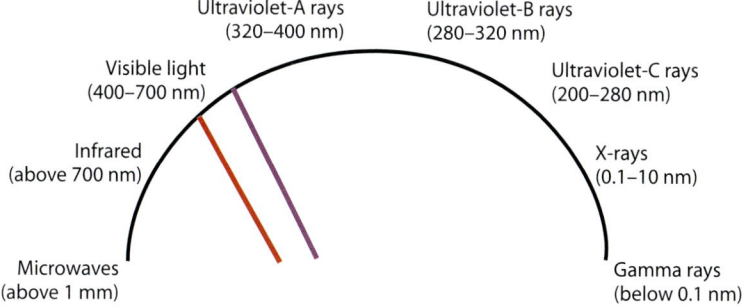

The wide spectrum of wavelengths of the sun's electromagnetic radiation.

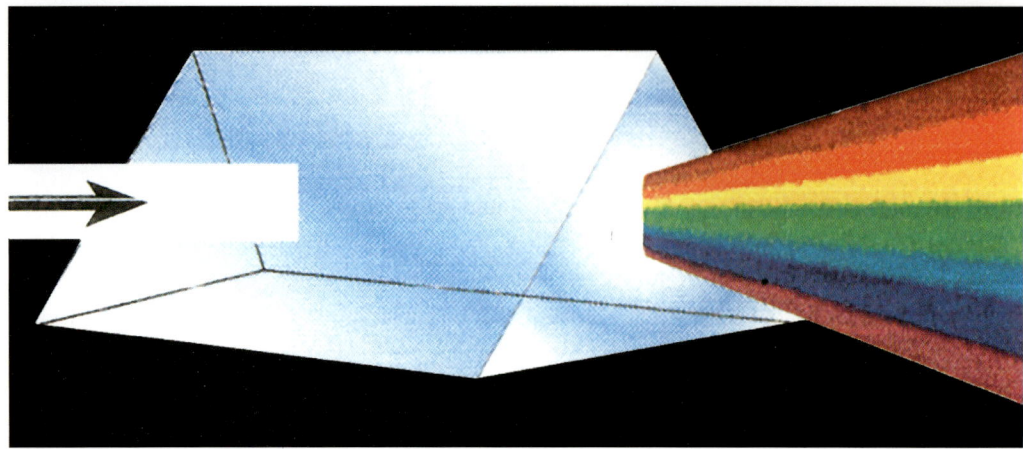

*A glass prism can split **visible light** into the familiar rainbow colors. At one end of the rainbow, the light is red, with a wavelength of about 700 nm. At the other end of the rainbow is violet light, with a wavelength of about 400 nm. In between lie the other colors of the rainbow. It should be remembered, though, that visible light is only a narrow band that makes up a small fraction of all radiation emanating from the sun. In the spectrum of electromagnetic radiation, those light rays whose wavelengths go beyond those of the visible violet light are called **ultraviolet rays**.*

The wavelength of ultraviolet radiation is adjacent to that of visible violet light. Ultraviolet-B (UVB) rays are high-energy emissions, which can cause significant damage to living tissues and cells. This is the main type of radiation that is responsible for:

- sunburn,
- tanning, and
- the appearance of skin tumors following prolonged, cumulative exposure to the sun.

The energy level of ultraviolet-A (UVA) rays is less than that of UVB rays, so they cause less skin damage. Until recently, UVA rays were thought to provide "safe" tanning, and most solariums still use lamps that emit UVA for achieving a tan. However, even UVA rays cause skin damage. Moreover, UVA rays penetrate deeper into the skin than do UVB rays, causing damage to the elastin fibers located deeper in the skin, and thus hastening skin aging.

Another fact that must be kept in mind is that UVB rays do not penetrate glass, while UVA rays do. Therefore, for example, when driving in a car with closed windows, skin damage can occur because of the UVA radiation. Hence, in an air-conditioned car, one tends to forget that the skin is still exposed to ultraviolet radiation. Therefore:

- It is not advisable to expose oneself to the sun—even through a glass window.
- Tanning at a solarium can damage the skin.

SHORT-TERM EFFECTS OF SUN EXPOSURE

What is Suntanning?

When we talk of "suntanning," we mean that the skin color darkens. From a medical point of view, suntanning is, in fact, the natural mechanism by which the skin protects itself. The sun's rays that reach the epidermis cause the **melanocytes**, that is, special cells in the epidermis, to produce **melanin**, which is the colored compound (pigment) that makes the skin darker. Melanin provides the skin with natural protection against solar damage. However, the amount of melanin that is produced in fair-skinned people following exposure to the sun is relatively low and does not afford them adequate protection, and they must take additional precautions against solar skin damage. In dark-skinned people, the amount of melanin produced is higher and is consequently more effective. That is why dark-skinned people often look younger than fair-skinned people of the same age—in the former, the skin changes less with age, and wrinkles and pigmented patches appear less frequently. Nevertheless, even dark-skinned people should avoid excessive sun exposure. In every case, the less the exposure, the less the damage.

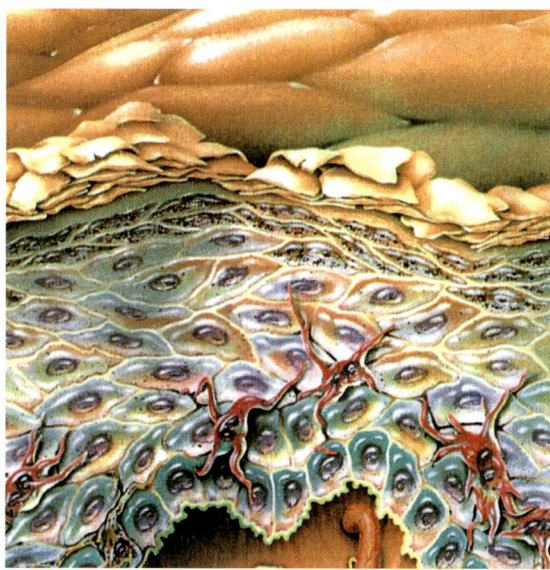
Melanocytes—the melanin-producing cells—at the base of the epidermis.

Summary
Tanning is the skin's defence against solar radiation. A tan is the result of the production of melanin in response to exposure to ultraviolet rays. Tanning does afford the skin a certain degree of protection, but usually not sufficient to prevent skin damage. Prolonged exposure will, over the years, result in the appearance of pigmented patches, abnormal skin texture, wrinkles and sagging of the skin. Later, skin tumors may appear, especially in those with risk factors.

Sunburn
Apart from tanning, ultraviolet radiation also causes redness. The medical term for this redness is **erythema**, and its appearance following exposure to the sun has nothing to do with melanin production. Erythema begins soon after excessive exposure to ultraviolet light—some four to six hours following exposure—reaching its peak around 24 hours thereafter. A mild burn (termed **first-degree**) is manifested by redness with pain and sensitivity of the skin. A deeper burn (**second-degree**) appears following more prolonged exposure to the sun and is manifested by the appearance of blisters, peeling, and severe pain. The treatment of first-degree burns is based on cooling the burnt area by rinsing with water. "Soothing" applications can also be used, such as those containing aloe vera. A second-degree burn (or a relatively severe or widespread first-degree burn) requires medical attention. In second-degree burns **antibacterial preparations**, which inhibit or kill bacteria and prevent infection of the burn, may be used. Silver sulfadiazine, an effective product for treating burns, is active against bacteria, and cools and soothes the burnt area. It may be used in cases of severe sunburn.

Other Immediate Complications of Excessive Exposure to the Sun
Other short-term risks of sun exposure are:

- dehydration, and
- heatstroke (sunstroke).

Although we draw attention to these risks, these problems will not be dealt with in this chapter.

Vitamin D and the Sun
Vitamin D is needed by the body to build and strengthen bones. Recent research studies have suggested that an appropriate amount of vitamin D may assist in preventing certain kinds of malignancies and certain disorders of the immune system. Exposure to sunlight stimulates the production of vitamin D in humans. It should be noted, however, that the amount of sunlight needed to produce the vitamin D required by the body is minimal. Exposing a few square centimeters of skin for a few minutes daily is sufficient. There are certain people who may lack

vitamin D, however, especially those living in northern countries, the elderly, the incapacitated, and people who intentionally avoid any exposure to the sun for religious, medical, or any other reasons. Absolute avoidance of sun exposure is definitely not desirable. On the other hand, worrying about an adequate supply of vitamin D is certainly no justification for excessive sun exposure. This is especially important in people with extremely fair complexions, those with a history of skin cancer, or those with evident sun-damaged skin. Low levels of vitamin D can be rectified by the injection of tablets, along with a proper diet including foodstuffs containing vitamin D.

LONG-TERM EFFECTS OF SUN EXPOSURE: SKIN DAMAGE

Cumulative solar radiation is a direct cause of skin damage. The changes that occur as a result of exposure to the sun are not the same as those processes that occur with natural aging of the skin. The former are known technically as **photoaging** and occurs in both skin layers, that is, the epidermis and the dermis.

Remember that exposure to the sun occurs not only at the beach or on hikes. In most people, certain parts of the body, particularly the face, neck, and backs of the hands, are exposed to the sun for more than an hour a day. We are talking of daily exposure over years, and it is clear that such cumulative exposure has detrimental effects on the health of the skin.

Effects on the Epidermis

Cumulative exposure to the sun leads to the appearance of wrinkles and an uneven distribution of pigment in the skin. This is caused by the exposure of melanocytes (the pigment-producing cells) in the epidermis to the sun. In young people, prolonged solar exposure may express itself in the form of freckles. In older people, the solar exposure leads to the appearance of **sun spots** (**solar lentigines**), which are brown blotches on the skin. In everyday language, these patches are often called "age spots" or "liver spots." One can see these lesions in older people in those areas usually exposed to the sun, such as the face and the backs of the hands.

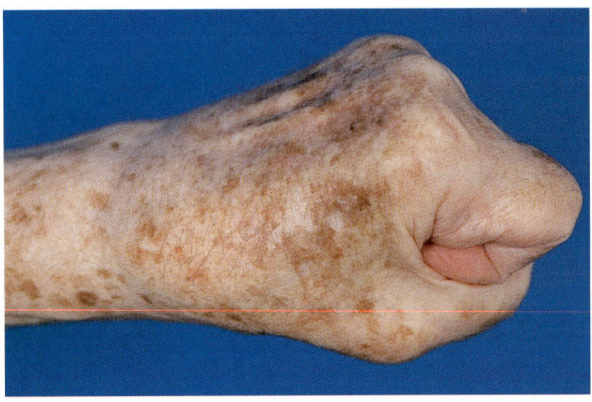

Sun spots (solar lentigines) on the back and side of the hand.

Other solar damage as a result of cumulative exposure to the sun includes the appearance of skin tumors—both benign and malignant (see chapter 15, "Skin Tumors"). Common tumors that result from cumulative solar exposure are:

- solar keratosis,
- basal cell carcinoma, and
- squamous cell carcinoma.

It is especially important to prevent excessive exposure to the sun in children. Current thinking is that the appearance of **malignant melanoma**, a particularly dangerous malignant skin cancer, is related to episodes of excessive exposure to the sun in childhood. In this particular case, we are not talking of cumulative exposure to the sun, but of episodes of excessive exposure resulting in severe sunburn.

Effect of Prolonged Sun Exposure on the Dermis

The changes in the dermis that occur as a result of prolonged sun exposure are as follows:

- The main damage to the dermis following cumulative exposure to the sun is the destruction of elastin and collagen fibers; these fibers confer upon the skin its elasticity and strength. If they are damaged, the skin loses its elasticity, becomes wrinkled, and can appear saggy.
- In addition, cumulative exposure to the sun damages the delicate blood vessels of the skin and the supporting tissues. The blood vessels become more fragile, making them more prone to hemorrhages (bleeding) following relatively minor injury.
- Similarly, the capillaries of the face may enlarge—a phenomenon known as **telangiectasis**.
- Excessive exposure to the sun dries out the skin. When there is constant dryness of the skin over a prolonged period of time, the skin's health and quality is affected.

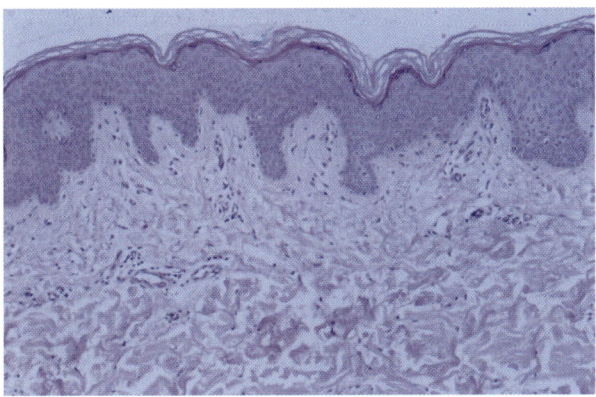

Healthy skin viewed through a microscope.

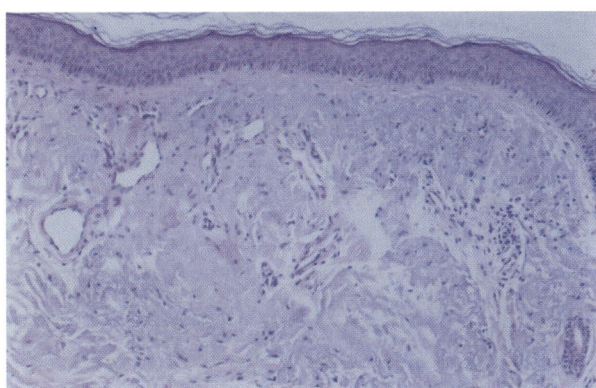

Photodamaged skin viewed through a microscope, showing thinning of the epidermis following long exposure to the sun.

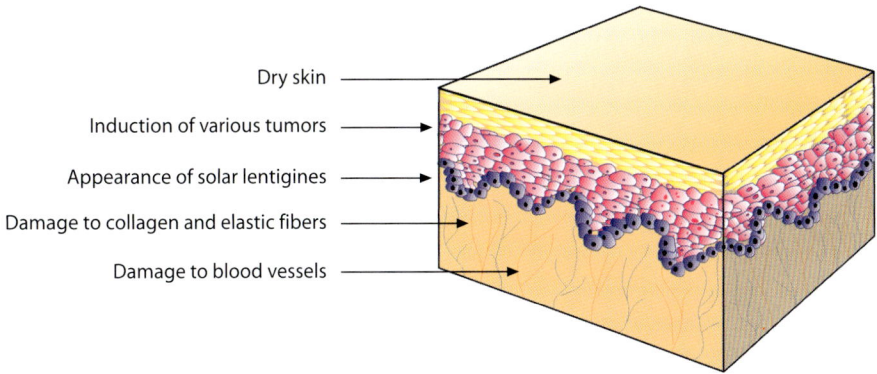

Illustration summarizing the effects of solar radiation on the skin.

The above points explain why, in older people with fair complexions, the skin in those areas exposed to the sun (face, neck, upper chest), looks "old" and wrinkled, while the skin that is not exposed to the sun (buttocks, abdomen, and inner part of the arms) looks smooth, clear, and younger.

Two Additional Comments
- Exposing the eyes to strong radiation, without adequate protection, can cause damage to the lens of the eye, with the risk of developing a cataract. There is also evidence suggesting that cumulative exposure to solar radiation may also damage the retina of the eye.
- Cumulative damage to the skin as a result of sun exposure can occur following many individual periods of exposure, each of which in itself is not sufficient to cause the skin to become red. Obviously, if a burn does actually occur, the damage is much more serious.

TYPES OF SKIN

The classification of skin into different types is based on the skin color, its propensity for developing sunburn, its tanning capability, and the degree of tanning. The parameters measured are the propensity for getting burned after 30 minutes of exposure to the sun at noon in early summer, and the tanning capability. Depending on these factors, one can determine the degree of protection needed against solar radiation.

Skin type 1
People with type 1 skin have pale skin, commonly blond or red hair, and light colored eyes. If these people are exposed to bright sun for 30 minutes, they will always get burnt. They never tan.

Skin type 2
Most of these people have a fair complexion and light-colored eyes. If a person with type 2 skin stays in the sun for about 30 minutes, his/her skin will usually develop redness and sunburn. Some of these people tan, but only after repeated sun exposures.

Skin type 3
In this group, there is a wide spectrum of skin complexions, ranging from relatively fair to relatively darker shades. After sun exposure of 30 minutes, they will tan, although the degree of tanning varies from one person to another. Following prolonged sun exposure, they may burn.

Skin type 4
People in this group generally have dark hair, brown or black eyes, and a relatively dark complexion. Most of the population of North Africa is in this category. They develop an even tan after 30 minutes of exposure to the sun, but will not burn.

Skin type 5
This group comprises dark-skinned people (e.g., people from India). They rarely get sunburnt, and always tan readily.

Skin type 6
People in this group (e.g., people of African origin) have skin that is dark even in areas never exposed to the sun. When exposed to the sun, their skin darkens to a deep brown/black shade. They do not get sunburnt.

Note: In order to identify types 5 and 6, there is no need to test the skin after 30 minutes of sun exposure—it is sufficient to observe the skin color.

PROTECTION FROM THE SUN

Protection is essentially based on avoidance of exposure. We emphasize that the same rays that cause tanning are the ones that cause damage. The lighter the person's skin, the more susceptible it is to solar damage. The purpose of a sunscreen is not to help tanning, but rather to block the sun's rays. In other words, one should ideally not be exposed to the sun. However, if someone is going to be exposed to the sun anyhow (at the beach, on a hike, or at work), he/she should at least make sure that his/her skin is protected by a sunscreen and appropriate clothing.

The typical advertisements for sunscreens generally show a suntanned model smearing a sunscreen preparation all over herself, then basking in the hot sun. That message is misleading:

- The belief that sunscreens help achieve a suntan is not correct.
- The belief that sunscreens filter out only the "harmful" rays is not correct.
- Harmful ultraviolet rays may definitely penetrate the skin despite application of sunscreen.

We stress that it is preferable to avoid exposure to the sun. However, if for any reason someone has to be in open area exposed to the sun then he/she should apply a sunscreen. Of the multi-billion dollar "beauty" market, and of all the products that promise to keep the face "young," there is nothing that comes anywhere near the simple act of avoiding exposure to the sun.

How to Minimize Sun Exposure

- Minimize the times of outdoor activities. Outdoor activities should be planned for those hours when the level of solar radiation is relatively low. Some define the peak hours as between 9:00 or 10:00 am and 4:00 pm. However, this depends on the geographical location and climactic conditions. Therefore, a good rule of thumb is to avoid exposure to the sun when the shadows are nonexistent or very short. UV exposure is less harmful when your own shadow exceeds your height, that is, in the morning or toward evening.
- During outdoor activities, it is important to keep to the shade as much as possible and to wear appropriate clothing. However, a large amount of solar radiation is reflected from water, sand, and concrete pavements—all of which a person may be exposed to even when sitting in the shade. A beach umbrella does not guarantee complete protection from the sun: ultraviolet rays are reflected from all sorts of surfaces, so that even under a beach umbrella one needs protection by wearing suitable clothing or a sunscreen preparation. For the same reason, a hat does not necessarily afford full protection against the sun.
- Cloudy days tend to be cooler and with relatively less sunshine, but a considerable percentage of the ultraviolet rays penetrate clouds, and even on cloudy days—especially relatively bright days—appropriate protective measures should be taken.
- Severe sunburn can occur in snow, because of reflection of a relatively high percentage of the sun's rays from the snow. Furthermore, the higher the altitude, the more solar radiation gets through to the earth, because the rays have to travel through a thinner layer of atmosphere (which filters the rays to some extent). Hence, when in an area of snow, it is important to protect the exposed areas, particularly the face and ears.
- Most clothing protects effectively against the sun's rays, because it either absorbs or reflects the ultraviolet rays. In general, the thicker the material, and the tighter the weave, the higher the level of protection it affords. The color of the material is also a factor: different colors absorb or reflect rays to different degrees, and the protective capabilities of a material are related to the chemical composition of the various dyes. Dyeing a cloth may raise its sun protection factor (SPF; see later) by 4 or more, compared with white cloth.

White material allows quite a lot of ultraviolet radiation to pass through it. If you wear a thin white T-shirt, you may still absorb about 20% as much radiation as if you had a bare torso. Wearing a thin shirt of that kind is approximately equivalent to using a sunscreen with an SPF of between 4 and 10, depending on the thickness, density of weave, and type of material of the shirt. Material such as that is not always sufficient for protection against solar radiation. Furthermore, if the shirt is wet, its protective capability decreases by 30% to 40% compared to when it is dry.

In addition, wearing tight clothes decreases the protective effects of the material, because stretching the material opens up the spaces between its threads in the weave. Thick woolen clothing, denim, and clothes made of polyester fibers afford good protection against solar radiation.

Sunscreens

Physical and Chemical Sunscreens

Until the 1970s, the attitude towards tanning preparations was that they were essentially cosmetic, that is, designed to increase tanning. Since the late 1970s, the importance of sunscreens in protecting the skin from solar damage has been more strongly emphasized.

Sunscreens may be physical or chemical. Most sunscreen preparations contain both physical and chemical sunscreens, and may be in the form of a cream, an ointment, an emulsion, a gel, etc.

Physical sunscreens prevent the sun's rays from reaching the skin by reflecting and dispersing them, as a mirror reflects light rays. The major component of physical sunscreens is a substance similar to talc called **titanium dioxide**.

Chemical sunscreens absorb ultraviolet rays, thereby preventing them from penetrating the skin. The degree of absorption depends on the particular substance used and its concentration. Substances used as chemical sunscreens are **oxybenzone, benzophenones,** and **para-aminobenzoic acid (PABA)**. These names can be found on the packages of different sunscreen preparations.

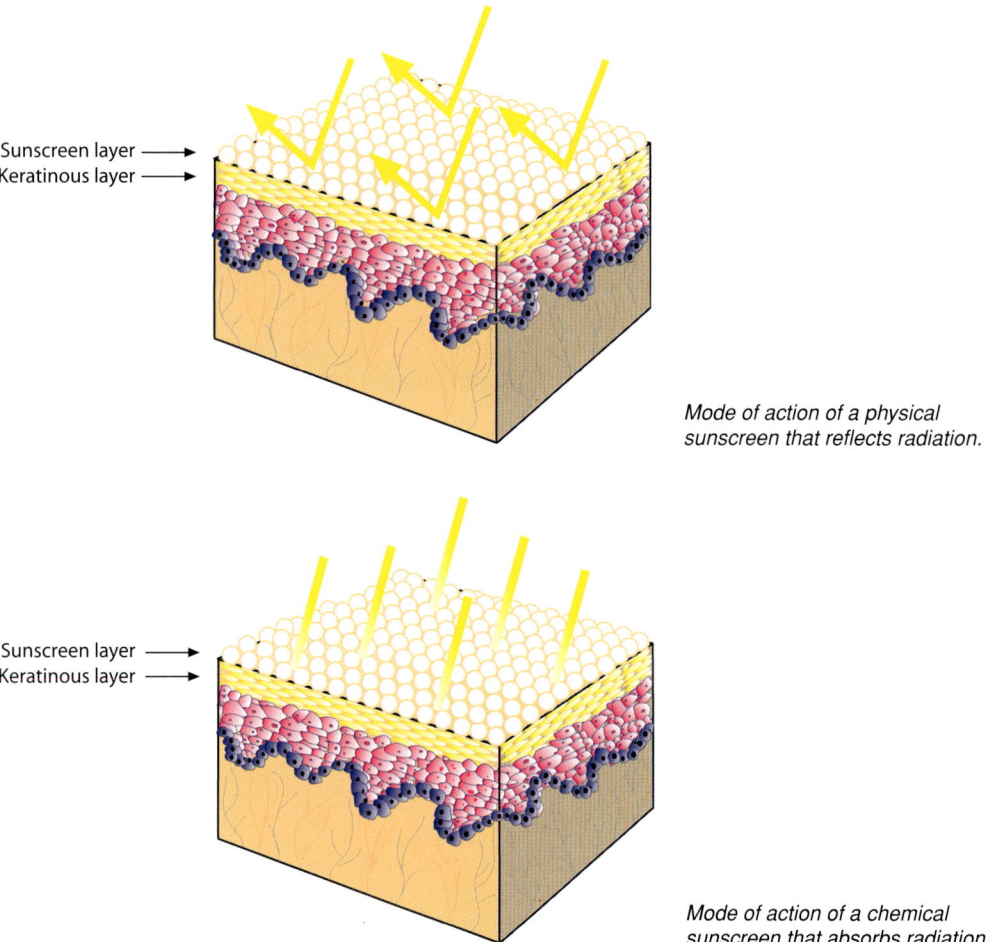

Mode of action of a physical sunscreen that reflects radiation.

Mode of action of a chemical sunscreen that absorbs radiation.

Blocking Ultraviolet Rays with Sunscreens

Most chemical sunscreens block 95% of the UVB rays, but most do not block UVA rays. Chemical sunscreens of the benzophenone group, as well as the physical sunscreens, block ultraviolet rays more completely, provided their SPF is above 15. In general, an ideal combination is a physical sunscreen combined with a chemical sunscreen.

What Does "Sun Protection Factor" Mean?

The term **sun protection factor** (**SPF**) was adopted by the US Food and Drug Administration (FDA). This measurement allows one to assess the degree of protection from ultraviolet rays provided to the skin by a sunscreen.

The effectiveness of a given SPF is measured in terms of the redness (erythema) that appears on the skin following sun exposure. The concept of a **minimal erythema dose** is an expression of the minimal amount of radiation that causes reddening of the skin. This radiation dose varies from person to person, depending on his/her skin shade and type. For example, if it takes someone, without any sunscreen, 10 minutes of sun exposure to develop erythema, exposure to that same strength of sunlight by using a sunscreen with an SPF of 15 will take 150 minutes (10 × 15) to develop erythema.

Considerations of Various Sunscreens

There are four main considerations when using a sunscreen:

- endurance on the skin,
- skin irritation,
- eye irritation, and
- SPF.

Endurance on the skin

According to the FDA's definitions:

- A **water-resistant** product provides skin protection even after 40 minutes of immersion in (fresh) water.
- A **waterproof** product retains its protective capabilities after 80 minutes of immersion in (fresh) water.
- A product that does not lose more than 25% of its effectiveness after a 40-minute swim is recognized as water-resistant.
- A product that loses over 25% of its effectiveness after a 40-minute swim is *not* water-resistant.

Skin irritation

Skin sensitivity tends to be more of a problem with chemical sunscreens. In the past, para-aminobenzoic acid was used in most sunscreens, but in recent years the trend has been to replace it with other sunscreens of the oxybenzone and benzophenone groups, which cause fewer skin irritations. Physical sunscreens, on the other hand, generally do not cause skin reactions. In many cases, skin sensitivity from contact with sunscreens is caused by other ingredients in the preparation, such as the perfumes or preservatives, and not necessarily by the sunscreen itself.

Eye irritation

Stinging of the eyes is a common side effect experienced after applying a sunscreen. The stinging sensation is most commonly related to irritation of the eyes from the fumes of the preparation. People who encounter this problem should change to a different sunscreen (preferably a physical sunscreen that contains titanium dioxide). In general, any sunscreen can cause irritation if it comes into direct contact with the eyes, as a result of the user rubbing the eyes after applying the preparation, or because the sunscreen is too runny. Water-resistant sunscreens tend to be less runny, and are recommended for the area around the eyes.

Sun protection factor (SPF)

While until recently, SPF of 15 was considered to be optimal, many doctors now recommend using preparations containing an SPF of 30 or greater. For people with skin type 1 or 2, and for certain people at high risk (such as those with an increased risk of skin tumors), a preparation with an SPF of over 30 may be necessary. The recommended SPF depends not only on people's skin types, but also on the length of time they intend to be in the sun.

Note: A sunscreen is considered to afford effective protection only if it has an SPF of 15 or greater. A sunscreen with SPF 15 blocks about 93% of UVB radiation. A sunscreen with SPF 30 blocks about 97% of UVB radiation. In sunscreens with SPF higher than 30, the additional improvement in the protection from ultraviolet radiation is minimal.

> **More on SPF ...**
>
> Recently there has been an increasing tendency to recommend higher SPF products, that is, 30 or more, especially for sensitive, fair-skinned people. The main arguments to support this recommendation are:
>
> - Even though increasing the SPF from 30 to 40 increases UVB protection by less than 1%, this increase may be significant for people who are sensitive to sun exposure.
> - Most people generally apply sunscreens too sparingly. Thus, the SPF number written on the label may not necessarily reflect the actual SPF in practical terms.
> - Following sunscreen application, there is gradual decrease in its effectiveness owing to factors such as swimming, sweating, washing, or the disintegration of the preparation due to the sun's rays.

How to Use a Sunscreen

Sunscreen should be applied to all exposed areas of skin, in particular the face, ears, neck, upper chest, backs of the hands, and, if necessary, bald areas of the head.

Note that sunscreen preparations dissolve in sweat, and, like other creams, come off following immersion in water or with rubbing. A water-resistant sunscreen should be re-applied every three to four hours; a sunscreen that is less water-resistant should be re-applied even more frequently. Every sunscreen should be re-applied after immersion in water, swimming, etc. During physical exercise, sport, etc., that causes sweating, it should be applied more frequently.

The accepted recommendation is to apply the sunscreen 15 to 30 minutes before going out into the sun (so that it has time to penetrate into the keratinous layer of the skin) and then once again, 15 to 30 minutes following exposure to the sun. It has been shown that most people use inadequate quantities of sunscreen and tend to apply it unevenly, leaving unprotected areas of skin. As the surface of the skin is nonuniform, applying two coats of sunscreen imparts better protection.

Note: We repeat that no sunscreen is 100% effective. Someone who stays in the sun for a long time exposes him/herself to sunburn and skin damage from cumulative exposure to ultraviolet rays.

Final Comments Regarding Sunscreens

Recent studies tend to show a statistical increase in the incidence of skin tumors among the general population, despite the increasing awareness and the use of sunscreen preparations. The main reason is apparently that these preparations, promoted extensively by advertising, have produced a feeling of complacency. They encourage their users to expose themselves to the sun, by giving a false sense of security and protection, which in fact does not exist. It must be remembered that, by staying in the sun for a lengthy period, even someone who religiously covers him/herself with a sunscreen will allow his/her skin to absorb a certain amount of radiation, which will cause skin damage.

Sunscreens are the last line of defence against the sun. They are designed to offer some protection to those areas of the body, such as the face and hands, that are unavoidably exposed to the sun. Sunscreen preparations offer some protection to those people who, for whatever reason (occupation or leisure activities) have no alternative but to be in the sun. Under those circumstances, they should use a sunscreen to minimize the damage. Advertisements that show people smearing themselves with a sunscreen preparation so that they can then frolic in the sun, with "safe, healthy suntanning," are misleading and deceptive. The first line of defence is to keep out of the sun as much as possible.

> **Does the SPF Really Measure the Effectiveness of Sunscreens?**
>
> Some criticism has been leveled against the use of the sun protection factor (SPF) as a measure of the effectiveness of a sunscreen preparation. The SPF of a sunscreen is determined by its ability to prevent the appearance of reddening of the skin (erythema) following exposure to the sun. This means that, by comparing one sunscreen with another in terms of their SPFs, one can tell how much each one delays the appearance of erythema. However, that does not necessarily tell us how effective the sunscreen is in preventing the appearance of malignant tumors on the skin, or its ability to prevent damage to the skin. Studies that have examined the effectiveness of sunscreens in the prevention of these phenomena have showed varying results. In any case, it is also necessary to be strict and to apply sunscreens together with avoiding exposure to the sun.

Additional Tips on Protection from the Sun

Protect the Nose
One needs to be particularly careful to protect the nose from the sun and to apply sunscreen more frequently. The nose receives the most exposure to the sun and is at particular risk of developing solar damage. Furthermore, if skin cancer develops on the nose, the tumor will have to be removed, and it should be noted that:

- Scars on the nose following removal of lesions always look more prominent because of the nose's central position on the face.
- The skin of the nose tends to form relatively thick, unsightly scars.

Keep Protection Consistent
There is no point in persisting with reasonable protective measures for months, and then one day at work or at some leisure activity, to be exposed to prolonged radiation and develop a burn. Under such circumstances, the damage will be even worse than usual, because the skin will not have been exposed to the sun previously, and will not have had a chance to develop natural protective means, in the form of melanin production.

Use Sunglasses
Sunglasses protect the eyes as well as the skin. The glasses should be of the type that screen out 100% of ultraviolet rays. It is wise to select sunglasses of a reputable, well-known make.

Note: Uncertified sunglasses should never be used. Simple plastic does not filter out ultraviolet light, but in fact blocks the visible light rays, so the damage is even worse! The pupils of someone using plastic sunglasses do not constrict, so an even greater amount of ultraviolet light can get into the eye and cause damage.

Sunglasses also prevent squinting in bright light. Repeated squinting may accelerate the appearance of wrinkles around the eyes, so sunglasses also help in preventing that from occurring. It is preferable to use sunglasses that are elongated and elliptical in shape, similar to the shape of the eye, or glasses with a wider side bar, to prevent rays reaching the eyes from the sides.

Wear a Wide-Brimmed Hat
Hats without a wide brim do not afford effective protection from the sun for the facial skin. Even wide-brimmed hats do not provide effective protection from the sun's rays (they are approximately equivalent to a sunscreen with an SPF of 3). Hence, even when wearing a wide-brimmed hat, additional protective measures should be taken, such as applying a sunscreen preparation onto the face and avoiding unnecessary exposure to the sun. For bald heads, which are at a high risk of developing damage, the hat plays much more significant role in protecting the skin. Bald people should wear hats during outdoor activities.

Protect the Lips
A sunscreen preparation should be used on the lips. Recent research has shown that tumors on the lips are more common in men than in women. The difference was attributed to the widespread use of lipstick by women. The lipstick acts as a filter for the sun's rays because of the dyes it contains, which function as a physical sunscreen and prevent penetration of the rays to the skin. Tumors of the lips are more common in women who do not use lipstick than in those who use lipstick regularly.

Protect the Neck
It would be advisable to wear clothing that covers the neck (don't forget to include the nape of the neck!) and the upper chest. Excessive sun exposure to these areas causes characteristic features of sun damage with wrinkling.

Shade the Car Windows
A sunshade should be placed inside car windows, since a certain percentage of ultraviolet rays gets through the glass, and may cause cumulative damage (UVA rays certainly penetrate glass). If necessary, special glass can be obtained that filters out most of the ultraviolet rays.

Note: Avoid using sunscreens for babies up to one-year old. The best would be, in this age group, to avoid exposing them to direct sun altogether.

Suntanning and Exposure to the Sun: How to Minimize Damage

For someone who still wants to acquire a suntan, despite everything that has been stated up to this point regarding the damage that exposure to sunlight causes to the skin, we can provide advice to minimize the damage:

- Even when staying in the sun, particular attention should be paid to protect those areas of skin that are normally exposed in daily activities—the face, backs of the hands, and especially the nose (even in the shade, they absorb ultraviolet rays). A sunscreen preparation should be applied more frequently and generously to those areas. A wide-brimmed hat should be worn to protect the face.
- Exposure to the sun should be avoided in the middle of the day, when the sun is strongest.
- Exposure to the sun should be gradual, so that the skin can build up a protective layer of melanin. Subsequently, once the desired level of tan has been achieved, exposure to the sun should not exceed 30 minutes per day (late in the afternoon), and should not exceed an hour or an hour and a half per week—depending on the type of skin. Furthermore, above a certain degree of tanning, increased exposure to the sun will not "improve" the suntan, but will merely cause skin damage. Having said that, it should be remembered that a suntan does not provide an adequate protective layer to the skin. It may reach a level of protection equivalent to a sunscreen with an SPF of 4 to 5, depending on the degree of tan and the type of skin.
- Exposure to the sun should be regular, and not just random. The damage to the skin is many times worse in someone who is exposed to the sun once for several hours compared to someone who is exposed for, say, a quarter of an hour a day once every two or three days, over a period of several weeks (despite the fact that in the latter case the total time of exposure to the sun is much longer). The most damage is caused by intermittent, irregular exposure to the sun. Dermatologists consider that many "beauty spots" (pigmented moles) on children's skins are due, apart from hereditary factors, to repeated, irregular exposure to the sun. Furthermore, it is possible that the statistical increase in the incidence of skin cancers despite the widespread use of sunscreens is related to irregularity in this use. The classic example of this is the person who is usually very strict and applies sunscreen daily, but forgets to apply it one day when hiking on a sunny day. The damage that is caused in that case may be much worse, because the skin is not protected and not ready for such a huge amount of solar radiation.
- Extreme care should be taken with children. Sun exposure should be for short periods only, so as not to induce redness.

People with a skin type that does not tend to tan should minimize sun exposure. Those with skin types 1 or 2 should totally avoid sun exposure.

Possible Advantages of Sun Exposure

In spite of the above, a reasonable amount of controlled exposure to the sun may have certain advantages such as the production of vitamin D, as mentioned earlier in this chapter. Also, being in a well-lit environment (where one is exposed to radiation in the visible range) improves one's mood. This is utilized in psychiatry, in the treatment of depression. Furthermore, some reports (albeit controversial) have appeared in the medical literature suggesting that controlled exposure to the sun may assist in the prevention, to some extent, of the development of various malignant diseases.

ARTIFICIAL TANNING AND ALTERATION OF SKIN COLOR

Artificial Tanning ("Sunless Suntan")

Dihydroxyacetone

Artificial suntanning preparations contain a substance called **dihydroxyacetone,** usually manufactured in concentrations of 3% to 5%. The accepted concentration is 5%. This substance reacts with amino acids in the keratin layer of the epidermis, which, it will be recalled, is made up of dead cells. Within a few hours, a suntan-like color appears on the skin, which may last for three to five days. This color disappears gradually, as the cells of the outer layers of the epidermis proceed towards the surface of the skin and are shed naturally. Until the outer cells are shed from the skin, the color resulting from the use of this substance cannot be removed. If a single application of the preparation does not produce a dark-enough tan, it may be re-applied a few hours later.

Artificial suntanning preparations may contain, apart of dihydroxyacetone, other ingredients such as sunscreens, bronzers (see later), certain vitamins (mainly those used as antioxidants), and various plant extracts.

Note: Dihydroxyacetone has no medical value. It does not protect the skin from the sun's rays, so an effective sunscreen must be used during exposure to the sun.

The earlier preparations based on dihydroxyacetone were not very effective. However, modern preparations are relatively effective in imparting to the skin a fairly uniform brown toning, which looks reasonably natural—depending on the normal skin coloring. The following precautions should be adopted when using these preparations:

- Care should be taken to avoid wetting the body for about an hour after applying the preparation, as this would prevent the appearance of the artificial tan.
- The preparation should not be allowed to get onto the scalp hair or the eyebrows, because it may change the color of the hair.
- The substance should be kept away from clothing because it leaves stains.
- Before using the preparation, it should be tried out first on a concealed area (that is not normally exposed) to check that there is no adverse reaction, and to confirm that the skin color is the desired shade (in some people, these preparations result in an unsightly pale-yellowish tinge).
- A thin, even layer of the preparation should be applied in order to avoid an uneven, blotchy effect, with patches of different shades of color.
- The hands should be washed after using the preparation to avoid staining of the palms.
- A basic soap (i.e., one with a high pH) should not be used to wash the body before applying the preparation, because the resulting color will tend to be more yellow, rather than the desired brown shade.
- Artificial tanning preparations without sunscreens do not provide adequate protection against sun radiation.

Note: The FDA approval for the use of dihydroxyacetone is restricted to external application only, as a color additive in artificial sunless tanning preparations. Some have pointed out the lack of recent safety studies. Therefore, it would be advisable to avoid its use in pregnant women.

Bronzers

These preparations contain a water-soluble pigment (color) that settles onto the skin. There is no chemical reaction between the pigment and the skin. If the end result is not what is wanted, the substance can be rinsed off with soap and water. These substances have no effect whatsoever in terms of protection from the sun. The main disadvantage of bronzing agents is that they have to be applied frequently, since they come off every time the skin is washed with soap and water. These preparations have no medical value. In fact, we are talking of a paint that is applied externally—basically a makeup.

Oral Medications That Alter Skin Color

Oral medications that alter skin color include:

- β-carotene,
- tyrosine, and
- "tanning accelerators"—psoralens.

β-Carotene

This substance is chemically similar to vitamin A. It is available as tablets, but is present naturally in large quantities in carrots, tomatoes, mangoes, and oranges. When large amounts are ingested, the skin changes color, becoming an orange-yellow. If that is combined with the exposure to the sun, the additional color imparted to the skin by the carotene may improve the tanning effect and darken the skin.

This preparation is available in Europe and Canada as "tanning pills"; it is not licensed for use in the United States. It should be taken after consultation with a physician, and it is important that the correct dosage be taken. If taken in excess (this applies also to people who eat excessive amounts of carrots or mangoes), **hypercarotenaemia** may occur, in which the skin turns a yellow-orange. If an even higher dosage of tanning pills is taken, it can actually result in poisoning.

> **Does β-Carotene Protect Against UV Rays?**
>
> In general, β-carotene has no effect in terms of protection against UV rays but it does block light in the visible spectrum to some extent. For most people, this is of no significance. However, certain skin diseases are caused by excessive sensitivity of the skin to sunlight, even within the visible light spectrum. In such cases, β-carotene is a useful medication for these diseases.

Tyrosine

At first glance, there appears to be a certain logic in using tyrosine, as it is the substance from which the pigment melanin is formed. Therefore, several preparations containing tyrosine, to be applied prior to exposure to the sun, have been produced. However, research has not shown any beneficial effect from the use of tyrosine-based preparations.

Psoralens

Psoralens are a group of substances that increase the sensitivity of the skin to ultraviolet radiation, causing faster tanning. They are used as medications in skin diseases (such as psoriasis or certain malignant skin diseases) but, as they accelerate tanning, they increase all the deleterious effects on the skin from solar exposure. Hence, they are definitely not approved for use as tanning agents.

Solariums

Tanning machines emit ultraviolet radiation. As stated above, this radiation causes skin damage—both damage that is seen in the skin tissue (the appearance of wrinkles and blotches) and a higher risk of developing skin cancers in later life. There are solariums that claim that their tanning is safe, since the machines emit only UVA rays. Remember, however, that this radiation also causes damage to the skin. UVA radiation penetrates deeper into the dermis and can damage the elastic tissue of the skin, which will accelerate the appearance of wrinkles. Another problem with solariums is that many people expose their *entire* body to the ultraviolet light, including the genitalia, which (one assumes!) have not been exposed to sunlight in the past. Those areas may be at higher risk of developing skin cancer following uncontrolled exposure to ultraviolet light in a solarium.

Tanning Oils

These are oils that are applied to the skin. There is a range of oily substances, from various sources—mainly vegetable, such as coconut oil, peanut oil, etc. These substances do not contain any sunscreen agent and do not protect the skin from the sun. On the contrary, they may actually concentrate the sun's rays on those areas of skin covered with them, and in that way result in even more severe damage.

- They may impede the normal function of sweat glands and sebaceous glands, which could result in the appearance or aggravation of various rashes, for example, a rash called **miliaria** ("**prickly heat**"). It may result in a rash of **acne**, manifested mainly by the appearance of comedones.
- Although manufacturers claim that these oils contain vitamins and various natural ingredients that "nourish" the skin, the beneficial effect on the skin is questionable (see chapter 16, "Active Ingredients in Cosmetic Preparations").
- The skin color achieved by using these oils is no different from the normal color that follows exposure to the sun, without any additional substance being applied to the skin.

11 | Networks of Blood Vessels on the Skin
Moshe Lapidoth

Contents Overview • Networks of blood vessels on the face • Treatment of telangiectasia on the face • Networks of blood vessels on the legs • "Spider" telangiectasia

OVERVIEW

The appearance of networks of fine blood vessels on the skin is common. Cosmeticians sometimes call this **couperose**, although the more widely used medical term for this condition is **telangiectasia**, which refers to the dilatation of fine, superficial blood vessels on the surface of the skin. These lesions are known as **telangiectases** (plural of **telangiectasis**). This chapter discusses:

1. the common appearance of telangiectasia on the face as a manifestation of cumulative damage to the skin,
2. appropriate treatment,
3. appearance of telangiectasia on the legs, and
4. other forms of telangiectasia.

NETWORKS OF BLOOD VESSELS ON THE FACE

Telangiectasia is a common phenomenon and is, in the majority of cases, the result of cumulative damage to the skin, leading to weakening of the walls of the blood vessels in the skin, and loss of the supporting tissue around the blood vessels.

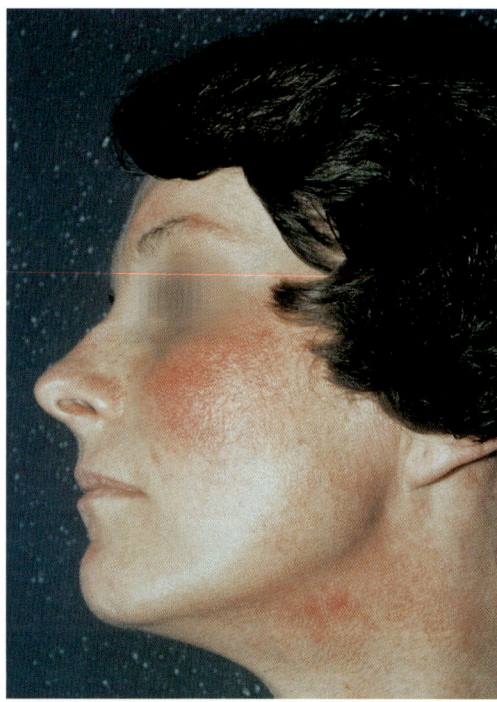

Telangiectasia on the face.

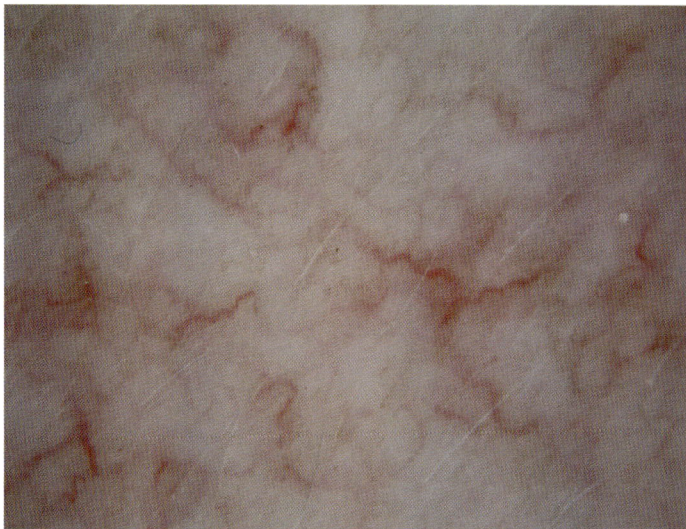
Telangiectasia under a magnifying glass.

Cumulative skin damage and the subsequent onset of telangiectasia can occur for the following reasons:

- skin aging because of cumulative sun exposure,
- prolonged exposure to cold weather and wind,
- exposure to irradiation (in patients with malignant disease),
- following mechanical trauma,
- prolonged application of corticosteroid-containing products to the skin,
- prolonged dilatation of the blood vessels of the face, for example, in alcoholism or in certain skin diseases (such as a condition known as **rosacea**), and
- pregnancy.

Telangiectasia that results from cumulative skin damage is usually in the form of lines. The lesions range in color from pink to dark red, and the diameter of the blood vessels is 0.1 to 1 mm.

TREATMENT OF TELANGIECTASIA ON THE FACE

The basic treatment of telangiectasia is aimed at the cause and its prevention. If the underlying cause is alcohol consumption then restricting alcohol improves the situation. If the underlying cause is rosacea, appropriate treatment of this disease by a dermatologist is required. In any case, exposure to the sun should be minimized, as should exposure to other environmental conditions that may be deleterious to the skin, such as cold or wind. The dermatologist has several treatment modalities.

Electric Cautery with a Needle

Electric cautery with a needle is an old method of treatment. It is insufficiently selective and may damage tissues around the blood vessels.

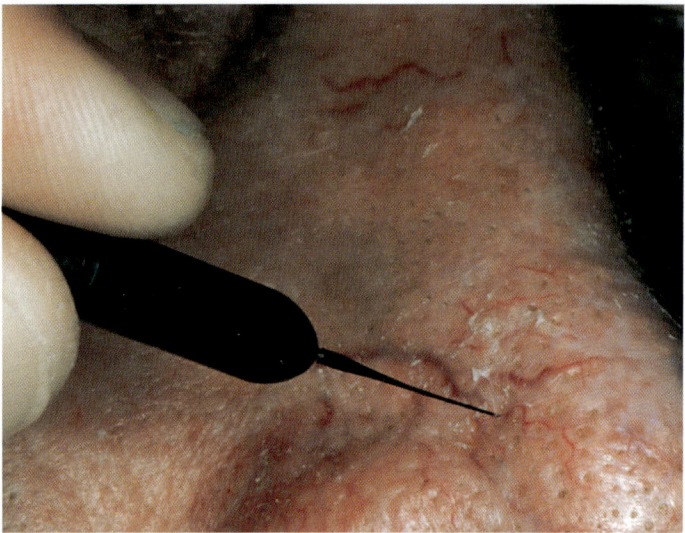
Treating blood vessels with an electric needle.

Laser Treatment
Currently, the most popular treatment of telangiectases is cauterization with a laser beam. A laser instrument is used that emits a ray with a wavelength precisely matched to the red color of the blood vessels. If a nonselective laser instrument is used, it may cause unwanted and excessive damage to the tissues around the blood vessels (see chapter 25, "Laser Treatment in Dermatology: Cosmetic Applications," for more information).

Other Treatments
Other modern instruments also work on the basis of **brief pulses of light rays** that are not laser rays (for example, the ESC "Photoderm" instrument), which are also selective for blood vessels. The physician selects the wavelength appropriate for the color and the size of the blood vessels.

The blood vessels that form telangiectases on the face are usually superficial (close to the surface), so that **skin peeling** (see chapter 24) may also solve the problem in some cases.

Make-up
Those who do not wish to undergo the above treatments may find that make-up to hide the lesions may be adequate (see chapter 29, "Camouflaging Skin Lesions and Other Disfiguring Conditions").

NETWORKS OF BLOOD VESSELS ON THE LEGS

Telangiectasia on the legs is related mainly to the problem of hydrostatic pressure, and is the result of poor function of the valves in the leg veins (the medical term for this problem is **venous insufficiency**). Because the valves in the veins do not function adequately, blood tends to pool in the lower part of the leg, and the veins become permanently distended with blood. At first, these veins appear as reddish lines in the skin, which turn blue with time. Telangiectasia of this nature is common in women older than 30 years, and tend to appear during pregnancy, so there is reason to believe that it is in some way related to hormonal influences. As mentioned above, telangiectases tend to appear as red or blue lines, sometimes in a lace-like pattern.

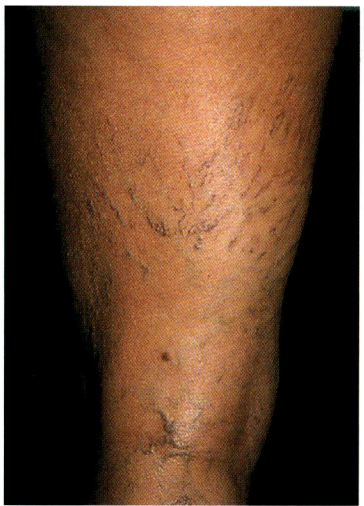

(A) *Arborizing telangiectasia.*

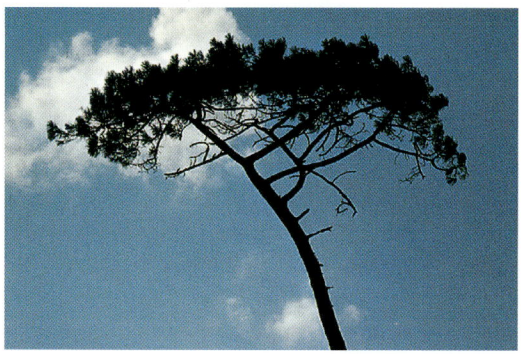

(B) *Maritime pine, a natural example of telangiectatic venous drainage and "feeding" vein.*

There is another form of telangiectasia that looks like the branches of a tree (**arborizing telangiectasia**); this usually occurs on the outer part of the thighs. Later this chapter deals in more detail with venous insufficiency and its treatment.

> **Other Forms of Networks of Blood Vessels on the Skin**
>
> In certain cases, telangiectasia can occur as a consequence of certain diseases that affect the connective tissue and blood vessels. These include, for example, diseases such as **lupus**, **scleroderma,** and **dermatomyositis**. In general, there is a long list of diseases—some genetically transmitted and some acquired during life—that can cause telangiectasia. In rare cases, the appearance of a network of blood vessels on the skin in children is a manifestation of a congenital syndrome. This topic is mentioned here to make the point that telangiectasia under these circumstances is not a cosmetic problem, and the patient should be referred to a dermatologist for the diagnosis and treatment.

"SPIDER" TELANGIECTASIA

Another form of telangiectasia is **"spider" telangiectasia**. These lesions tend to occur mainly on the upper half of the body—face, neck, and arms. They are usually approximately 1 to 1.5 cm in size. Tiny blood vessels radiate from a central artery, as shown in the sketch. If you press exactly on the center of the lesion with a pencil or pen point, you can see how the entire lesion "disappears." If you then release the pressure from the central artery, the blood vessels all then "reappear" (in fact, they now fill up with blood and become visible). If you press lightly with a glass slide on the central artery, you can see pulsation of the artery corresponding to the patient's heartbeat.

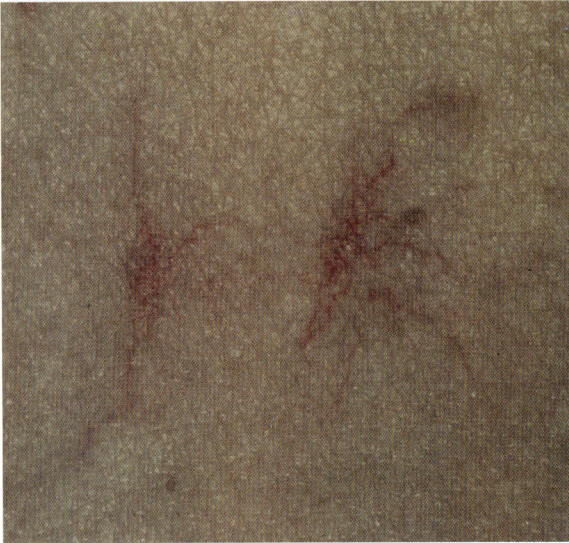
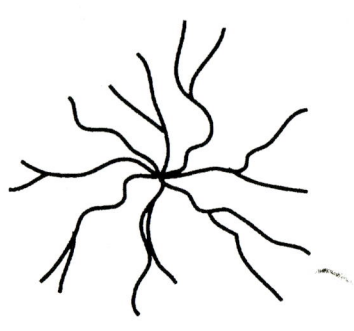

Spider telangiectasia.

Spider telangiectases normally appear in approximately 10% to 20% of the population, and can also be seen normally in children. They occur particularly in women and are considered to be related to high levels of estrogen hormones, so they tend to appear under those circumstances when there are high levels of estrogen, for example, in pregnancy, or in patients with certain liver diseases. With regard to pregnancy, more than 50% of pregnant women may develop spider telangiectases. The lesions tend to grow during the pregnancy, and usually disappear within a few weeks after delivery. In terms of the aesthetic management, these lesions are treated in the same way as other telangiectases.

Venous Insufficiency in the Legs

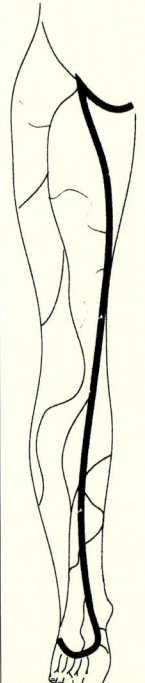

Venous insufficiency in the legs leads to varicose veins—relatively large, dilated blood vessels in the lower limbs—as well as to a network of fine blood vessels (telangiectases).

The blood drains from the legs via the veins. There is a system of valves in the veins that ensures that this blood flow is in one direction only (from the feet toward the heart). With age, there tends to be a weakening and decrease in efficiency of the venous drainage system. This leads to a tendency to dilatation (widening) of the veins. In larger blood vessels, this dilatation results in varicose veins. Since many small veins drain into the larger veins, there is also a "banking up" of blood in the smaller vessels, which also become dilated and appear as telangiectases. The problem is more common in women.

The reasons for abnormal blood flow in the legs are partly hereditary and partly hormonal (including the effects of pregnancy). Prolonged standing may induce and aggravate the condition. The problem can also appear following thrombosis of the veins.

Venous insufficiency leads to swelling of the legs, pain when standing for long periods, and dilatation of superficial veins on the surface of the skin. With more severe venous insufficiency, particularly in old age, the skin around the problem areas may become inflamed. This is a condition known as **stasis dermatitis**, in which the skin appears thicker, becomes dark, and tends to itch.

Blood flow along the leg veins.

What Can Be Done to Alleviate Venous Insufficiency?

- The problem is more severe in people who stand up for long periods so, as far as possible, one should avoid standing for prolonged periods. Furthermore, when sitting, one should not sit with the legs dangling down, rather the legs should rest on a stool or chair (ideally, the feet should be at the height of the buttocks).
- Walking is beneficial, since activating the muscles of the legs helps propel the blood upward.
- Elastic stockings may be helpful.
- If the problem is one of fine telangiectases on the legs, the treatment is the same as for telangiectases elsewhere on the body, and includes cautery with an electric needle, laser treatment, or treatment with light rays.
- Larger veins may be treated by injecting sclerosing agents into the vein. These substances in fact "solidify" the vein so that it can no longer function.
- In more severe cases, a surgical procedure is carried out to remove the problem vein entirely.
- Each case of problem veins in the legs must be treated according to its specific clinical characteristics following medical consultation.

12 | Cellulite

Ron Yaniv

Contents What is "cellulite"? ● Prevention of cellulite ● How NOT to treat cellulite ● Cosmetic preparations for cellulite ● Surgical methods for removing excess fat: liposuction ● Other technologies to treat cellulite

WHAT IS "CELLULITE"?

The term cellulite is widely used in everyday speech, but it has no scientific basis, and is not an accepted medical term. The reason the term cellulite has a medical ring about it is that it sounds like the medical term "cellulitis," but there is no connection between the two; **cellulitis** describes a bacterial infection of the skin. So then, what does the term cellulite mean?

Cellulite refers to an unsightly distribution of fat under the skin, in certain areas of the body—especially the thighs and buttocks. The subcutaneous fat is distributed in a manner that creates hollows and bumps in these areas.

Cellulite is definitely not an abnormal medical condition. Although its appearance may be disturbing, it only represents the pattern of distribution of body fat. Being actually a normal phenomenon, it is infrequently referred to in scientific/medical journals. Cellulite is much more common in women than in men, affecting 80% to 90%, especially older than 35 years. The high prevalence among women suggests that it may be related to hormonal factors.

Why Does Cellulite Appear?

Under the dermis lies a layer of fat, called the **subcutis**. This layer is made up of many fat cells that coalesce to form fatty tissue. These lumps of fat are surrounded and separated from each other by rigid strands, as illustrated.

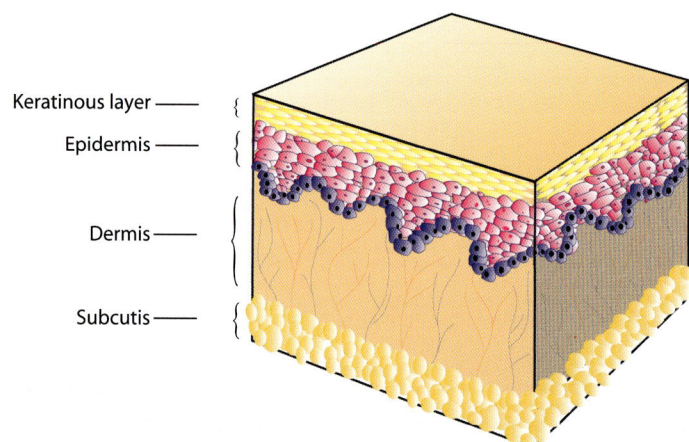

Layer of subcutaneous fat (subcutis).

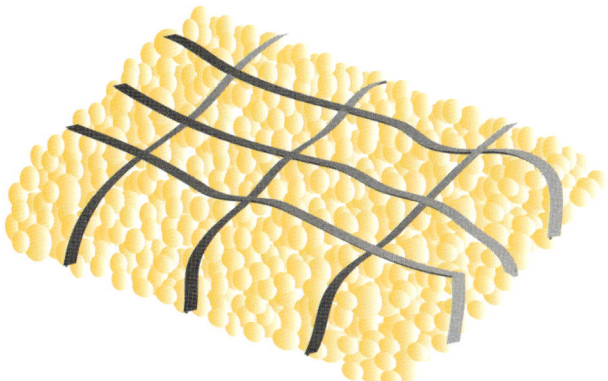

Subcutaneous fat divided into lumps by rigid strands.

If there is a high dietary intake of fats or carbohydrates (which are converted to fat in the body), the fat cells fill up with fat, swell up, and may grow to three or more times their normal size. At the same time, the rigid strands cannot stretch beyond a certain amount. Thus, the fatty tissue bulges out from the strands around it.

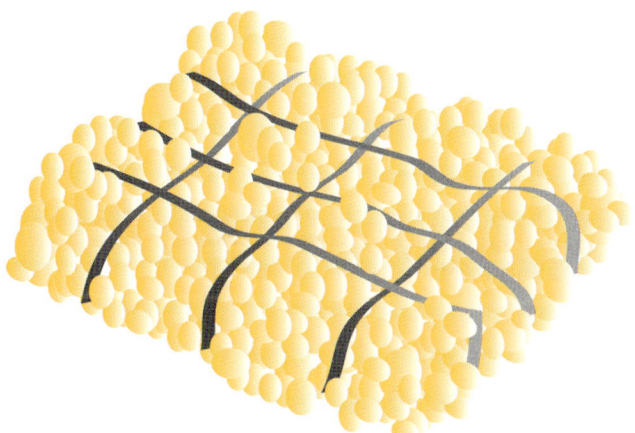

Fatty tissue bulging out from the rigid strands that surround it.

PREVENTION OF CELLULITE

Attention to Diet and Avoiding Weight Gain

Since good dietary habits prevent an increase in the amount of subcutaneous fat, there is certain logic to the suggestion that one should avoid gaining too much weight. Nevertheless, it must be remembered that cellulite has a significant hereditary factor. There are some thin women who take great care with their diet but who still have cellulite. Remember that:

- A woman who has excess fat in the thighs and buttocks and goes on a reduction diet to lose weight may not necessarily lose fat from those particular areas.
- The loss of fat from areas that were bulging for a long period may result in **excess skin** that had previously been stretched over the fatty areas.

It is important to adhere to sensible dietary habits over many years, to maintain a stable weight and to avoid weight gain. A "crash" diet losing, say, 20 kg in 10 days is in any case undesirable, not only for the reasons mentioned above but also for other medical reasons.

Physical Exercise

Physical exercise can further improve the appearance

- by converting fat tissue to energy with subsequent decrease in excess fatty tissue, and
- by increasing the bulk of the muscles—instead of the fat accumulating in large "lumps," muscle tissue tends to grow in a uniform, smooth, more aesthetically acceptable manner.

HOW *NOT* TO TREAT CELLULITE

- It has not been demonstrated scientifically that any dietary product can "burn" and get rid of excess fat.
- "Exercise" machines that cause passive repeated movements of the fatty tissues of the thighs and buttocks so as to "burn up" the fat have not proven to be effective.

COSMETIC PREPARATIONS FOR CELLULITE

Cosmetic products to treat cellulite are supposed to penetrate through the keratin layer, the epidermis, and the dermis and "dissolve" the excess fatty tissue. The active ingredients commonly present in these preparations are methylxanthines, various plant extracts, and vitamin A derivates. Recently, some of these compounds have been combined with liposome technology, being a good delivery system that may assist in deeper penetration of the active ingredients into the skin. The effect of this combination is still to be assessed.

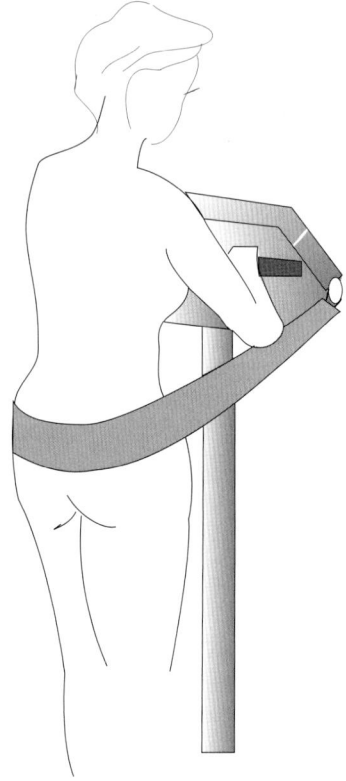

Exercise machine that causes passive movements of the fatty tissue.

Methylxanthines

Methylxanthines are known to have a certain effect on fat cells. They are supposed to break down and dissolve the fat in the cells. Substances in this group include:

- **theophylline**, derived from tea leaves, or produced synthetically,
- **caffeine**, present in coffee, tea, cola, and guarana, and
- **aminophylline**, used as a medication in asthma.

Thus far, there is no concrete scientific proof that any product containing any of these substances can, when applied onto the skin, penetrate the subcutaneous tissues, dissolve the fat, and improve the texture of the tissues. From time to time, conflicting reports on the use of these substances are published.

Some doctors claim that preparations containing methylxanthines reduce the amount of water between fat cells. This may give the impression of firmer tone in that area, since the skin is attached somewhat tighter to the tissues underneath. Yet, this effect is only temporary.

Plant Extracts

Some plant extracts contain substances similar in their chemical structure to the methylxanthines. Every now and then, a new product appears on the cosmetic scene, only to be supplanted by the next fad.

Retinoids and Vitamin A Derivates

Topical agents containing retinoids and vitamin A derivates also are used as optional treatments for cellulite. For the time being, there is no substantial scientific evidence to support their efficacy.

These creams may induce a smoother texture of the skin, but they do not seem to affect the fat cells directly.

SURGICAL METHODS FOR REMOVING EXCESS FAT: LIPOSUCTION

In cases where the accumulation of subcutaneous fat is extreme and causes psychological distress, one may consider referral for **liposuction**. In this procedure, a small incision, a few millimeters long, is made in the skin, a thin tube is inserted into the subcutaneous fat layer, and the fat cells are sucked out through the tube. Following liposuction, new fat cells will not grow or multiply in the area. If there is excessive plumpness in the area, it will be due to the growth of those fat cells left behind.

Not everybody is suitable to undergo liposuction, and an appropriately trained surgeon should be consulted with regard to the suitability for the operation, its advantages and disadvantages, and the expected outcome. It is difficult to predict the exact results following liposuction and, to a large extent, the outcome depends on the skill of the surgeon.

OTHER TECHNOLOGIES TO TREAT CELLULITE

There have been new technological developments for treating cellulite. These involve measures such as the use of laser devices, light sources, and the application of high-energy radiofrequency. Certain types of laser/light devices at present have received FDA approval as being safe and effective in the treatment of cellulite. For the time being, however, because of a relative lack of clinical research in this field, it would be difficult to provide an accurate assessment of their effectiveness. Their long-term effects (if any) are still to be examined.

Injection lipolysis is a new method using an injected compound into the subcutaneous tissue that dissolves undesirable small accumulations of fat (see chapter 13, "Injection Lipolysis—A New Method of Body Contouring," for further information).

13 | Injection Lipolysis: A New Method of Body Contouring

Franz Hasengschwandtner

Contents Overview • The substance used • The procedure

OVERVIEW

Injection lipolysis is a new method using an injected compound into the subcutaneous tissue that "dissolves" undesirable small accumulations of fat. This method is experiencing growing worldwide popularity in the field of aesthetics. Injection lipolysis was first reported on in 1988. Originally criticized by established cosmetic surgeons, it has now gained a foothold due to very good results and almost hardly any unwanted side effects.

THE SUBSTANCE USED

The injected active agent is a substance called phosphatidylcholine, a lecithin extracted from the soy plant. Phosphatidylcholine is, in fact, also found in all bodily cell membranes, and is highly concentrated in the membrane of liver cells and fat cells (adipocytes). It occurs naturally, for instance, in the lungs of embryos from the fourth month on, enabling the inflation and deflation of the lungs, preventing them from sticking together. It performs a similar function as a lubricant in the intestines to avoid adhesions.

Phosphatidylcholine is not only used for aesthetic purposes. It has been already widely accepted in intravenous and oral treatment of certain medical conditions such as fatty embolism, certain liver diseases, and severe disturbances in fat metabolism. For these purposes, the daily-administered intravenous dose is many times higher than the dose used in "lipodissolving" treatments. Furthermore, various research studies are being conducted in order to examine the potential of phosphatidylcholine for use in the fields of neurology, cardiology, and antiaging medicine.

THE PROCEDURE

To make phosphatidylcholine injectable for the purpose of lipolysis, a solvent is required that also needs to be a detergent substance. In the case of phosphatidylcholine, it is deoxycholic acid. To achieve the desired effect, both detergent substances (phosphatidylcholine and deoxycholic acid) are necessary.

First step:
Lipolytic agents are injected into the subcutaneous tissue at a depth of approx. 10 to 12 mm.

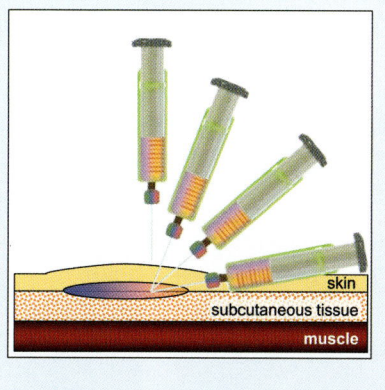

Second step:
Lipolytic agents are injected through the dermis to a depth of approx. 6 mm

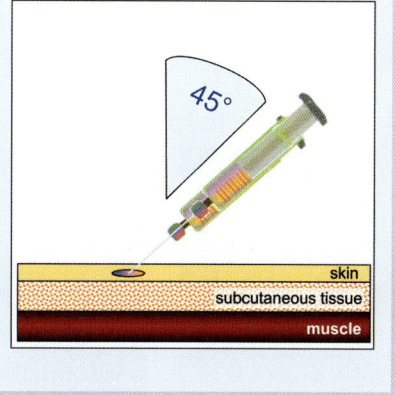

Third step:
Lipolytic agents are injected intradermally to a depth of around 1 mm, at an angle of 45 degrees, about 3 mm apart

"The three-step cellulite cure"—injecting phosphatidylcholine for treating cellulite.

In addition to phosphatidylcholine and deoxycholic acid, benzylalcohol, in small concentrations, is used as a preservative. The compound (i.e., phosphatidylcholine, deoxycholic acid, and benzylalcohol) is injected into the subcutaneous fatty tissue with very thin needles.

The agent, functioning like a detergent, dissolves the double layer of the fat-cell membranes, which results in the production of tiny little fat particles of nano size (one millionth of a millimeter). Simultaneously, enzymes stored in the fat cells are released, which gradually break down the lipid content of the tissue over a period of around eight weeks. This period of eight weeks is known as a "melting cycle." The breakdown products are transported to the liver, where they are metabolized. Depending on the body region injected, one to four sessions are necessary. The desirable time gap between sessions is approximately eight weeks. The majority of patients need only one or two sessions to achieve the desired results.

In the use of phosphatidylcholine for aesthetic medicine, one has to be aware of the bounds of possibilities to melt fat accumulations. The ideal patients are of almost normal weight, exercise, and watch their diet. They have small problems with fat accumulations that refuse to disappear through the measures just mentioned.

The lipolysis method is intended for the treatment of jowls, double chins, excessive fatty tissue in the axillary folds, backrolls, upper arms, abdominal fat protrusions, outer and inner thighs, and the region above the knees. It is implemented in the treatment of "cellulite," and for lipomas (benign growths containing fatty tissue).

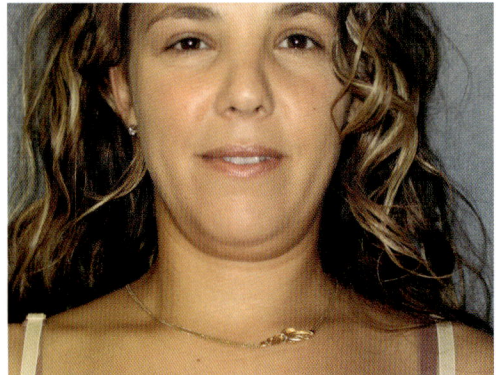 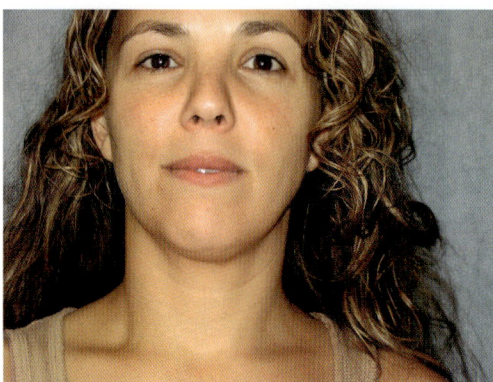

Eliminating "double chin." Before (left) and after (right) treatment.

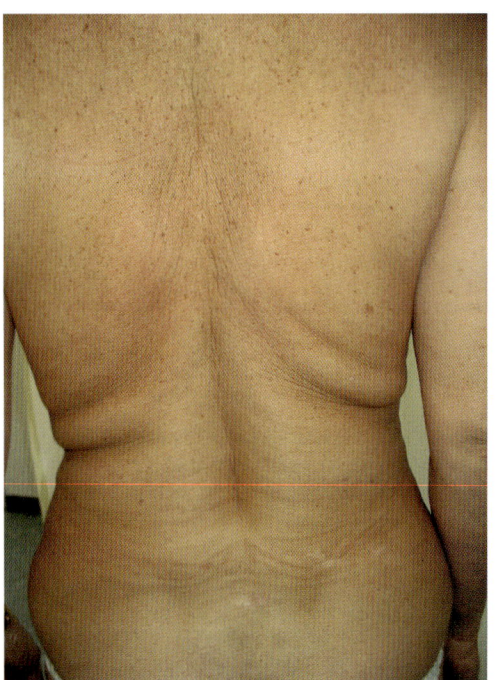 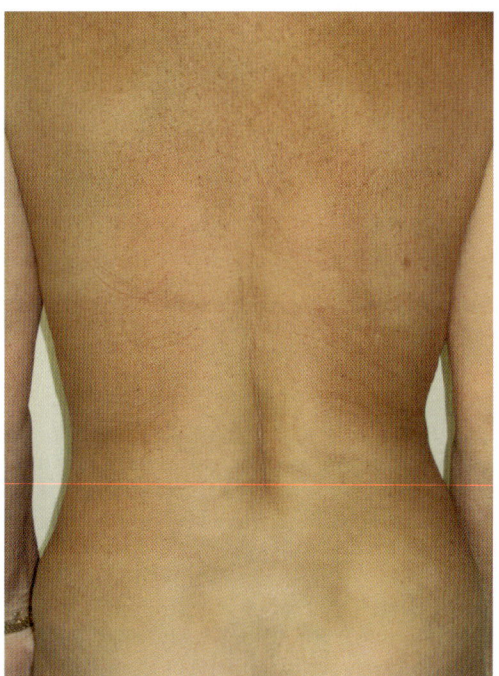

Eliminating undesirable accumulation of fat in the back. Before (left) and after (right) treatment.

Lipolysis is a good method to correct slight unevennesses following liposuction procedures, and sometimes preceding them to pretreat known problem areas around the umbilicus or the inner thighs. Only in approximately 1% of all cases, lipolysis treatment does not reach the desirable outcome. In these cases, further measures such as surgical intervention may be required.

The known side effects after injection lipolysis are swelling, reddening, bruising, slight circulatory problems, and increased stools during the first days after the injections. More threatening side effects are not expected to occur if accepted standards are undertaken. Thus far, more than 60,000 patients have been treated without any severe adverse effect having been documented.

In summary, injection lipolysis using phosphatidylcholine may be regarded as a highly effective and safe technique in the treatment of unwanted fat accumulations, and has rightly won its acclaimed position in aesthetic medicine.

14 | Inflammation, Dermatitis, and Cosmetics
Arieh Ingber and Avi Shai

Contents Overview • Definitions: inflammation and dermatitis • Stages in the development of skin inflammation • Causes and types of skin inflammation • Contact dermatitis • Types of contact dermatitis • Hypoallergenic preparations • Diagnosis • Principles of treatment

OVERVIEW

Cosmetics are a relatively common cause of skin inflammation. The inflammation results from exposure of the skin to a specific component of the cosmetic preparation. In many cases, certain tests need to be performed in order to identify the offending component. To make this subject more easily understood, we first clarify what the term **inflammation** means and then we discuss the common types of skin inflammation. Finally, we discuss skin inflammation that results from contact with specific substances, including components of cosmetics.

DEFINITIONS: INFLAMMATION AND DERMATITIS

The term **inflammation** can be defined simply as the defensive response of the body to various processes, including infections (bacterial, viral, or fungal) and many other injuries. A chain of events, mainly involving the white blood cells (leukocytes), results in the appearance of the inflammatory process. Inflammation is characterized by:

- **warmth** in the inflamed area,
- **redness** caused by the dilatation of blood vessels,
- **swelling** caused by an increase in the permeability ("leakiness") of the blood vessels, with leakage of fluid,
- **pain** or **itching** due to irritation of nerves, and
- **loss of function** (partial or complete) of the involved organ or limb.

The term **dermatitis** means inflammation of the skin. The term **eczema** means the same as "dermatitis"—they are synonymous.

Note: In medical terminology, any inflammation is usually given the suffix -**itis**; for example, inflammation of the appendix is called **appendicitis**, inflammation of the meninges (the coverings of the brain) is called **meningitis**, and inflammation of the dermis (skin) is called **dermatitis**.

STAGES IN THE DEVELOPMENT OF SKIN INFLAMMATION

Any inflammation, regardless of cause, may appear at various stages. The accepted medical approach differentiates **acute** inflammation from **chronic** inflammation. An acute illness, in medical terminology, is one that progresses rapidly and does not last a long time (it either subsides or moves into a chronic phase), whereas a chronic illness is prolonged.

Acute Inflammation
In the skin, acute inflammation manifests itself as red and swollen areas. In severe conditions, the skin may weep and blisters may appear.

INFLAMMATION, DERMATITIS, AND COSMETICS

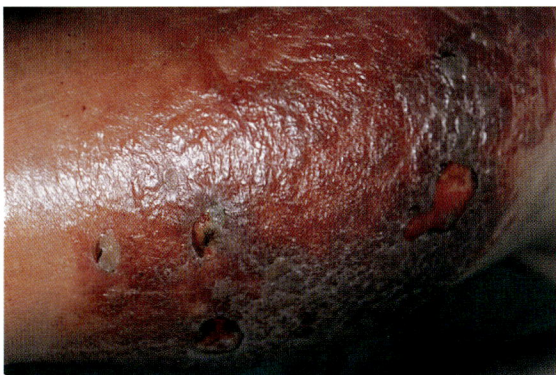

Acute skin inflammation.

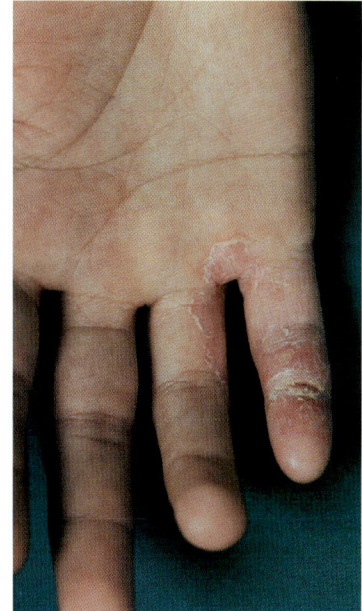

Chronic skin inflammation of a mechanic's hand following exposure to motor oils.

Chronic Inflammation

The skin in chronic inflammation is dry, thickened, and scaly, with accentuation of the normal skin markings. Sometimes the skin is cracked.

> ### Subacute Inflammation
>
> Another stage in the development of inflammation is the subacute phase. This is an intermediate stage between acute and chronic inflammation. In subacute skin inflammation, the skin is still red and swollen to a certain extent, but less so than in acute inflammation. There may be slight weeping. In certain areas, the skin begins to peel.

CAUSES AND TYPES OF SKIN INFLAMMATION

Skin inflammation can be due to:

- infection,
- diaper dermatitis,
- seborrheic dermatitis,
- atopic dermatitis, or
- contact dermatitis

This chapter concentrates on contact dermatitis, since it is the type that may result from the use of cosmetic preparations.

> ### Various Types of Skin Inflammation
>
> - **Skin infection**: Any infection of the skin, be it bacterial, viral, or fungal, produces a defensive response from the body, resulting in the appearance of inflammation.

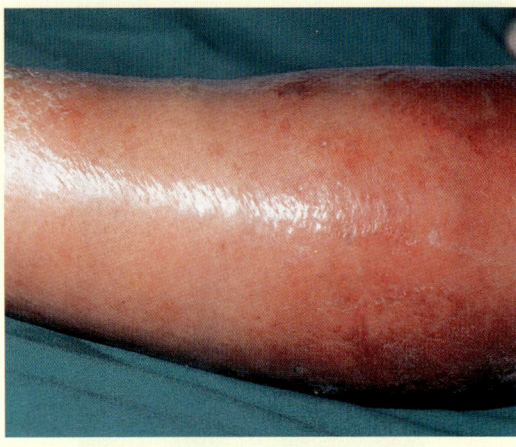

Infection in the leg: In the infected area, there are signs of inflammation, such as redness and swelling.

- **Diaper dermatitis**: This inflammation occurs in babies in the diaper area as a result of prolonged contact with urine and stool, or with remnants of soap or other substances that were applied to the area.
- **Seborrheic dermatitis**: This is an inflammatory process characterized by redness and scaling in certain areas. The areas that are usually affected by seborrheic dermatitis in adults are the scalp, the folds alongside the nose, and the eyebrows.
- **Atopic dermatitis**: This is a chronic skin inflammation that is related to hereditary factors, and manifested by dry skin, with marked itching. Atopic dermatitis is related to the group of allergic diseases called **atopic diseases**, which include asthma, allergic rhinitis ("hay fever"), and allergic conjunctivitis (allergic eye inflammation).

We do not discuss the treatment of these conditions in this chapter. In all such cases, the patient should seek medical attention.

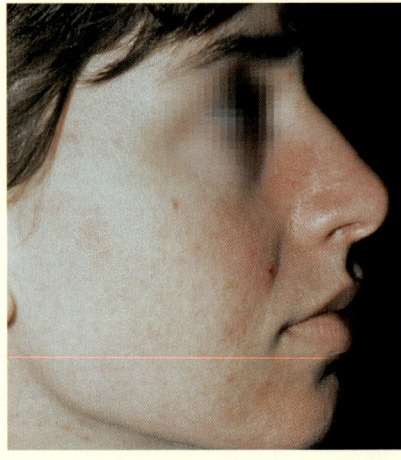

Seborrheic dermatitis.

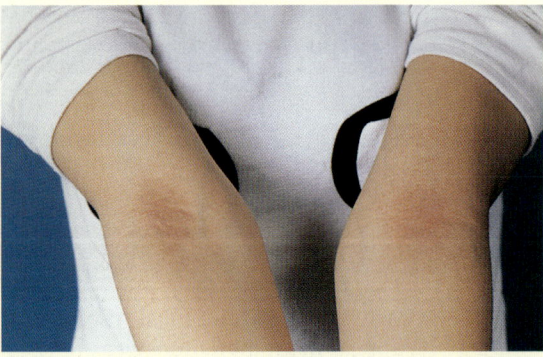

Atopic dermatitis.

CONTACT DERMATITIS

Overview

Contact dermatitis is a common form of skin inflammation caused by contact of certain substances with the skin. The skin is normally in contact with numerous substances, almost any of which can cause inflammation

- by direct irritation of the skin—**irritant contact dermatitis**.
- by an allergic mechanism—**allergic contact dermatitis**.

Irritant Contact Dermatitis

In irritant contact dermatitis, the offending substance has a direct toxic effect on the skin. Hence, the severity of the reaction depends on the concentration of the irritant substance and the period of exposure. This is not a specific sensitivity of a particular person to the substance. Anybody coming in contact with that substance, above a certain concentration, and for a long enough time, will develop inflammation of the skin. For example, contact with various acids causes irritant contact dermatitis.

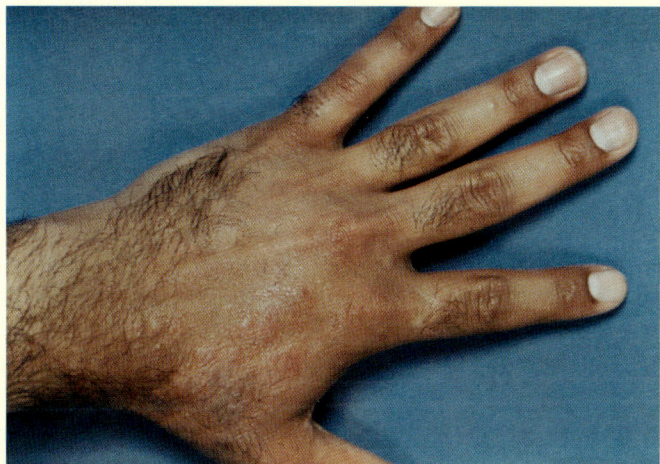

Irritant contact dermatitis following exposure to moderate concentrations of hydrochloric acid.

Allergic Contact Dermatitis

Allergy is a state of hypersensitivity arising from an immune response of the body to a particular substance. This can follow exposure to the substance by inhaling it, by swallowing it, or by direct contact of the substance with the skin. In allergic contact dermatitis, the allergic reaction occurs because of hypersensitivity to substances in direct contact with the skin.

Allergic contact dermatitis does not occur in everyone exposed to the specific substance. For some reason, partially due to a hereditary factor, there is a fault in the patient's immune response. In an allergic patient, the immune system is triggered by a substance that normally has no adverse effects, but in that specific patient causes an inflammatory response of the skin. In the classic and most common form of allergic contact dermatitis, the patient has been exposed to the same offending substance for long periods in the past without developing any reaction. During this period, however, an unnoticed process occurred and an allergic response developed in the body's immune system. At a certain stage, the response becomes manifest and, from then on, every exposure to the substance may be followed by an allergic response.

The offending substance may be a cleansing agent, any cosmetic preparation, a metal such as nickel or chrome, glues, etc. Once the immune system has identified and reacted against a certain substance, the allergic reaction can occur following exposure to minute amounts of the substance. The patient does not need to come into contact with a large amount of the substance to trigger an allergic reaction. Furthermore, there does not have to be daily exposure to the substance to produce an allergic reaction; infrequent exposure—even once every few weeks or years—to small amounts of the substance may be sufficient to trigger such a reaction.

TYPES OF CONTACT DERMATITIS

Hand Eczema

Hand eczema is a common problem and is the result of prolonged exposure to water and cleaning agents, to which housewives and other workers (e.g., food handlers, florists) are frequently subjected. Prolonged exposure to cleaning agents removes the oily layer of the skin surface. The combination of this loss of the oily protective layer with frequent exposure to cleaning agents that may contain irritant and/or allergenic substances results in hand **eczema** (or "hand dermatitis"), sometimes called "**housewife's eczema.**" The chronic form of hand eczema is manifested by the appearance of scaling and fissures. From time to time, there may be flare-ups of acute inflammation, with reddening and swelling of the skin.

This inflammation occurs on the palms, backs of the hands, webs of the fingers, and underneath rings, bracelets, and watch straps, because remnants of cleaning agents and other offending materials tend to remain there, with subsequent prolonged contact with the skin. Usually some improvement can be observed if the patient refrains from cleaning activities. However, the inflammation will recur on resuming these activities without appropriate protection.

Nickel and Other Allergens

In many cases, contact sensitivity may be triggered by nickel—a metal that is a common component in rings, bracelets, and watch straps. Wetting the skin (or sweating) results in the release of small quantities of nickel, which contacts the skin and causes allergic contact dermatitis. In addition, skin exposure to certain common foodstuffs, especially vegetables and fruits, may provoke allergic reactions.

Prevention of Hand Eczema

Contact with water and detergents should be avoided as much as possible. As explained in chapter 4 on skin moisture and moisturizers, repeated exposure to water effectively dries the skin. In addition, detergents are designed to remove the layer of grease from the dishes but, by the same token, they remove the protective oily layer that coats the skin and protects it. To minimize contact with water and detergents, it is advisable to adopt the following measures:

- Gloves should be worn. Note that the rubber of normal gloves may actually contain substances that can trigger an allergic skin reaction. Furthermore, so long as one wears rubber gloves, the hands are constantly moist as a result of small amounts of water that may have got into the glove and from perspiration. Use gloves that have an inner lining made of cotton, or to wear an inner set of cotton gloves underneath the rubber ones. In any case, the rubber gloves should be worn for as brief a period as possible (no longer than a few minutes). If it is felt that the hands are perspiring, the gloves should be removed and the hands aired.
- Advantage should be taken of appliances such as dishwashers and washing machines (or other members of the family!).
- Occlusive ointments should be applied frequently to isolate the skin from cleansing agents. Silicone-containing preparations may be used as well. Details of silicone preparations appear in chapter 4 on skin moisture and moisturizers. However, if there is skin inflammation, protective preparations should not be applied. In this case, the first thing to do is to seek medical advice to treat the inflammation. Only after the inflammation has disappeared should protective cream be applied.
- In cases where an association between hand dermatitis and certain foodstuffs is identified, contact with these substances should be avoided as much as possible.

Phytodermatitis and Phytophotodermatitis

Contact dermatitis can be caused by contact with plants, flowers, or fruit juices. This phenomenon is called **phytodermatitis** (Greek: *phyton* = plant).

In other cases, the actual contact with the plant does not cause skin inflammation by itself. The allergic reaction occurs only after the skin has been exposed to sunlight as well. This phenomenon is known as **phytophotodermatitis**.

Plants known to cause these reactions include chrysanthemums, celery, mango, citrus fruits, figs, and others. In such cases, a typical rash is manifested by a linear distribution of blisters.

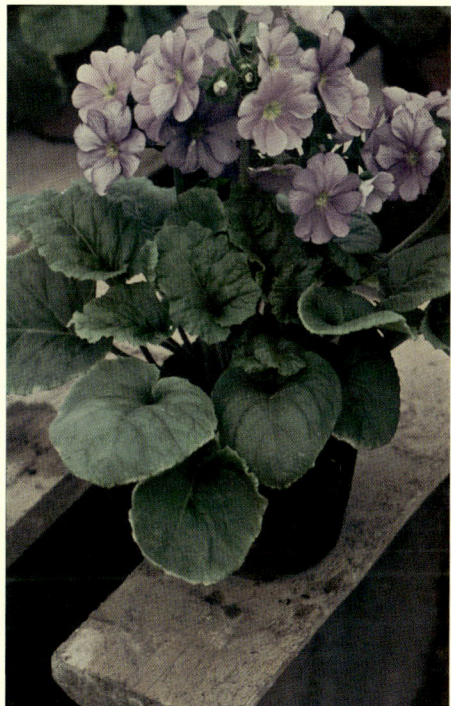

Primula obconica: Skin inflammation may appear after touching the dry petals of the plant.

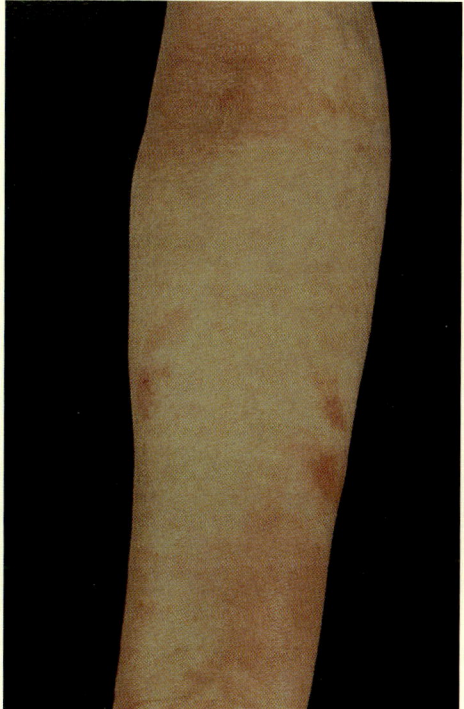

Skin inflammation following exposure to Primula obconica.

Hand Eczema Can Be a Form of Atopic Dermatitis

Note that hand eczema is not always related to contact with offending substances. Sometimes, it represents a unique form of **atopic dermatitis**. These cases are much more difficult to deal with, and the conventional modes of prevention and treatment are not so effective.

Cosmetics and Dermatitis

Cosmetics can cause contact dermatitis. The chances of this happening are relatively low, considering the number of people using cosmetics, but it does occur. It is estimated that approximately 10% of women who use cosmetics develop contact dermatitis from some cosmetic preparation at least once in their lives.

Cosmetic preparations contain several components, any one of which could potentially cause skin inflammation:

- the active ingredient of the preparation,
- the vehicle (base) that contains the active ingredient, or
- additional components that may be present, such as fragrances or preservatives.

Before using any cosmetic preparation, establish that the user is not allergic to one of its components. Before using some cosmetic for the first time, a small amount should be applied to a small area of skin that is not exposed (usually behind the ear) for a few days. Only after confirming that there is no intolerance should the preparation be used regularly. Remember, however, that sensitivity can appear with time, even to a substance that has been used frequently.

If sensitivity to a specific preparation appears,

- use of the preparation should be discontinued, and
- a dermatologist's advice should be sought, and he/she should be consulted as to how the particular component of the preparation that was responsible can be identified. Subsequently, preparations containing that specific chemical should be avoided.

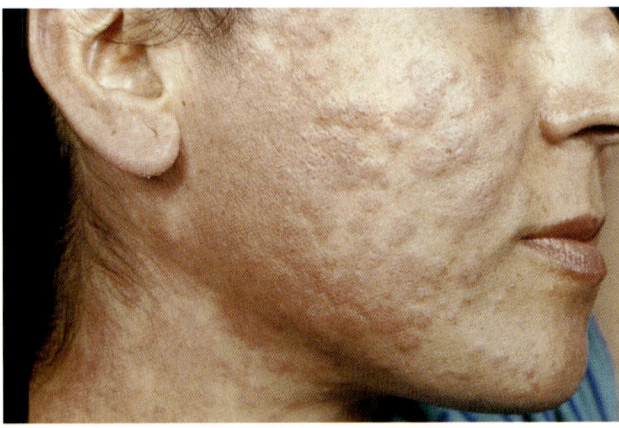

Allergic contact dermatitis following exposure to fragrance in a facial moisturizer.

HYPOALLERGENIC PREPARATIONS

Hypoallergenic preparations do not usually contain components such as perfumes or certain preservatives that are known statistically to have a higher than average risk of causing allergic reactions. Remember, however, that hypoallergenic preparations can still cause allergy. Sensitivity to a particular substance is an individual characteristic. In practice, there is no cosmetic preparation that can never cause an allergic reaction in someone.

The term "hypoallergenic" may be misleading. Many people mistakenly believe that such preparations do not contain any substance that can cause an allergic reaction. However, hypoallergenic preparations can also contain fragrances, preservatives, and other components that may also induce an allergic reaction. Nevertheless, statistically, the likelihood of a hypoallergenic preparation causing an allergic reaction is certainly less than that of a normal preparation.

DIAGNOSIS

Usually, the most efficient way of diagnosing the cause of an inflammation is by questioning the patient carefully. In some cases, the patient has a fairly good idea what caused the problem, and will tell you that the rash appeared after using a certain cosmetic or medical preparation. However, the offending agent may be present in many cosmetic preparations. Therefore, avoiding the use of one particular preparation and replacing it with another may not necessarily solve the problem. To identify precisely to which particular component the patient has reacted, there is a special test kit called a **"patch test."**

INFLAMMATION, DERMATITIS, AND COSMETICS

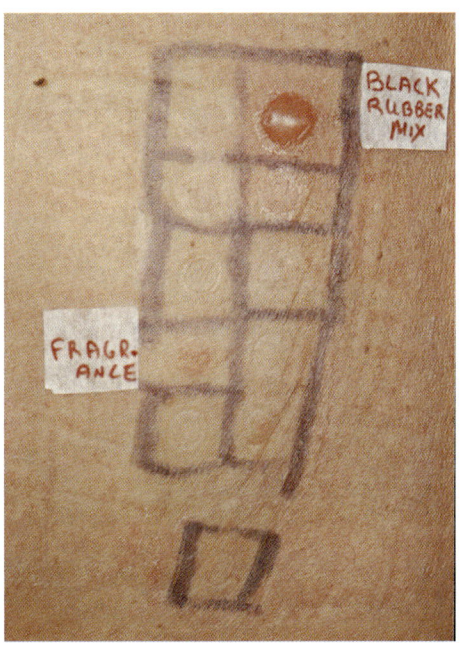

Patch test demonstrating sensitivity to black rubber. In this case, the patient should avoid contact with rubber products.

In patch tests, substances known to commonly cause allergic reactions are applied to an area of clean, unaffected skin (usually the skin of the back). The substances are applied on small discs that are held against the patient's skin with special adhesive plaster. From 48 to 96 hours later, if the patient is indeed allergic to one or more of the test substances, a skin inflammation will appear at the area of contact (under that specific disc). The inflammation is manifested by redness, itching, and sometimes the appearance of blisters, depending on the level of sensitivity to the material being tested.

Skin allergy to cosmetics can be a prolonged, frustrating problem. Treatment requires patience. Having diagnosed the offending substance by the patch test, one then has to embark on a process (sometimes lengthy and tedious) of finding cosmetic preparations that do not contain that substance or other substances that are chemically similar to it.

PRINCIPLES OF TREATMENT

Prevention
Treatment of allergic contact dermatitis is based on prevention. If it is known what the substance is that caused the reaction, then contact with that substance should be avoided.

Corticosteroids
The most effective treatment for dermatitis involves the use of corticosteroid preparations for application to the skin. Steroids are effective at suppressing inflammation. The dermatologist has a wide range of such preparations at his/her disposal, of varying strengths for differing degrees of inflammation. These preparations should never be used for self-medication; most are only available on prescription. Only preparations that contain low concentrations of hydrocortisone (0.5–1%) may be purchased over-the-counter in the United States. In more severe cases of inflammation, oral medications containing corticosteroids are sometimes necessary, and may even be given by intramuscular injection. The use of corticosteroids is discussed in detail in chapter 22 on preparations used in dermatology.

Antihistamines
Allergic skin reactions involve the release of **histamine** in the affected tissues, with subsequent exacerbation of the inflammatory reaction; therefore, **antihistamines** may be used to lessen the allergic response. Antihistamine preparations may be applied to the skin in the form of creams

or gels. However, these preparations themselves may cause allergic reactions. Hence, some physicians recommend patients to avoid the use of topical antihistamines.

Oral antihistamine preparations are used in various inflammatory situations, including allergic processes that occur in the skin. These medications usually require a doctor's prescription.

Note: Some antihistamine medications may cause drowsiness and fatigue. Therefore, there are strict restrictions regarding driving a motor vehicle after taking them. This also applies to engaging in any other activity for which decreased alertness may be dangerous.

Other Treatments

Other types of treatment are available, such as phototherapy (in which the skin is exposed to ultraviolet rays), and may be used at the physician's discretion.

15 | Skin Tumors
Avi Shai and Daniel Vardy

Contents Overview • Basic definitions • What types of tumors occur in the skin? • Skin tumors that originate in the keratinocytes • Skin tumors that originate in the melanocytes • Prevention • Self-examination • Regular medical examinations • Management of possibly cancerous lesions

OVERVIEW

It is important for a cosmetician to have a basic knowledge of skin tumors. Clients ask cosmeticians questions relating to skin tumors, and in the course of their professional work cosmeticians may observe a variety of skin lesions and growths. This chapter defines some basic terms related to tumors in general, and presents the main features of some of the more common skin tumors.

Note: The purpose of this chapter is not to qualify cosmeticians to treat skin tumors. However, a better knowledge and understanding of this topic can provide the reader with the tools to recognize abnormal lesions and tumors that require referral of the client to a dermatologist.

A skin lesion refers to any abnormal condition that appears on the skin. Dermatology is the science of diagnosing and treating skin lesions. There are many reasons for lesions to appear on the skin such as due to infection (viruses, bacteria, or fungi), inflammation, or various types of abnormal growth. This chapter deals with these abnormal growths of the skin.

BASIC DEFINITIONS

Below are some of the basic definitions in the field of skin tumors. A **tumor** (**growth** or **neoplasm**) is a lesion that represents an abnormal overgrowth of body tissue. This overgrowth is caused by an uncontrolled proliferation of tumor cells.

What Is a Tumor?
A tumor may be benign or malignant. A **benign tumor** does not spread aggressively. It remains limited to the region in which it was formed. It has defined borders that can be clearly distinguished from its surroundings.

The Formation of a Malignant Tumor

The tumorous process results from a change in the genetic features of a certain cell. A change in the genetic content of a cell can lead to repeated divisions and replications. This results in an abnormal proliferation of that cell.

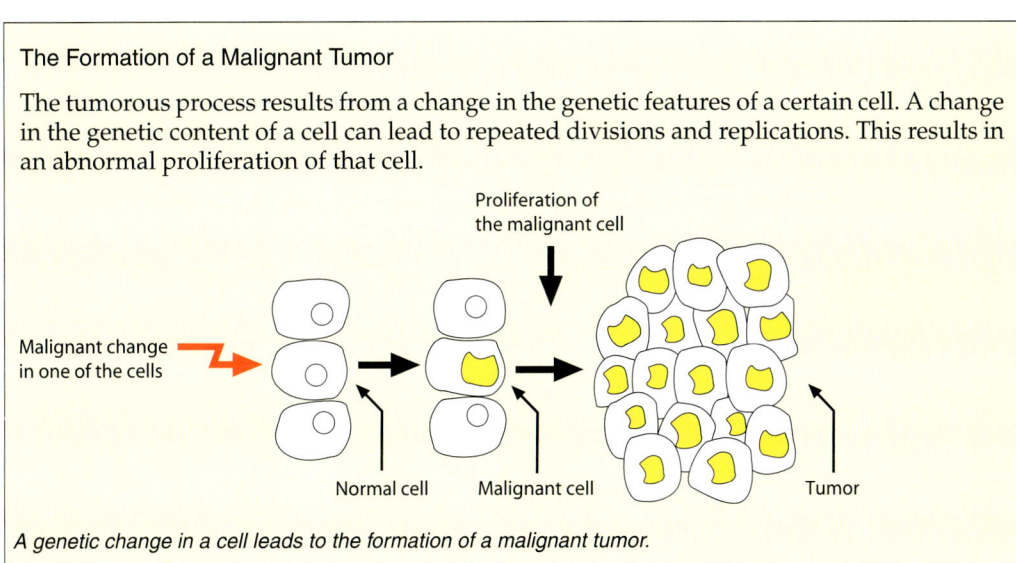

A genetic change in a cell leads to the formation of a malignant tumor.

Note: While the word "tumor" or "growth" in everyday use has a frightening connotation, in medical/scientific terminology, a wide range of lesions are classified as benign tumors. For example, in medical/scientific terminology, a melanocytic nevus ("mole," "beauty mark") is defined as a benign tumor. Despite the frightening-sounding name, moles are considered common skin lesions that have no particular medical implications. Nevertheless, the presence of moles requires regular medical follow-up in order to ascertain that they remain benign and will not develop any suspicious changes.

In contrast, a **malignant tumor** tends to spread aggressively. The tumor cells divide and replicate uncontrollably, and the body's defence mechanisms are unable to halt or control the cell division. The edges of a malignant tumor are not well defined, and cannot be clearly identified, because the tumor cells invade and destroy the surrounding tissues.

Tumor cells that spread to distant areas of the body, remote from the primary tumor, are called metastases.

What Are Metastases?

A **metastasis** (plural: **metastases**) is a group of malignant cells that have broken away from the primary, original tumor and have found their way to other tissues in the body. In those tissues, which may be close to the original (primary) tumor or far from it, the malignant cells continue to divide and cause destruction. The tumor cells can spread, for example, by way of the lymphatic system or the bloodstream. In this way, malignant cells originating in a tumor can reach various organs in the body via the bloodstream. They can reach, for example, the liver, brain, lungs, bones, and other organs. The cause of death from malignancies is frequently related to the presence of metastases in various internal organs and the damage they wreak. The development of metastases is, therefore, the hallmark of malignant tumors; **there are no metastases from benign tumors**.

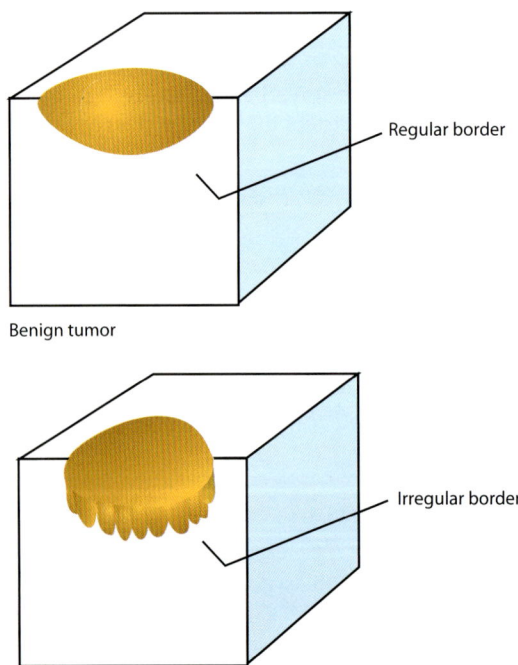

Benign versus malignant tumor: graphic representation.

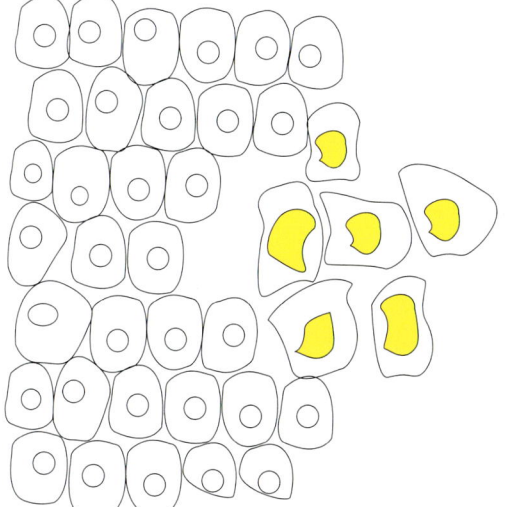

Local spreading of a malignant tumor: direct extension of the malignant cells (marked in yellow) into the surrounding tissues.

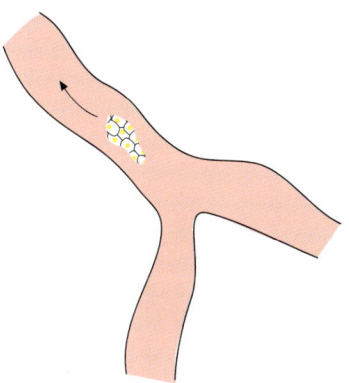

Tumor cells are carried in the blood vessels to distant sites (metastases).

The Progress of a Malignant Tumor at a Glance
- A genetic change takes place in a single cell.
- Repeated cell divisions of that particular cell will result in a malignant tumor that continues growing, until it may eventually become visible to the naked eye.
- Cells from the tumor can break away from the original mass, and establish themselves (as metastases) in distant tissues, and destroy them.

The Term "Cancer" Means Exactly the Same As "Malignant Tumor"
The word "cancer," which is Latin for "crab," is apparently related to the resemblance of the malignant cells spreading out of the primary tumor in the shape of a crab. Although the term "cancer" is widely used in everyday language, "malignant tumor" is the accepted medical/scientific term.

What Is the Source of Tumors in the Human Body?
Every cell in the body, including skin cells, can potentially develop into a tumor. In any cell, a possible "fault" may occur, which will trigger an abnormal division of that particular cell. This abnormal cell division may be limited, in which case a benign tumor results, or it may be uncontrolled, overwhelming the body's defence systems, and results in a malignant tumor.

WHAT TYPES OF TUMORS OCCUR IN THE SKIN?

A skin tumor may develop from any of the living cells present in the skin. The source of the tumor may be in the epidermis, dermis, or the subcutis. In this chapter, we discuss only the relatively common skin tumors.

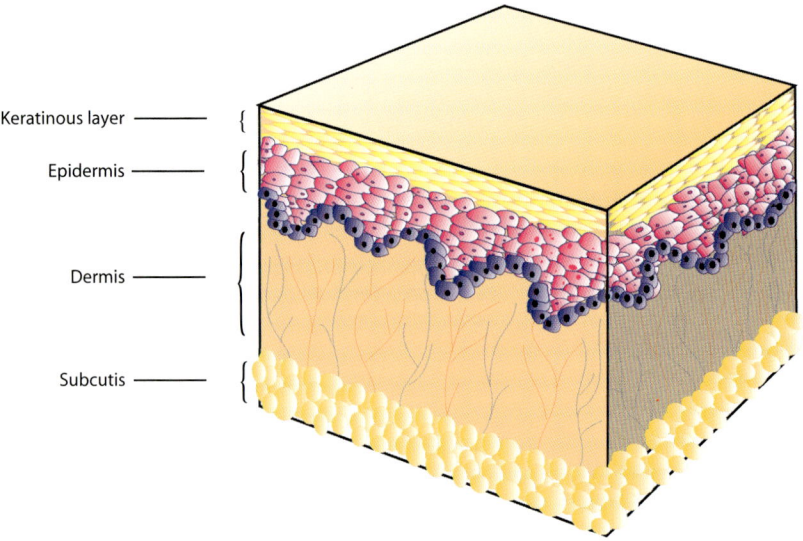

Diagram of the structure of the skin.

Epidermis

Most of the skin tumors to be described in this chapter arise from the epidermis, that is, the outer layer of the skin. The main types of cells in the epidermis are the **keratinocytes** (**squamous cells**), which may be the origin of a tumor. In addition, there are other cells in the epidermis, for example **melanocytes**. These latter cells produce the pigment melanin (you will recall that melanin is the major determinant of skin color). Melanocytes can be the source of various growths as well.

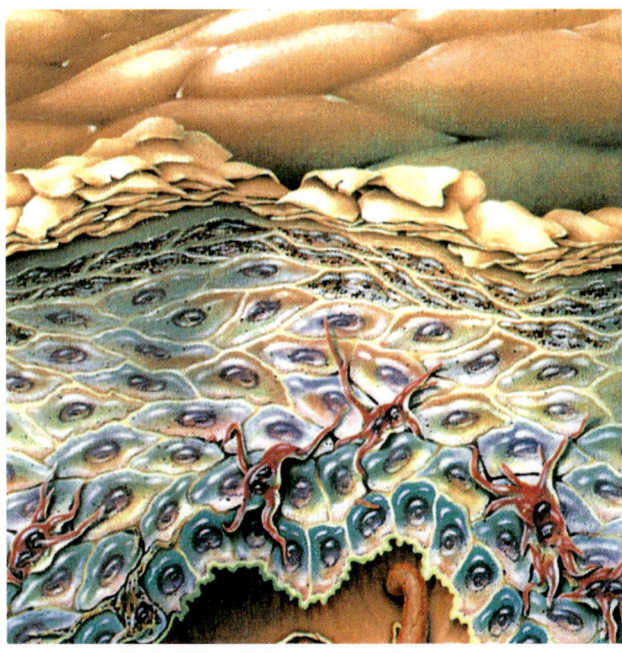

Melanocytes (red) in the basal layer of the epidermis.

Dermis

The dermis contains:

- sebaceous glands,
- sweat glands,
- nerve cells,
- blood vessels,
- muscle cells, and
- other types of cells and tissues.

Any of these elements may be the source of a skin tumor. Such tumors may be benign or malignant. In addition, metastases from primary malignant tumors in other parts of the body may get to the skin. For example, a malignant tumor of the lung or the breast may seed metastases that will get to the skin and present as lumps in the skin.

SKIN TUMORS THAT ORIGINATE IN THE KERATINOCYTES

Tumors that originate in the keratinocytes are:

- solar keratosis (a precancerous lesion),
- squamous cell carcinomas, and
- basal cell carcinomas.

Note: Both basal cell carcinomas and squamous cell carcinomas are defined as "cancerous" growths. The term **carcinoma** covers a wide range of malignant tumors of various types.

Solar Keratosis

In general, the term **keratosis** means a thickening of the keratinous layer of the skin. This thickening is seen in various inflammatory processes that occur in the skin, and can also be a cancerous or precancerous condition, as in solar keratosis. These lesions usually occur in fair-skinned people older than 40 years. They appear in areas exposed to the sun—the face and the backs of the hands. They are slightly raised, dry, rough, reddish-pink lesions with a slightly scaly surface. These lesions originate from the keratinocytes in the epidermis. Keratinocytes are also called **squamous cells**.

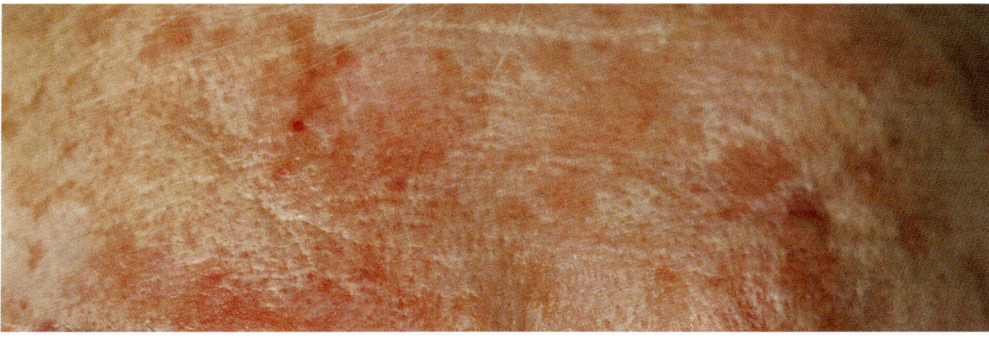

Solar keratoses on sun-damaged skin.

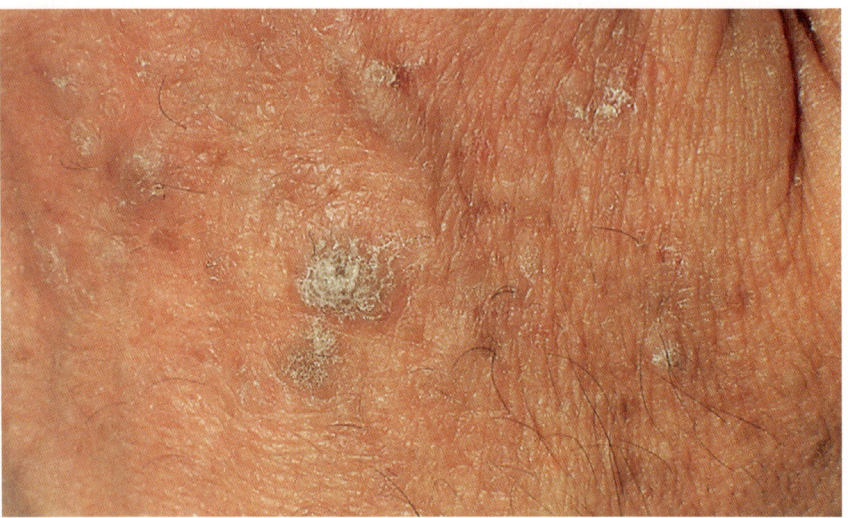

Several small keratoses on the back of the hand of an elderly man.

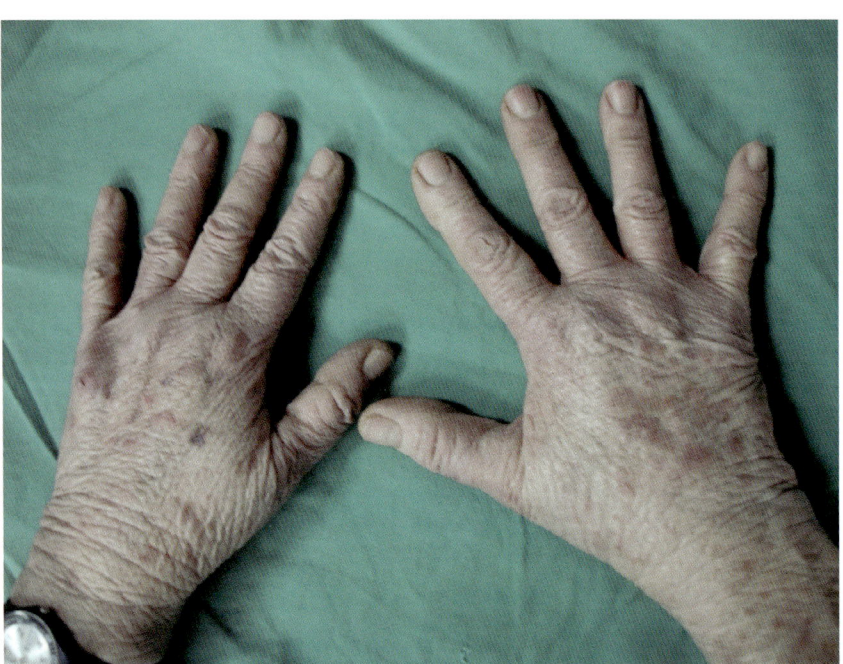

Solar keratoses on the backs of the hands of an elderly woman.

A solar keratosis is a **precancerous lesion,** that is to say, it is still not considered malignant. Having said that, if the lesion extends beyond the epidermis and reaches the dermis (see the next illustration), it becomes a **squamous cell carcinoma** and is then defined as a cancerous skin lesion. The likelihood of such transformation to occur is very low. Nevertheless, it may happen, and this justifies appropriate treatment of a solar keratoses.

SKIN TUMORS

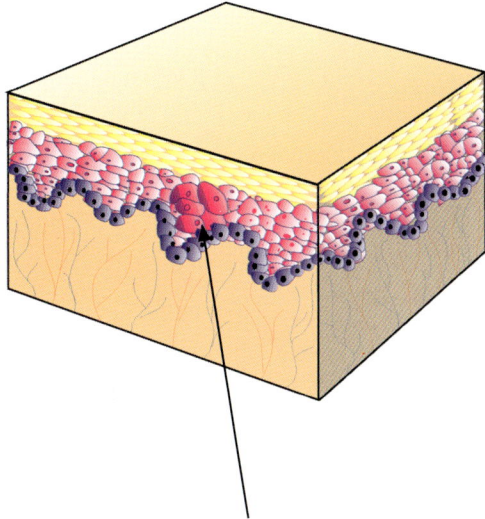

Development of solar keratoses from epidermal keratinocytes.

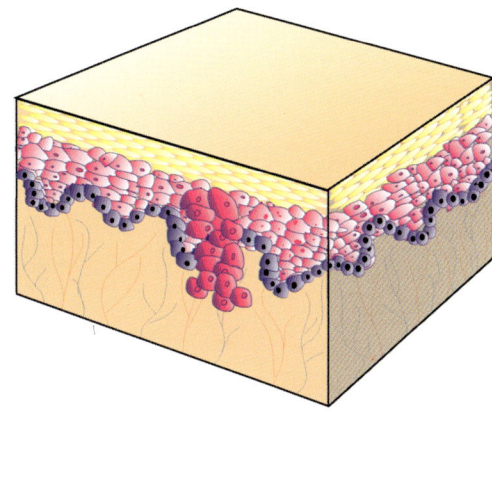

Some cells of the solar keratosis have broken through into the dermis. The lesion is now considered a **squamous cell carcinoma**.

Treatment of Solar Keratosis
Although the likelihood of a solar keratosis turning into a cancer is statistically extremely low, the lesion must be treated by a physician. The treatment is based on destroying the lesion—there is usually no need to excise it surgically. There are a number of methods available to the doctor. The most widely used are as follows:

- freezing the lesion with liquid nitrogen, which destroys the cells of the lesion,
- treatment with a preparation for local use, called 5-FU (5-fluorouracil), which is available as a cream and solution, and specifically targets the abnormal cells and destroys them,
- applying a topical medication called Imiqimod.

Note: Sometimes the lesion cannot be exactly identified, and the doctor may not be fully convinced that it is indeed a solar keratosis. If there is any doubt, and the lesion may be some other skin tumor, it should be excised in its entirety and examined under a microscope.

Squamous Cell Carcinoma

As in solar keratosis, squamous cell carcinoma arises from keratinocytes (squamous cells) in the epidermis except that, in this case, the tumor does not remain confined to the epidermis, but spreads into the dermis (as shown in the previous illustration). Sometimes the tumor spreads even further, into deeper tissues, and may even seed metastases to internal body organs.

Squamous cell carcinoma may appear on normal-looking skin, or it may arise from solar keratoses.

This tumor usually appears in later life. In most cases, it arises in areas of skin exposed to the sun, but it can appear in areas that are not normally exposed. Indeed, squamous cell carcinoma can arise inside the mouth.

The tumor usually looks like a "sore" on the skin; in other words, in the area of the tumor the normal skin is absent, exposing the underlying tissues to varying degrees. Since the tumor tissue has destroyed the normal protective skin layers, the area of the tumor may become infected with bacteria and a purulent (pus) discharge may appear. The characteristic feature that helps to distinguish this tumor from an innocent sore is the time factor. Any

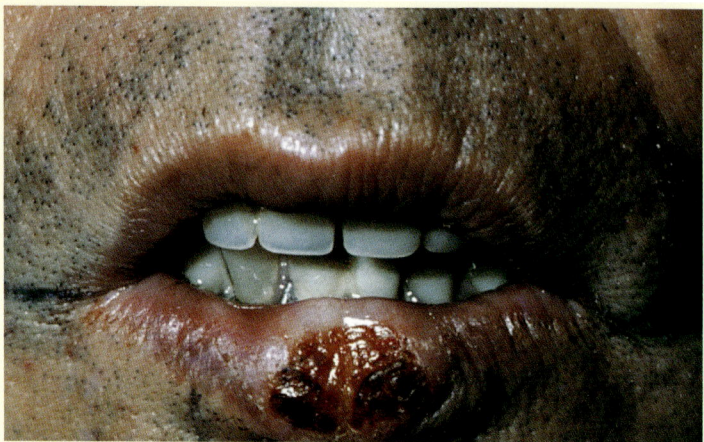

Squamous cell carcinoma of the lower lip—this is a very common site for squamous cell carcinoma to appear.

sore that does not heal within a reasonable time—a few weeks—requires urgent referral to a dermatologist.

This tumor can also appear as a lump above the skin level, commonly slightly damaged on its surface. Other forms of squamous cell carcinoma may occur as well.

Basal Cell Carcinoma

In basal cell carcinoma, the renegade cells that have multiplied and produced a tumor originate from the keratinocytes in the basal layer of the epidermis.

Basal cell carcinoma is a common skin tumor. As with solar keratosis and squamous cell carcinoma, the direct cause of this tumor is prolonged, cumulative exposure to the sun. The lesions usually appear in people of light complexion, older than 40 years, and in areas exposed to the sun, including the nose, ears, bald areas of the scalp, neck, upper chest, and back. Basal cell carcinoma has a low degree of malignancy. It is rare for a basal cell carcinoma to seed metastases. Although it grows slowly, it may cause marked destruction of the surrounding tissues. After a long time, the tumor may penetrate the soft tissues under the skin and may even penetrate underlying bones. Hence, if a basal cell carcinoma is not treated early and completely excised, it will continue to grow and treatment will involve the removal of a much larger area of skin.

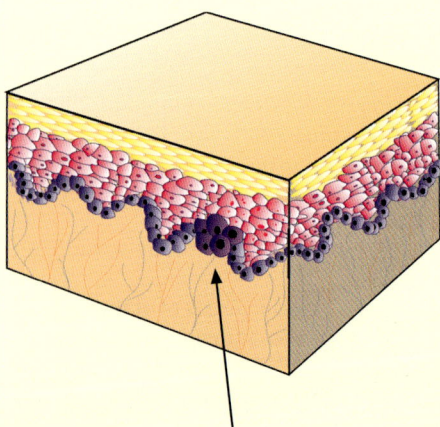

The basal layer of the epidermis, where basal cell carcinoma starts to develop.

A basal cell carcinoma is most commonly manifested as follows: a small, shiny swelling appears in an area exposed to the sun. The lesion slowly grows larger. Usually, there are tiny blood vessels visible over its surface. A typical lesion usually develops elevated margins, whose color is commonly referred to in medical texts as "pearly." Later, the tumor tissue destroys the normal skin tissues in the area, and a sore appears in the center.

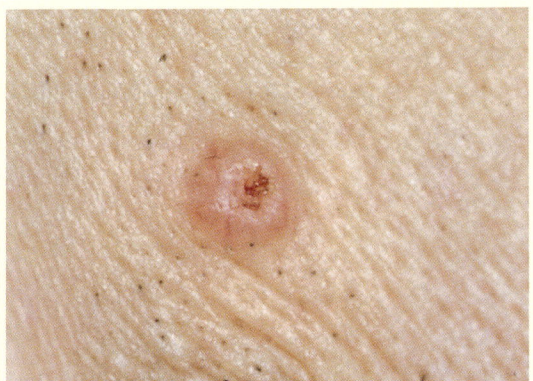

Basal cell carcinoma—the "pearly" margins surround a typical sore.

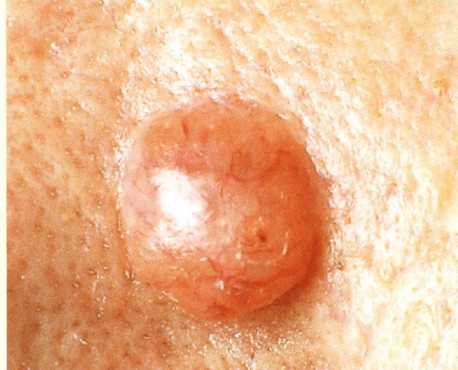

Basal cell carcinoma; blood vessels are seen over its surface.

Although the above is the commonest presentation of basal cell carcinoma, other forms may occur.

Note: Whenever a skin "injury" or sore does not heal for a relatively long time (several weeks), the possibility of basal cell carcinoma or squamous cell carcinoma should be considered, and the client should be referred to a physician as soon as possible.

TUMORS THAT ORIGINATE IN THE MELANOCYTES

Tumors that originate in the melanocytes (the cells that produce melanin) include:

- melanocytic nevi (commonly known as moles or beauty spots), and
- malignant melanoma.

A nevus is a common benign skin lesion. As long as the nevus remains "normal," there is no medical problem (this will be discussed in more detail later). On the other hand, a melanoma is an aggressive malignant tumor. If not identified and treated early, melanoma tends to metastasize throughout the body, and it is considered a highly dangerous and potentially disastrous lesion. In recent years, the incidence of malignant melanoma has been increasing.

Note: Skin tumors originating from melanocytes are usually dark in color—brown, bluish, or black. However, a few cases are not pigmented. On the other hand, tumors arising from keratinocytes are usually light-colored and rarely dark.

There are other skin lesions derived from melanocytes: solar lentigines ("sun spots") and freckles (detailed in chapter 20 on bleaching).

Melanocytic Nevus (Mole)

This lesion originates from the melanocyte, the cell that produces the pigment melanin in the epidermis.

In this case, the growth and proliferation of the melanocytes is **controlled**. The lesion is benign—scientifically, a mole is by definition a benign tumor. Because it is such a common lesion, the connotations of the term "tumor" do not really apply to a mole.

In general, moles develop gradually, usually within the first 20 years of life; only 3% to 4% of newborn infants have moles. The number of moles gradually increases until about the age of 25 so that most people have some moles somewhere on their skin.

There are several different types of moles. They may be raised or flat, and their color may vary from light brown to dark brown. If a lesion is indeed benign, it is expected to have a regular, clearly defined edge and uniform color over its entire surface. It is important to be sure that a lesion is, in fact, a benign mole, and one must distinguish an innocent, normal mole from one where atypical changes are taking place or one that shows unusual features. Changes in the appearance of a mole could suggest the diagnosis of malignant melanoma, which necessitates the removal of the mole so that it can be examined under the microscope.

There are certain signs or changes in a mole that are suggestive of malignancy, and should turn on a warning light. These include:

- irregular, poorly defined edges,
- nonuniform coloration,
- asymmetry,
- rapid growth,
- bleeding or discharge from a mole, and
- the appearance of a "sore" within a mole.

These changes do not necessarily mean that the mole (nevus) is malignant. There are perfectly innocent moles whose coloration is not uniform, and similarly a lesion may bleed for any one of a number of simple, banal reasons. Nevertheless, if there is any doubt, the patient must be referred urgently to an experienced physician.

The above changes are detailed below.

Malignant Melanoma

This is the most aggressive skin cancer, with the highest mortality rate. There has been a gradual increase in its incidence worldwide. The likelihood of a light-skinned person developing malignant melanoma in his/her lifetime is estimated today at almost 1%. There is substantial evidence that someone who was exposed intensively to sunlight in the past, such as to have caused sunburn, is at much higher risk of developing melanoma. We are not only referring to prolonged, cumulative exposure. A severe case of sunburn in childhood or adolescence significantly increases one's risk of developing melanoma later in life.

The source of melanoma is the cell that produces melanin in the epidermis—the **melanocyte**. Hence, a melanoma can be (but not necessarily) brown, or black, or blue in color, or a mixture of all.

If the tumor is diagnosed at an early stage and is completely removed, with an adequate safety margin of surrounding healthy skin, complete recovery can be expected. On the other hand, if the tumor is not diagnosed in time, and has penetrated deeper into the skin, it has higher likelihood to metastasize to other areas of the patient's body, and the outcome will be fatal.

Medicine has yet to find a cure for melanoma with malignant metastases. In such cases, melanoma cells seed to distant tissues of the body, which will eventually result in death.

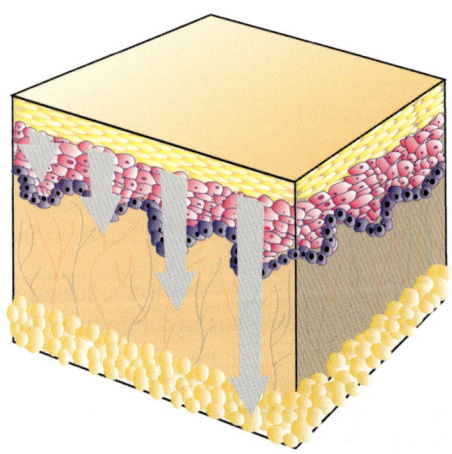

The deeper the melanoma penetrates into the dermis, the worse the outcome.

SKIN TUMORS

A malignant melanoma can develop from a melanocytic nevus ("mole") or from skin that has been damaged by cumulative exposure to the sun, or it may appear "de novo," from healthy skin.

What Characterizes a Potential Melanoma?
There are certain things that characterize a potential melanoma such as irregular, poorly defined edges; nonuniform coloration; asymmetry; unusually rapid growth; and bleeding or discharge.

Irregular, Poorly Defined Edges
When the edges of the lesion partly blend into the surrounding skin, and you cannot see a definite border between the mole and the healthy skin, as well as any change in the appearance of the border, such as from a round border to a jagged one, should arouse suspicion.

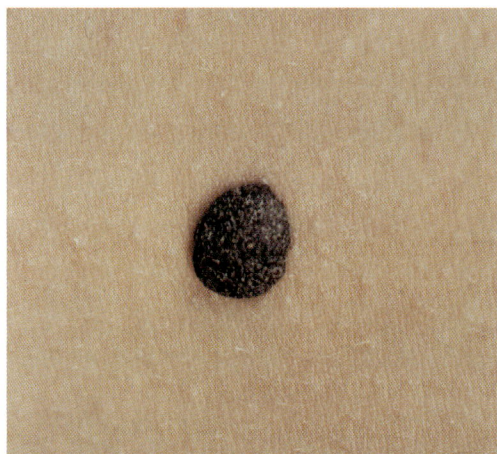 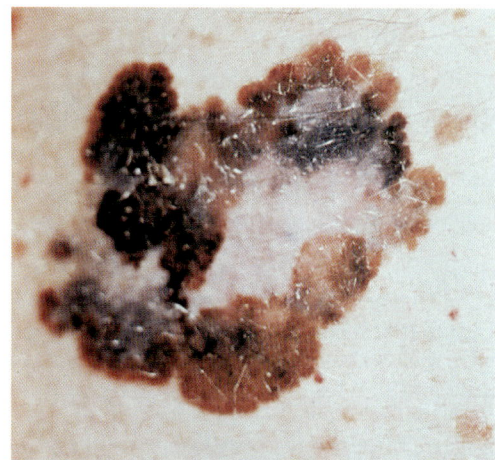

Note the poorly defined border of the lesion shown on the right, which was diagnosed as melanoma. Compare that with the clearly seen sharp border between the skin and the lesion shown on the left, which is of a benign mole.

Nonuniform Coloration
A nonuniform color of the lesion, or the development of other colors within the lesion—blue, gray, red or, in particular, a deep, black hue—indicates that it is developing abnormally. Also, the appearance of islands of normal looking skin within a dark lesion should arouse suspicion.

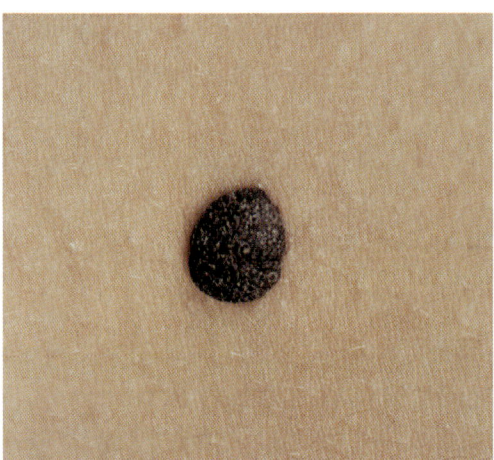 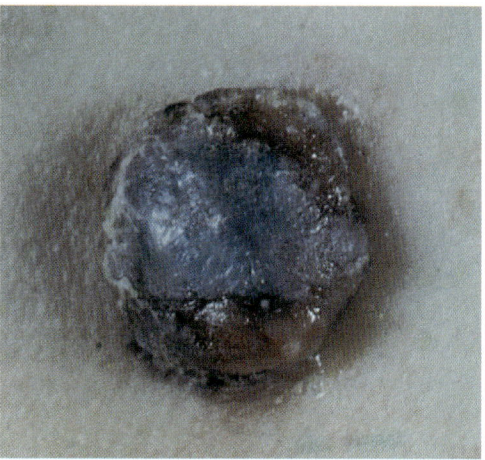

Note the nonuniform color of the lesion shown on the right, which was diagnosed as melanoma. Compare that with the uniform coloration of the lesion shown on the left, which is a benign mole.

Asymmetry of the Lesion
Asymmetry is a suspicious sign; in contrast to the symmetric, regular shapes of benign moles.

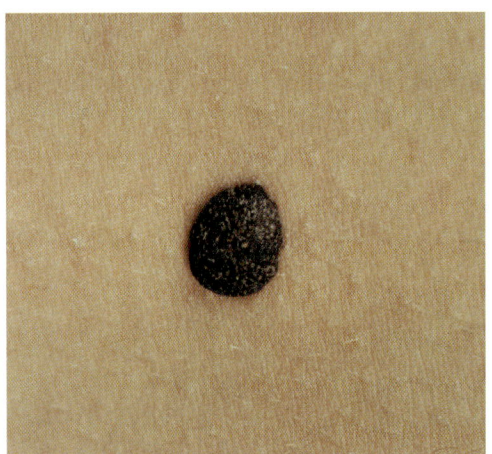 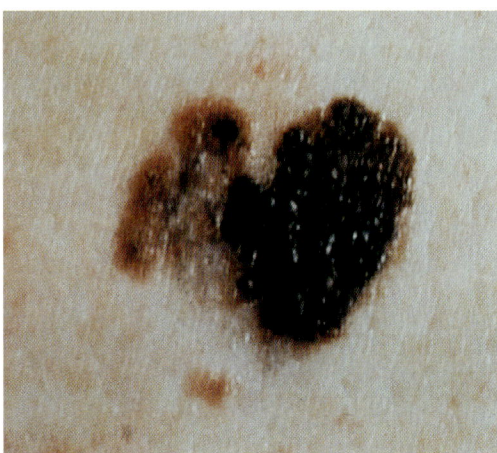

Note the asymmetric shape of the melanoma shown on the right, in contrast to the symmetric shape of the benign mole shown on the left.

Unusually Rapid Growth
In children and adolescents, moles generally grow in parallel to the overall growth of the child. A lesion that seems to be growing out of proportion to the child's general growth should arouse suspicion. Therefore, a sudden acceleration in the growth rate of a lesion is worrisome. In an adult, any skin lesion that seems to be growing should be seen by a doctor.

Bleeding or Discharge from a Mole or the Appearance of a Sore Within It
Any abnormal, uncharacteristic course of a nevus (including the onset of itching or pain) should arouse suspicion, and the patient should be examined by a physician.

Note: The appearance of a relatively large lesion (above 6 mm diameter) is also considered to be a suspicious sign. However, that does not mean that "small" lesions may be ignored. There have been melanomas as small as 2 or 3 mm. **In any case of a suspicious lesion, refer the client urgently to an experienced physician!**

PREVENTION

Early detection is of paramount importance. The simplest way to diagnose a malignant lesion early is by self-examination.

SELF-EXAMINATION

Self-examination is performed in front of a mirror. It must include all areas of the body, including "hidden" areas that one tends to overlook, such as the buttocks, soles of the feet, and the genital region.

Self-Examination
There are various ways to best carry out self-examination. With the help of mirrors, or a second person, one can usually cover hard-to-see areas.

In Front of a Mirror
This part of the examination covers the face (including inside the mouth), the neck, and the chest; women should examine the skin underneath the breasts. The armpits should also be examined. The mirror is used to examine all the areas of the upper arms, forearms, thighs, and lower legs.

SKIN TUMORS

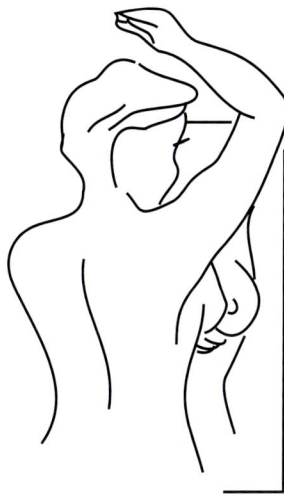
Self-examination in front of a mirror.

Using a Second Mirror
The ears, behind the ears, the back of the neck, shoulders, and upper back should be examined. The second mirror should also be used to examine the lower back, the buttocks, and the back of the legs.

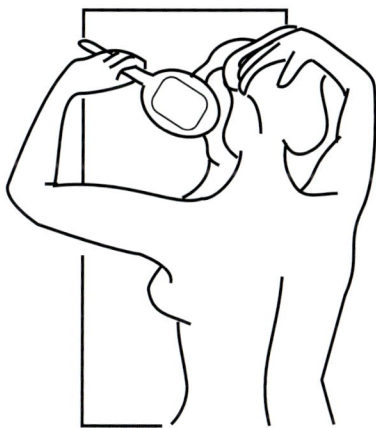
Using a second mirror.

The Scalp
The scalp can be examined with the assistance of a second person—a friend or member of the family. A hairdryer is useful to spread the hair out and expose all areas of the scalp.

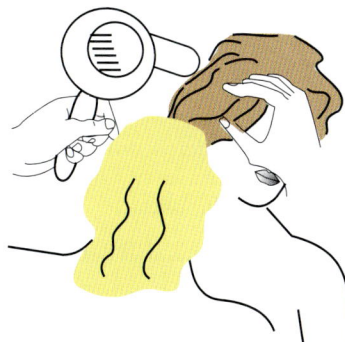
Examining the scalp by using a hairdryer.

The following areas should be carefully examined:

- hands—palms and backs of the hands, between the fingers, and under the fingernails,
- genitalia, and
- the legs and soles (it is easiest to do this while sitting, using a stool).

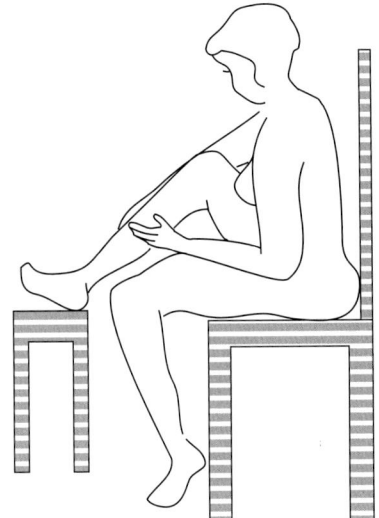

Examining the soles.

REGULAR MEDICAL EXAMINATIONS

A regular checkup by a doctor should be scheduled every few months. The more risk factors a person has for skin malignancies, the more frequent these examinations should be. The major risk factors requiring more frequent checkups are

- fair complexion,
- a past history of a melanoma or skin cancer, and
- a family history of melanoma or skin cancer.

MANAGEMENT OF POSSIBLY CANCEROUS LESIONS

If any of the lesions described above—squamous cell carcinoma, basal cell carcinoma, a suspicious mole or malignant melanoma—are found, the physician must remove it in its entirety, with a safety margin of surrounding normal-looking skin.

Note: A lesion suspected of being cancerous should not be treated by methods that will destroy it and not enable it to be examined under the microscope, such as "freezing" the lesion with liquid nitrogen, burning it off (cauterization) with an electric needle, or destroying it by using local chemical preparations. A skin lesion may only be treated with one of those techniques if an experienced doctor has diagnosed it and determined that cauterization is the appropriate treatment (for example, solar keratoses may be treated by liquid nitrogen).

Every lesion that is suspected of being cancerous must be examined microscopically. The removal of any piece of tissue from the body, including skin, for the purpose of laboratory examination is called a **biopsy**. There are several reasons for performing a biopsy:

1. to make a definitive diagnosis regarding the type of tumor (as this diagnosis will determine the proper treatment),
2. to confirm that the tumor has been completely removed, and that no tumor tissue (or malignant cells) remains in, or under, the patient's skin,

3. to determine the depth to which the tumor has reached: in many cases, the depth of the tumor has prognostic implications, that is, it allows prediction of the probable future course of the illness; the depth is also a factor that determines the proper treatment.

Note: The pharmaceutical industry produces chemical substances that cause localized destruction of skin tissue. These substances can only be purchased with a prescription, and only a physician may use them. If a tumor has been cauterized (burnt off) or treated by local application of a chemical substance, or not removed in its entirety, the area of the lesion may heal, and may be covered by scar tissue—**but underneath the scar there will still be tumor cells**. These residual tumor cells may proliferate and give rise later to a cancerous state, with severe consequences for the patient. Therefore, **only an experienced physician can determine the type of treatment that is appropriate for skin lesions**. In any case, "amateur" treatment of skin lesions with chemicals should be avoided. Such treatment may only be carried out by an experienced physician.

How Does a Surgeon Remove a Suspected Cancerous Lesion from the Skin?

In the case of a skin lesion that is suspected of being malignant (such as a basal cell carcinoma, squamous cell carcinoma, or malignant melanoma), an **excisional biopsy** is performed—that is, the surgeon biopsies the lesion after removing it in its entirety. Steps in the procedure are as follows:

1. **Anesthesia**: Local anesthetic is injected into the area of the lesion.

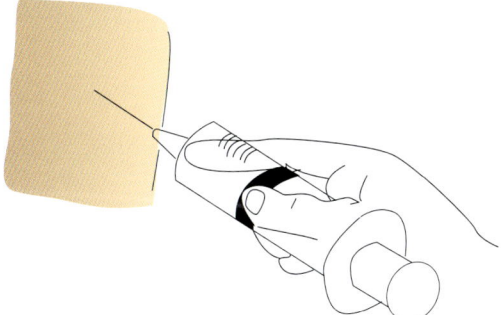

Anesthetizing the area of the lesion.

2. **Excising the lesion**: The physician uses a **scalpel**—a surgical knife. The commonly used incision is lens-shaped, which is usually the most effective and easiest shape for total removal of a lesion. The incision should include a rim of healthy tissue around the lesion, so as to ensure total removal of all the cells of the lesion. Sometimes, because of the shape or location of the lesion, a lens-shaped incision cannot be used, and some other shape of incision is required.

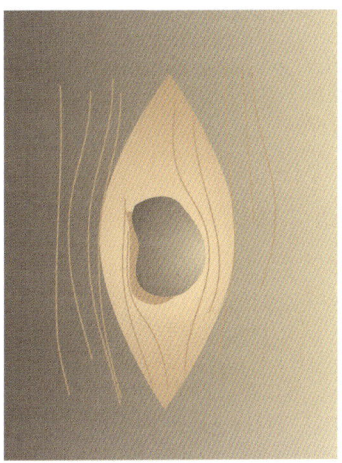

"Lens-shaped" incision around a lesion.

3. **Suturing the surgical wound**: Sutures are used for sewing up the incision. The stitches are removed some days later, the exact time depending mainly on the size and location of the incision. In places where the skin is delicate and cannot be put under tension, such as the skin of the face, the stitches are removed after five to seven days. In places where the skin is thick (areas where the skin is normally subjected to various forces in the course of normal activities), such as the back or the limbs, the stitches are removed after 10 to 14 days.

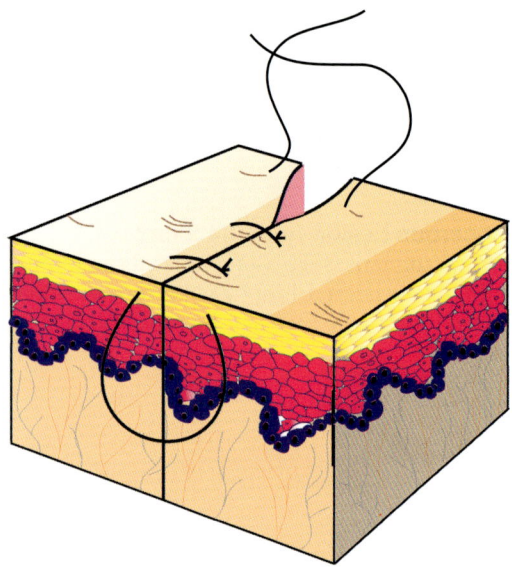

Suturing the surgical incision.

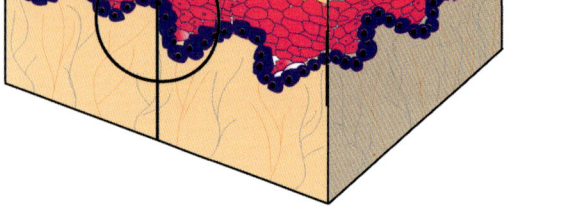

After suturing the surgical incision.

4. **The excised skin is sent for microscopic diagnosis of the lesion**: Once the type of lesion and its depth have been determined, it is possible to determine if the excisional biopsy that was carried out will suffice, or whether further treatment may be necessary.

In the case of a malignant melanoma, further excision of the skin surrounding the excised lesion creating wider "safety" margins may be performed. Removal of adjacent lymph nodes may be considered and, in severe cases, chemotherapy, that is, anticancer drugs may be given in an attempt to destroy tumor cells in distant areas.

SUMMARY

The treatment of skin lesions suspected of being cancerous is based on total removal of the lesion, with safety margins of normal skin surrounding the lesion. Such lesions must never be burnt off with an electric cautery needle, or destroyed by the application of chemical substances. Every case of a suspected cancerous skin lesion must be referred to an experienced physician.

16 | Active Ingredients in Cosmetic Preparations
Gil Yosipovitch

Contents Overview • Naturally occurring substances extracted from animal tissues • Plant extracts • Aromatic oils • Vitamins • Common foodstuffs • Some additional comments

OVERVIEW

During the last decade, there have been significant developments in the cosmetics industry. The trend today is toward improving the health of the skin generally, and not merely improving its appearance temporarily. Many preparations for skin care lie in the gray area between what are considered to be cosmetics and what are considered to be drugs. This chapter examines the various active ingredients in cosmetic preparations, and what we know regarding their actions and effects, based on the accredited scientific research and what has been published in the scientific and medical literature. Research is also performed by leading cosmetics companies; however, the results are rarely published and the information is not readily accessible—neither to the scientific community nor to the general public.

As long as there has been no reliable, reproducible (meaning that if the experiment is repeated by other researchers, similar results are obtained) scientific research performed on the product, its efficacy cannot be established. Nevertheless, it is likely that there are many substances whose potential has not yet been identified, and about which no studies have been published in the accredited medical literature as yet. These substances may eventually find their way into the cosmetics industry.

The active ingredients of cosmetic preparations can be classified into animal-derived substances, plant extracts, vitamins, and foodstuffs.

Animal-Derived Substances
This group includes proteins such as collagen and elastin, amino acids, nucleic acids, hyaluronic acid, placental extract, amniotic fluid, and ceramides.

Plant Extracts
This group includes substances obtained from a wide range of plants, such as aloe vera, lavender, chamomile, calendula, echinacea, jojoba oil, and tea-tree oil. The **aromatic oils** also belong to this group. They are derived from eucalyptus, camphor, mint, jasmine, chamomile, and lavender plants. The **phytosterols** include extracts from cocoa butter, coconut, olives, avocado, sesame, sunflower seeds, and soya oil. γ-**Linoleic acid** is derived from the oils of the evening primrose and foxtail plants. α-**Hydroxy acids** are derived originally from fruits and vegetables, so they can also be included in this category. These are discussed in detail in chapter 18. **Allantoin** is included here because in the past it was extracted from plants, although it is now produced synthetically from uric acid.

Vitamins
These include vitamins C and E, β-carotene, and provitamin B (pantothenic acid).

Foodstuffs
Many cosmetics in use for centuries in various cultures are based on foodstuffs, such as milk, eggs, honey, and propolis.

NATURALLY OCCURRING SUBSTANCES EXTRACTED FROM ANIMAL TISSUES

Collagen

This protein is a major component of the skin. Many consumers mistakenly believe that the collagen in cosmetic preparations can penetrate the skin and replace the "old" collagen. This, of course, is incorrect. Because of its high molecular weight, collagen cannot penetrate the keratinous layer of the skin and enter into the "living" skin layers.

The only way in which collagen can effectively penetrate the skin is by injection into the deep layers of the skin, in order to treat depressed scars or wrinkles. In this case, collagen provides no benefit other than to "raise" the wrinkles or depressed scars, and even then its effect is only temporary because the injected collagen is absorbed within months.

Collagen, as it absorbs water effectively, serves to increase the moisture content of the skin. The feeling of improvement in the skin's appearance after applying cosmetic products containing collagen is probably due to this increased moisture in the skin. In addition, collagen may be used in hair-care products, especially those intended for hair that has been damaged by incorrect treatment (see the section on protein conditioners in chapter 32).

Amino Acids, Elastin, and Other Proteins

Like collagen, these substances cannot penetrate the keratinous layer of the skin and do not reach the epidermis. Some of them absorb water, so they increase the moisture level of the skin. There is no scientific evidence that these substances can delay skin aging or the appearance of wrinkles.

Nucleic Acids

Various combinations of nucleic acids form DNA—the genetic material in all living cells that contains the genetic code. There is no proof that nucleic acids or DNA have any effect on preventing skin aging. However, these substances do absorb water, and can increase the moisture content of the skin to a certain extent.

Hyaluronic Acid

The dermis is largely made up of an amorphous intercellular substance (i.e., a substance that has no defined shape or structure), which serves as "cement" for all the components of the dermis. One of the substances making up the intercellular material in the dermis is hyaluronic acid, which is an efficient water-absorbing substance. Hyaluronic acid is widely used in moisturizing compounds.

Amniotic Fluid

The concept of using amniotic fluid, which surrounds the developing fetus in the womb, has connotations of "rejuvenation" and prevention of skin aging. Amniotic fluid used in the cosmetics industry comes from pregnant cows and is obtained by puncturing the amniotic sac with a needle inserted through the cow's uterus. The beneficial effect of these products has not been proven.

Placental Extracts

As with amniotic fluid, the fact that the placenta (the afterbirth) is intimately bound up with fetal development leads some consumers to feel that it influences rejuvenation and prevents aging of the skin. This has not been proven.

There are cosmetic products containing complex mixtures of various placentally derived enzymes and other proteins, which differ according to the industrial processing of the extracts from animal and human placentas (note that in most countries the use of human tissue for cosmetics is forbidden). This processing involves rinsing the tissues (to remove blood), and then extracting the clean placental tissue.

It appears, however, that this process is now being used less and less. One possible reason is that placental tissue is particularly well supplied with blood vessels. In recent years the use of any product related to blood has become anathema to consumers because of possible contamination by viral or bacterial diseases. Although the transmission of infectious diseases by placental extracts has never been documented, the market for these products is on the decline.

Ceramides

Ceramides are lipid compounds found in high concentrations in the membranes of cells of human body and are a significant component of the keratin layer. They are important in protecting its integrity. Applying products containing ceramides to the skin of animals creates an impermeable, insulating layer. Ceramides are not only structural components of cell membranes, but also actively participate in a wide range of cellular functions and processes. Hence, some researchers assume that preparations containing ceramides may not only serve as a coating on the skin's surface, as in many other oily moisturizers, but also assist in replenishing interstitial lipids within the skin. However, there is currently no concrete evidence to support this claim. Cosmetics companies have developed ointments containing ceramides in various concentrations—both as moisturizing preparations and as protective substances to prevent and repair skin damage resulting from exposure to various chemicals (including soaps that damage the keratin layer of the skin).

PLANT EXTRACTS

Plant extracts have a wide range of effects. Some provide a pleasant scent or attractive color to cosmetic preparations; some provide moisture to the skin and act as "skin softeners" (usually the fattier extracts). Certain extracts are known for their soothing properties (such as chamomile or aloe vera extracts), and others, such as witch hazel extract, as astringents (astringents are discussed in detail in chapter 21).

In general medicine, drugs of immense value have been produced from plants. Digoxin or quinidine serve as good examples of such medications. Many studies have been conducted to assess the efficacy of plant extracts for medical purposes. Some of these studies have been performed under high standards of scientific accuracy. From time to time, however, articles are published indicating that some herbal extract may have beneficial effects on the skin. In most cases, these reports require further verification. In the field of cosmetics, on the other hand, many studies lack sufficient scientific quality and are of little use for assessing the possible benefits of the examined herbal extract.

Not all the extracts derived from a given plant are uniform or identical. There may be subtypes or different varieties of a plant, whose extracts may have quite different pharmacological properties from one another. Sometimes the extracts vary depending on the season of the year during which the plant was picked, and sometimes their pharmacological properties depend on the method of extraction used. In certain cases, the main effect of the final product actually depends on other substances present in the product containing the plant extract.

Some plants have antibacterial or antifungal properties. When dealing with skin that is infected or irritated, it is preferable to use accepted medical preparations (after consulting a physician) rather than plant extracts: conventional medicine has a wide range of dermatological medications that have been proven to be effective against bacteria and fungi and are known to be safe.

The following pages give details of plant extracts in common use in the cosmetics industry. The discussion here is largely based on accepted, widely known information; but most of the available information is not definite, and further scientific research is needed to verify it.

Aloe Vera

Aloe vera is widely used both as a cosmetic and as a home remedy for simple cuts and burns and for skin irritation. In cosmetics, it is present in every conceivable product: creams, ointments, soaps, shampoos, tanning lotions, cleansing lotions, and others.

The soothing effect of aloe vera has been known for many years. The aloe vera plant was already known for its medicinal properties in antiquity in Mesopotamia and Egypt. The ancient Chinese used it for the relief of abdominal pain (it has a cathartic effect when taken by mouth); the Indians used it for treating urinary problems. Throughout the whole of history, extracts of this plant have been used for skin treatment. The aloe vera plant has yellow flowers, with fleshy leaves arranged in a rosette pattern. The leaves of the aloe vera contain two main pharmacological extracts: (*i*) a yellow fluid, which is extracted from certain areas in the inner leaf, has a bitter taste, and some laxative effect; and (*ii*) a gel produced from the inner parts of the leaves. This gel is the substance intended for cosmetic and dermatological applications. There are specific subtypes of the plant in which the composition of the substance may vary chemically and pharmacologically.

Some compounds contained in the aloe vera plant such as carboxypeptidase, magnesium lactate, and lectin-like substances, are considered to have anti-inflammatory effects. The plant also has an antibacterial effect, perhaps because of a component known as saponin. Aloe vera is well known, however, for its apparent ability to accelerate wound healing. This may be attributed to its antibacterial properties, or perhaps to the increase in blood flow to the area following application, or both.

The results of experiments examining the use of aloe vera compared with conventional treatment for skin infections and burns have been inconclusive, and at times contradictory. However, the general impression is that aloe vera extract indeed has a soothing effect on the skin. One may consider its use in certain mild cases of skin inflammation, wounds, and superficial burns. In a few research studies, aloe vera extracts have been shown to have some beneficial effect in the treatment of radiation burns.

Oral ingestion of aloe vera is not recommended. Systemic use in pregnancy has been associated with premature delivery.

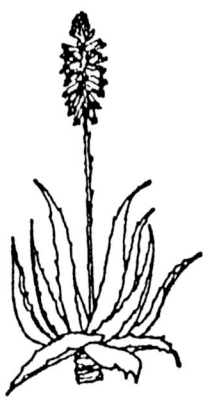
Aloe vera.

There are many different subtypes of aloe vera, each with its own pharmacological effect. The nature and composition of the extracts also vary, depending on the season in which the leaves are picked. Sometimes the other components in the preparation in which the substance is found can change and neutralize the effect of the active ingredient. Different methods of extraction can produce differences in the composition and effects of the extracts. Hence, one product containing aloe vera may have a beneficial effect on the skin, while another product may be useless. The major ingredient responsible for the various effects (anti-inflammatory, antibacterial) has not been definitively identified, so further research is needed to determine the efficacy of the substance and the purposes for which it is best suited.

Lavender

Lavender is extracted from the flowers of *Lavendula officinalis*; the oil derived from it has a pleasant scent. Some claim that the substances extracted from lavender for use on the skin have antioxidant properties. Other lavender extracts are used for soothing skin irritation and inflammation. The lavender flower is used mainly for producing various fragrances.

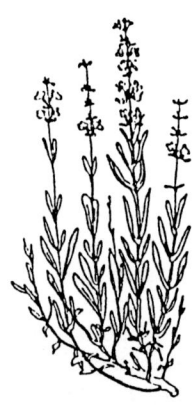
Lavender.

Chamomile

Chamomile is derived from the flowers of two plants: *Anthemis nobilis*, known as Roman chamomile, and *Matricaria chamomilla*, known as German chamomile. The extracts from both of these plants have a pleasant fragrance. Drinking chamomile extract is said to have soothing effects on the digestive system. Those products derived from the chamomile plant for use on the skin are claimed to possess anti-inflammatory effects and are able to constrict blood vessels—properties that help to soothe skin irritations. Tea made from chamomile (after it has cooled down) is used widely in dermatological practice as a mouthwash in cases of painful mouth sores. In addition, a recommended treatment for swelling around the eyes is to place cotton compresses soaked in chamomile extract (or cooled chamomile tea) on the swollen area for a few minutes several times a day. In a few isolated cases, chamomile extract has been found to have a certain effect on the healing of wounds—but this has never been confirmed scientifically.

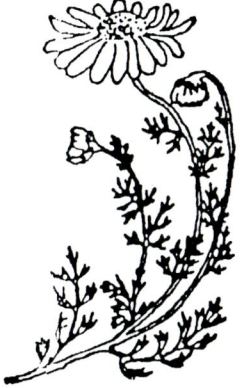
Anthemis nobilis (Roman chamomile).

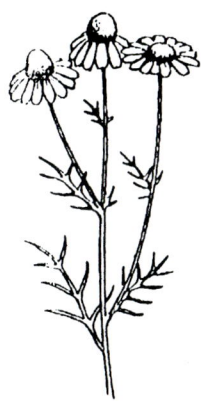
Matricaria chamomilla (German chamomile).

Calendula (Marigold)

The extract derived from the petals of *Calendula officinalis* is said to have anti-inflammatory properties, and is used for the treatment of mild skin irritation. The extract also is said to be a mild astringent. Some have suggested that it also has antibacterial and antifungal properties.

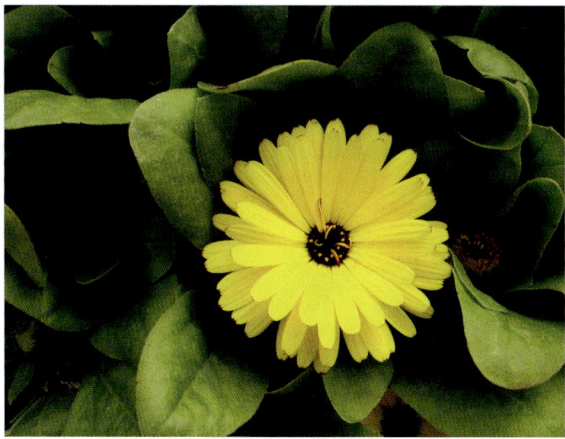
Calendula.

Although the value of calendula extracts has not been supported by high-quality research studies, it seems to possess an anti-inflammatory effect, to a certain degree. Hence, it is commonly marketed in nappy creams and ointments. In addition, some researchers have suggested that calendula extracts may have some beneficial effect in patients undergoing radiation therapy.

Echinacea

Echinacea, a medicinal herb grown in North and South America, has been used for centuries. The extract is usually obtained from the root of the plant. Yet, there are different species of echinacea, and the source of extracting depends on the specific species.

In general medicine, echinacea extracts are said to enhance the activity of the immune system, thereby helping to prevent and heal upper respiratory infections such as the common cold.

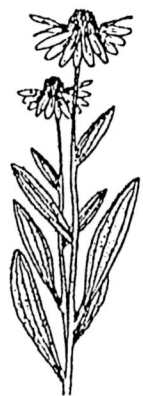

Echinacea.

Results of most experiments examining the use of echinacea compared with conventional treatment for upper respiratory infections have been inconclusive or contradictory. In 2005, a large-scale, controlled study published in the *New England Journal of Medicine* showed that echinacea is not effective in preventing the common cold, nor has any influence on the severity and/or duration of the infection.

As to the effect of echinacea on the skin: the extract is said to be effective mainly against infections—bacteria, fungi, and viruses. This effect may be related to the ability of the extract to neutralize a substance called **hyaluronidase**, which is secreted by bacteria. There have not been any reports in the scientific literature of controlled studies performed on echinacea extract to document this effect. Echinacea has never been proven to be as effective as the antibiotic medications.

Hyaluronidase

Hyaluronidase, an enzyme secreted by bacteria, is able to dissolve and break down **hyaluronic acid** which, as mentioned earlier in this chapter, is part of the intercellular material in the dermis. The assumption is that by neutralizing and blocking hyaluronidase, echinacea extract prevents possible damage to bodily tissues caused by bacteria or fungi. This has not been proven in controlled research studies thus far.

Australian Tea Tree Oil

The oil of the Australian tea tree (*Melaleuca alternifolia*) is extracted after distilling its leaves. It is a colorless to clear-yellow liquid, which has a characteristic scent that is generally considered to be pleasant. This substance has been used for centuries by Australian aborigines. It is marketed as an antibacterial and antifungal preparation and does have some antiseptic properties. Tea tree oil is also said to have a soothing effect on the skin. It is meant to be used on skin inflammations, bacterial or fungal infections, and minor cuts or burns. It appears in several forms—as an emulsion, a cream, or an ointment. In a scientific study published in Australia in 1990, the substance was found to have a beneficial effect on acne. In recent years, other research studies have been published, indicating the efficacy of Australian tea tree oil on fungal infections of the skin.

Jojoba Oil

Jojoba oil, derived from the crushed bean of the jojoba shrub, a plant that grows in Mexico and southwestern North America, is widely used as a folk remedy. Being an oil, it is applied onto the skin to moisturize and soften it. Jojoba oil penetrates the keratinous layer of the skin, and is considered to have higher penetration into the skin as compared to other plant oils. Several researchers have demonstrated that it reaches the dermis, and attempts have been made to use it as a carrier to deliver other substances deep into the skin. Currently, it is used in a wide range of cosmetic preparations, including moisturizing creams, shampoos, and hair conditioners. In addition, it has been suggested that jojoba oil can decrease excessive sebaceous gland secretion, and that it has certain beneficial effects on mild skin inflammation and irritation.

Phytosterols

Phytosterols have a similar chemical structure to cholesterol and are extracted from various plant sources, such as cocoa butter, coconut, olives, avocados, sesame, sunflower seeds, and soya oil. Their major biological effect is anti-inflammatory, and their use in cosmetics is mainly related to this property. Phytosterols are usually present in anti-inflammatory creams for people with dry skin, in sunburn creams, and in creams for the treatment of various inflammatory conditions of the skin, including diaper rash in infants (which results from skin contact with various irritating substances contained in the urine and stool). It is usual to include a mixture of phytosterols, such as avocado oil or similar compounds, in hair-care products. These combinations act to condition and soften the hair; the lowering of the electrostatic charge of the hair by these compounds prevents the shapeless wispy look.

γ-Linoleic Acid

γ-Linoleic acid is a fatty acid said to have anti-inflammatory properties. It also acts as an insulating, impermeable substance in the keratin layer of the skin, thereby improving the skin's protective qualities. In cosmetics, γ-linoleic acid is used mainly as an ingredient in various moisturizing compounds.

In dermatology, there have been reports (albeit controversial) of a beneficial effect in the treatment of atopic dermatitis by using **evening primrose oil**, which contains a high concentration of γ-linoleic acid.

Another oil that contains large amounts of γ-linoleic acid is **borage oil**. The regular application of cosmetics containing borage oil for several weeks or more lessens the amount of moisture lost through the skin. Skin damage with dryness and roughness of the skin, resulting from the frequent use of detergents such as sodium lauryl sulfate (a common ingredient in soaps and shampoos), has been successfully treated by the regular application of preparations containing borage oil.

Allantoin

Allantoin used to be extracted from various plants, mainly from the *common comfrey root*. Today, in the cosmetics industry, it is made synthetically from uric acid. It appears as a white crystalline powder, which may be incorporated into a wide range of cosmetic preparations. Allantoin is considered a soothing substance for irritated skin, and it is claimed to have some effect on the repair of wounds, but there is no scientific substantiation to these claims. Allantoin is a **keratolytic** substance, which means that it is able to soften and dissolve the keratin (horny) layer of the skin, by virtue of its action on the keratin protein that makes up this layer. It is a common ingredient in moisturizing substances and products used to diminish skin irritation. It is used, for example, in treating thickened, dry skin, and cracked lips, and it is a common ingredient in shampoos for the treatment of dandruff.

Other Herbal Extracts

In recent years, other herbal extracts from plants such as thuja, sarsaparilla, gotu kola, and ginkgo-biloba have been used in dermatological and cosmetic preparations, the indications for and beneficial effects of which remain to be studied and defined.

AROMATIC OILS

Aromatic oils have been used for millennia, by the ancient Greeks and Egyptians, for pain relief and as sedatives. These oils, derived from various plants, are volatile liquids with a characteristic fragrance. They may be extracted from different parts of plants—not just from the flowers and fruit, but also from the roots of certain plants and the trunks of some trees. The pharmacological effect is achieved by inhaling the vapor (after warming) or by massaging the substance into skin. Aromatic oils are reputed to possess anti-inflammatory and antibacterial properties. Some have analgesic (pain relieving) properties and some, such as menthol and camphor, have a cooling effect on the skin.

Aromatherapy is used as a tool in the holistic approach to medicine for achieving an improved sense of well being. Because of their unique fragrances, some of the aromatic oils are said to affect emotional and psychological processes to some extent, with the ability to influence mood and to enhance the healing potential of the body. These effects may be related to a central mechanism in the brain that is connected to the sense of smell. Some of these substances (e.g., mint oil) have a stimulatory effect, while others (e.g., rose oil and jasmine oil) have a calming, soothing effect. There is a wide range of uses of aromatic oils in the cosmetics industry:

- in shampoos, hair conditioners, and hair curling preparations,
- in soaps, such as chamomile soap, which increases the moisture content of the skin and gives a feeling of "smooth skin" during and after bathing; similarly, adding aromatic oils in a concentration of about 1% to soaps provides a degree of antibacterial effect,
- in deodorants, because of their fragrance and the antibacterial effect, and
- in insect repellents.

Recently, more use is being made of the mood-altering properties of aromatic oils—for relaxation and also for stimulation. Several cosmetics companies produce an "energizing shampoo" and also a shampoo with a soothing fragrance. The energizing shampoo contains stimulatory oils, such as camphor and mint, whereas a shampoo with a soothing fragrance may contain jasmine or rose oils.

In summary, the use of aromatic oils is not expected to independently cure any existing disease. It may, however, improve the general sense of well being.

Under no circumstances should aromatic oils be orally ingested.

VITAMINS

Vitamins, by definition, are organic compounds of various types, present in small amounts in food, and whose presence is essential for the normal physiological function of the body.

The term "vitamin" holds a special marketing magic in the cosmetics industry, but in fact the beneficial effect of some vitamins on the skin remains unproven. The last decade has seen enormous interest in vitamins with antioxidant properties. These include vitamin C, β-carotene, and vitamin E. The assumption is that these vitamins can trap oxygen free radicals, which cause damage to bodily tissues.

What Are Oxygen Free Radicals?

Oxygen free radicals, by-products of chemical changes in the oxygen molecule, are continuously being produced in body tissues. The production of oxygen free radicals increases in response to certain situations, such as exposure to the sun and to X-rays, smoking, and environmental pollution.

Oxygen free radicals damage cell walls in the body, damage the genetic material (DNA) in the cells, and may alter various biochemical compounds within cells. It appears that oxygen free radicals play a significant role in heart and blood vessel disease, and in the development of malignancies. Scientists believe that the gradual, cumulative effect of oxygen free radicals accelerates the aging process in the various body systems (including the skin). Also, solar skin damage is largely thought to be due to the effect of oxygen free radicals.

The discussion below refers to two main points: (*i*) if there is any benefit in the addition of vitamins to the diet and (*ii*) if there is any value in their applying them to the skin.

Is There Any Benefit in the Addition of Vitamins to the Diet?

Many studies have been performed to determine whether, in fact, the addition of antioxidant vitamins to the diet can decrease the incidence of heart disease, blood vessel disease, and cancer. It is also said that they may strengthen the immune system, and may improve cognitive functions. Although some studies seem to support this, the topic is still controversial. Furthermore, the question of whether the addition of these vitamins improves the quality of the skin, and slows down the process of skin aging, remains unanswered.

The current line of thinking is that healthy individuals who consume balanced diets do not need extra vitamin supplementation. On the other hand, there exist many research studies that seem to support its use in certain cases, provided that the dosage does not exceed the recommended daily allowance.

1. Some claim that in the preparation of many foodstuffs, they undergo various processes (including exposure to pesticides, addition of preservatives, etc.) that decrease their quality and reduce the bioavailability of the vitamins.
2. Recent evidence has indicated that the diet of many people, especially among the elderly, does not provide optimal amounts of all vitamins. Although this rarely manifests clinically in the form of classical vitamin deficiency syndromes, many people only consume sub-optimal levels of certain vitamins in their diet.
3. The genetic profile of individuals may be used in the future as a guide to individual tailoring of vitamin supplementation. For example, researchers have recently suggested that supplementation of vitamin E may prevent heart diseases in diabetic patients with specific genetic characteristics.

In any case, excessive intake of vitamins should be avoided. A physician or a dietician should be consulted as to the desirable dosage of vitamin supplementation, in order to avoid toxicity.

What Do We Know About the Use of Vitamins When Applied to the Skin?

Until recently, the classic argument of those who denied the effectiveness of products containing vitamins when applied to the skin was that the vitamins are unable to penetrate the keratinous layer, and hence cannot reach the epidermis or dermis. However, recent research has shown that vitamins C and E, when present in some skin preparations, do in fact penetrate the epidermis and are absorbed. The degree of penetration depends in the specific chemical form used of the vitamin, its concentration, and the presence of other constituents in the preparation. Remember, however, that although these vitamins can penetrate the epidermis and dermis, this still does not mean that they necessarily have any beneficial effect on the skin, or that they act as antioxidants and trap oxygen free radicals, and in that way improve the quality of the skin.

In recent years, there has been an accumulating number of studies indicating that preparations containing antioxidants may benefit the skin. However, it is difficult to plan and conduct a high-quality study that examines the precise benefits of any topical preparation on the quality of the skin, or its exact role in anti-aging. When dealing with creams based on certain vitamins, the effect, if any, is slower as compared to compounds such as retinoic acid or α-hydroxy preparations, and certainly less dramatic than the impact of a skin peeling.

In some cases, the addition of vitamins to certain preparations is done mainly in order to increase their marketing appeal. However, certain vitamins can exist in various chemical forms. Some preparations do not always contain the specific chemical form, or the required concentration, of a certain vitamin that has been shown to be preferable in research studies. It is, therefore, advisable to purchase products of reliable manufacturers.

In some cases, certain vitamins, such as vitamins A and C, being antioxidants, may also be used as preservatives in the cosmetic industry. They are considered to be more gentle than other preservatives and seem to cause fewer irritations or allergic reactions.

Vitamin C

The assumption is that vitamin C in skin preparations has antioxidant properties that protect the skin from damage caused by ultraviolet radiation, air pollution, and smoke. In view of these properties, it is said to have some anti-aging effect, by preventing the appearance of fine wrinkling on the skin. Vitamin C also plays a role in stimulating cells in the dermis to produce collagen, so that applying skin preparations containing this vitamin may be of some value.

Note: When we talk of function of vitamin C in protecting the skin from the sun and ultraviolet radiation, we are not implying that it is acting as a screen that filters out or reflects the damaging rays. What we mean is that apparently it has some effect on the repair of pre-existing sun and radiation damage.

Vitamin C, in its natural form, is a rather unstable compound. It is easily oxidized and destroyed in response to exposure to heat, air, or light. Hence, some products containing vitamin C in its natural form may not only lack any beneficial effect, but may even be harmful when applied to the skin.

The desirable forms of vitamin C are fat-soluble, which do not tend to easily oxidize. When vitamin C is combined with palm oil to form a synthetic ester, it becomes fat-soluble and less acidic. Common forms of vitamin C in cosmetic products are *ascorbyl palmitate* and *magnesium ascorbyl phosphate*.

Ascorbyl palmitate has photo-protective effects. In one study, when applied to sunburn, it reduced redness by 50% as compared to the untreated areas.

L-Ascorbic acid is a water-soluble form of vitamin C that has been found to benefit the skin. It must be formulated at a low pH in order to ensure its stability. It has been shown that only relatively high concentrations—of more than 10% of the preparation—are able to penetrate the skin.

β-Carotene and Vitamin A

β-Carotene (provitamin A), being the chemical precursor of vitamin A, is a proven antioxidant. In the diet, it is found mainly in tomatoes, carrots, and yellow-orange vegetables. However, it is a rather unstable chemical compound, unsuitable for use in cosmetic preparations.

Similarly, in the standard scientific literature there is no proof that topical preparations containing vitamin A have any beneficial effect on the skin. On the other hand, retinoic acid, a compound similar in chemical structure to vitamin A, has been proven to have a beneficial effect. Retinoic acid and its effects are discussed in detail in chapter 17.

Provitamin B (Panthenol)

This substance is claimed to be able to aid in the healing of wounds and to lessen skin inflammation. It is, therefore, a common ingredient in products designed for treating diaper rash in infants.

Other Compounds

Some physicians and dermatologists advocate enthusiastically the use of topical creams containing other compounds, such as α-lipoic acid or dimethylaminoethanol. For the time being, there is no concrete scientific evidence to support their topical use.

Vitamins in Summary

So far, there have been no high-quality research studies on humans that have unequivocally confirmed that skin preparations containing vitamins have a beneficial effect on the skin. Nevertheless, more and more observational evidence is starting to accumulate that suggests that they may do so. Further research is needed to verify that vitamins in cosmetic products benefit the skin.

COMMON FOODSTUFFS

Eggs and Milk
Apart from their nutritional value, there is no evidence that cosmetic preparations containing eggs or milk have anything to contribute to skin care, other than perhaps improving the moisture content of the skin and thereby imparting a smooth texture to it. Even if they do, the same results can be obtained from standard moisturizing substances.

Honey, Propolis, and Royal Bee Jelly
Substances such as honey, propolis and royal bee jelly have long been in use in folk medicine—mainly for healing wounds. Honey has been found to have certain beneficial properties in the treatment of burns. This effect, it is presumed, is related to the high concentration of sugars in honey, which prevents the growth of bacteria on the injury. Nevertheless, with regard to the healing of burns, honey has never been proven to be as effective as the standard substances used in these cases. No other beneficial effect of honey or propolis on the skin (such as prevention of skin aging) has been proven.

SOME ADDITIONAL COMMENTS

The Meaning of the Word "Natural" in Cosmetics
We stress that not everything that has the label "natural" should automatically be used or recommended. Indeed, various medications used for treating serious diseases are manufactured by a completely synthetic process. And without doubt, treatment with these synthetic substances is by far preferable to the course (totally natural) of illness, or of death. Thus, by the same token, a baby hair shampoo made of a synthetic substance is generally less harmful and less irritating to the skin than normal soap, which is derived from "natural" animal fats. Not only that, not all preparations marketed as "natural" are indeed such. In the course of the manufacture of so-called natural products, there is usually a whole chain of processes—sterilization, alcohol disinfection, and the addition of preservatives, artificial coloring agents, and fragrances. As the product reaches the consumer it is usually totally different from its natural, basic form, although it too, may be marketed as "natural."

Hence, the label "natural" should be viewed with circumspection. More important than the degree of "naturalness" of a product are factors such as the following: What is known about its side effects? How irritating or damaging to the skin is the substance? To what extent has its efficacy been proven?

Preparations Purporting to "Enrich the Skin with Oxygen"
Some cosmetic preparations are advertised as "providing oxygen to the skin." However, the skin receives its oxygen through blood vessels in the dermis, and, provided there is no damage to that blood supply, the skin needs no alternative source of oxygen. Not only that, today considerable research is being devoted to the question of possible damage caused by oxygen and its by-products (free oxygen radicals) to various tissues, including the skin. Indeed, there are products (such as certain vitamins) that are used specifically because of their antioxidant effects (see above).

The Concept of "Skin Nutrition"
When a cosmetic product is said to "nourish the skin," this usually means that it contains ingredients that have a biological effect on skin cells. All the substances covered in this chapter come into this category—some have scientific backing for their biological activity, while others have no scientific proof of their beneficial value or their biological effect on the skin. In general, the skin (epidermis and dermis) obtains its nutrients via the blood vessels in the skin, and not from substances applied to its surface. Preparations said to nourish the skin are generally fatty substances that are relatively impermeable to water. They are usually applied at night and are meant to remain on the skin for several hours. They contain various active ingredients supposed to benefit the skin after penetrating deeply. Remember that in terms of "nutrition," in most cases, cells and tissues do not take up substances in their original forms. Proteins are broken down in the digestive system to amino acids, which are then absorbed into the bloodstream; fats are

broken down to fatty acid units; most sugars are broken down to single-sugar units. Thus, the bodily tissues, including the skin, are neither "used to" nor able to take up complex molecules such as proteins.

Penetration of Substances into the Skin Cells

The cell membrane represents the outer surface of the cell. It acts as a selective barrier that regulates the entry and exit of substances in and out of the cell. The cell membrane is made up of phospholipids (fatty compounds containing phosphorus), proteins, and polysaccharides (complex sugars).

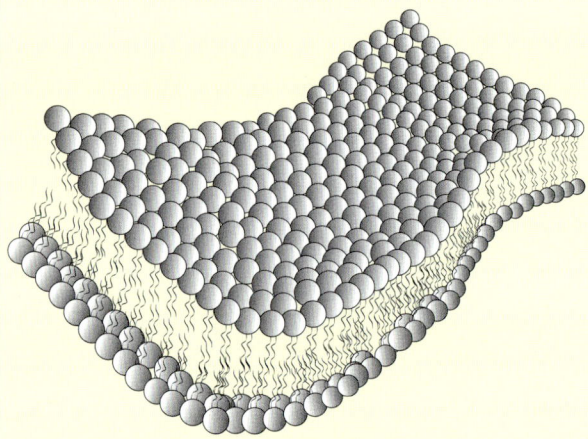

Microscopic structure of the cell membrane, made up of a double layer of phospholipids.

As can be seen in the illustration, the phospholipids are organized in a double layer. This arrangement of the cell wall prevents the unwanted passage of fatty substances or water-soluble substances in or out of the cell.

Liposomes were developed in order to allow the penetration of substances into the epidermis and dermis, and thence into the skin cells. The logic behind the development of liposomes is that, just like the cell wall, they are made of phospholipids. The assumption is that they will therefore be able to become attached to the cell wall and penetrate it.

The use of liposomes enables various active ingredients to penetrate the keratin layer of the skin, which is made up of closely packed layers of cells. This is discussed in detail in chapter 23.

Recently, cosmetic preparations containing various vitamins, particularly vitamins C and E, have been developed. A certain level of these vitamins can get to the cells of the epidermis and dermis, so one could regard this as a certain form of skin "nourishment."

17 | Retinoic Acid
Avi Shai, Howard I. Maibach, and Robert Baran

Contents Overview • Beneficial effects of retinoic acid • Who may benefit from retinoic acid? • Guidelines for use • Side effects • Warnings • Retinol and other retinoids • Conclusion

OVERVIEW

An important turning point in the world of cosmetic dermatology occurred with the development of retinoic acid, a synthetic retinoid compound. Retinoids resemble vitamin A in their chemical composition and are used in the treatment of several skin diseases.

The regular application of products containing retinoic acid improves, to a certain extent, the signs of **photoaging**, i.e., skin damaged by exposure to the sun, and **chronological skin aging**, related to increasing age.

Retinoic acid was originally intended for acne treatment. Dermatologists observed its beneficial effect on the skin when treating adult women with acne. These patients reported that their skin became somewhat smoother, and fine wrinkles flattened and nearly disappeared. Dark facial blemishes were lightened, and some vanished. Subsequently, the efficacy of the product was compared to creams with similar ingredients but without retinoic acid. Both creams were applied for prolonged periods, each on a different side of the face. The studies demonstrated the efficacy of retinoic acid, both in the prevention of skin aging and in improving pre-existing damage.

Some Preparations Containing Retinoic Acid in Various Countries

- Airol®
- Avita®
- Locacid®
- Renova®
- Retin-A®
- Retisol-A®
- Vesanoid®

BENEFICIAL EFFECTS OF RETINOIC ACID

Retinoic acid lessens the consequences of photoaging. In addition, there are some beneficial effects of retinoic acid on chronological skin aging:

- At the microscopic level, retinoic acid enhances cell division in the **epidermis**, replacing damaged and unorganized cells with new, organized cells. It also reduces melanin production. In the **dermis**, new collagen and elastic fibers are formed.

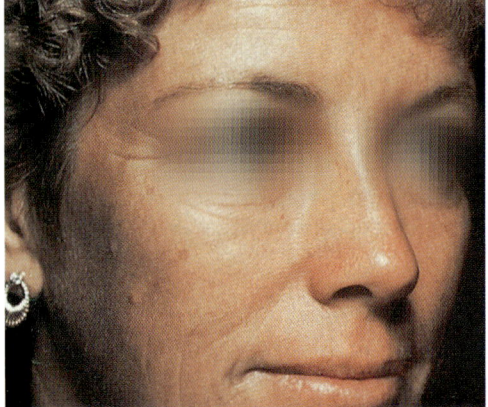
(A) Wrinkles before treatment.

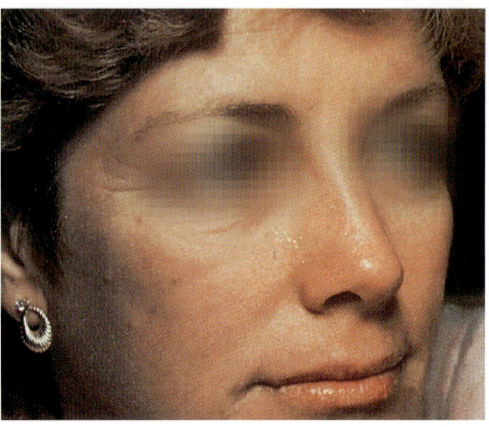
(B) Wrinkles 24 weeks after treatment with retinoic acid.

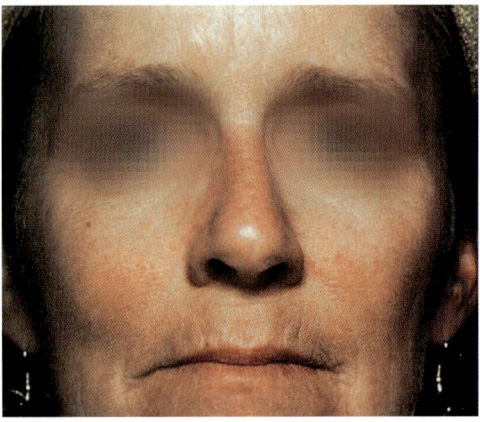
(A) Before treatment.

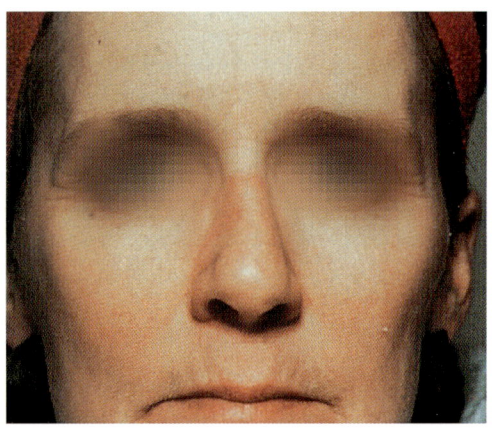
(B) 24 weeks after treatment with retinoic acid.

- The skin becomes visibly smoother and thicker. Retinoic acid can cause significant flattening, diminishing, and even the disappearance of fine wrinkles in the skin.
- Dark blemishes on the face (brownish-yellow or light-brown lesions, often referred to as **age spots** or **liver spots**) can lighten and sometimes disappear. (The precise medical term for "age spots" is **solar lentigines**, also referred to as **senile lentigines**. Further details are provided in chapter 20, "Bleaching and Bleaching Preparations")
- Regular application of retinoic acid may cause the regression or disappearance of precancerous lesions such as **solar keratoses**, although this is not necessarily the sole or preferred treatment for such lesions. The treatment of solar keratoses should only be carried out by a physician.
- Retinoic acid increases the blood flow in the skin, producing a healthy rosy color.

The beneficial effect of treatment with retinoic acid is gradual and prolonged, and significant improvement may be apparent only after several months. Maximal improvement occurs within the first year of treatment. In the first year, the aging process is delayed, and even somewhat reversed. If treatment is continued for more than a year, the delaying effect continues, but further repair of already-damaged skin cannot be expected.

Prolonged, severe damage caused by the sun cannot be fully corrected. Nevertheless, many patients are pleased with the results. Expectations should be realistic. The product is not a substitute for relatively aggressive treatments, such as chemical peeling or surgical interventions. Neither deep wrinkles nor expression lines can be corrected by such treatment—the results are apparent only on fine wrinkles. Nor will all dark facial blemishes be lightened by the product, so alternative regimens should be considered for these types of skin lesions.

Certain types of retinoid compounds affect the sebaceous glands by decreasing their size. The beneficial effect of isotretinoin, another retinoid, on acne, has been documented (see chapter 9, "Acne," for more information). With increasing age, the sebaceous glands tend to increase in size with subsequent widening of the skin's pores, and gradual thickening and enlargement of the nose. Some physicians suggested that continuous and prolonged use of retinoic acid preparations onto the skin of the nose may prevent these changes. However, thus far this has not been proven.

WHO MAY BENEFIT FROM RETINOIC ACID?

Retinoic acid is beneficial primarily for individuals older than 35 years with evidence of photoaging caused by excessive sun exposure manifested by the appearance of fine wrinkles and dark blemishes. Patients with skin damage due to chronological aging also benefit from treatment with retinoic acid.

Mechanism of Action of Topical Retinoic Acid

Initially, retinoic acid binds to a specific protein found within cells of the skin. This protein (**cellular retinoic acid binding protein**) transports retinoic acid into the nucleus of each cell. The next stage is within the nucleus. By binding to specific nuclear proteins, retinoic acid modulates the expression of genes, thus altering the processes of growth and maturation of the cells in the epidermis and the dermis.

GUIDELINES FOR USE

Retinoic acid can only be purchased with a physician's prescription, and precise directions must be followed. The treatment is tailored to each individual patient, according to age, skin type, history of sun exposure, and possible sensitivities to specific medications.

Retinoic acid is marketed in three concentrations:

- 0.025%,
- 0.05%, and
- 0.1%.

Treatment should be initiated with the lowest concentration, and increased gradually as necessary. The product is usually applied as a cream but, in the case of very oily skin, a gel may be favored. The face should be washed with a gentle soap prior to the application of retinoic acid. The product should be applied at night and washed away in the morning, since it increases sensitivity to the sun. The product is intended to be applied to the

- face,
- upper chest,
- outer arms, and
- backs of the hands.

A small amount of the product should be applied. Dermatologists state that a small quantity (a pea-sized amount) should suffice for an area of skin the size of the forehead. At first, retinoic acid should be applied nightly. For sensitive skin, application should be started with once every other night, and gradually increased to nightly application. After one year, when maximal improvement has been attained and the condition of the skin has stabilized, application of the product two or three times weekly may be sufficient for continued preventative treatment.

During treatment, activities that damage the skin, such as sun exposure or smoking, should be avoided. In the daytime, the face should be protected with appropriate sunscreen and moisturizers. The purpose of moisturizers is to avoid dryness of the face, resulting from the application of retinoic acid. Retinoic acid should not be applied at the same time as moisturizers, since this combination may cause adverse effects.

SIDE EFFECTS

When first applied, retinoic acid reduces the thickness of the outer epidermal layer as well as the keratinous layer. Only at a later stage does the product affect cell division in the epidermis and cause epidermal thickening. Consequently, most patients will initially notice a dry sensation with slight scaling. This occurs within two weeks to three months from the beginning of treatment. Therefore, a cream-based product is preferable to a gel-based one, since gel tends to dry skin to a greater extent. The gel form is recommended only for oily skin. If necessary, moisturizing cream can be applied to the face during the day. Another possibility is to use the retinoic acid preparation every other night, combined with a moisturizer on the alternate nights.

Also, within two weeks of beginning treatment, the skin may become slightly red and there may be a sensation of mild stinging which usually disappears within two to three months. If, however, the redness or stinging becomes irritating, a physician should be consulted. Consider

- temporary discontinuation of treatment,
- a reduction in the concentration of active ingredient,
- reducing the amount of cream or gel applied, or
- reducing application of the product from every day to only every second or third day.

Note: The stinging and/or burning sensation is not related to the therapeutic effect. In any case, any patient with a reaction that is more pronounced than slight stinging should follow the guidelines above.

WARNINGS

When using retinoic acid, one should

- minimize sun exposure,
- avoid using other cosmetic products at the same time,
- not use retinoic acid during pregnancy,
- avoid physical contact with eyes or mouth,
- avoid combining retinoic acid with certain medications, and
- avoid hair removal by wax or laser.

Minimizing Sun Exposure
Retinoic acid increases sensitivity to the sun, so application must be at night, and the face washed in the morning. The product should not be applied at all during the day, and sun exposure should be minimized. A moisturizer should be applied during the day, with an adequate sunscreen. In any case, there is no point in treating sun-damaged skin while at the same time exposing the skin to the harmful rays of the sun.

Avoiding Simultaneous Use of Other Cosmetic Products
Retinoic acid should not be applied to the skin at the same time as any other cosmetic product. It is not stable when combined with other products. However, it is possible and quite acceptable to combine the use of retinoic acid preparations in parallel with other cosmetic products. For example, a sunscreen may be used in the morning while retinoic acid is intended for nighttime use. By the same token, retinoic acid preparations may be combined with antibacterial preparations to increase the efficacy of treatment of acne. However, concomitant use of retinoic acid with cosmetics that may cause skin irritation, such as astringents and strong soaps, should be avoided.

Retinoic Acid and Pregnancy
Oral retinoids have a **teratogenic effect**, causing birth defects in the fetus. As to retinoic acid, intended for external use only, there is no clear scientific proof for its association with birth

defects. Nevertheless, dermatologists do not recommend the use of topical retinoic acid at all during pregnancy.

Physical Contact with Eyes or Mouth
A small amount of the product can be applied near the lower eyelids or lips. A certain beneficial effect is produced by applying around the mouth and at the outer edges of the eyes. Nevertheless, it is best to be cautious and avoid direct contact of the product with eyes or mouth.

Retinoic Acid with Certain Medications
Topical retinoic acid can be combined with most medications. However, it is best not to combine it with medications that may increase the skin's sensitivity to the sun. A dermatologist should be consulted in any case of oral drug ingestion concomitant with the use of topical retinoic acid.

Avoiding Hair Removal by Wax or Laser
As with other retinoid compounds, the use of retinoic acid increases skin's fragility. One should avoid hair removal by laser or by wax, or using abrasive facial cleansers during treatment with topical retinoic acid for a certain period thereafter on the treated areas.

RETINOL AND OTHER RETINOIDS

The labels of many cosmetic products contain the names of compounds that are chemically similar to retinoic acid, such as retinol (vitamin A alcohol), retinyl palmitate, retinyl acetate (vitamin A esters), and retinal (vitamin A aldehyde). The fact that these compounds can be sold without a doctor's prescription allows them to be marketed freely.

Retinol, as opposed to retinoic acid, is the pure form of vitamin A. It is reasonable to assume that after its penetration into the skin, it is converted chemically to retinoic acid. However, only small quantities of retinoic acid are produced leading to decreased efficacy with less adverse effects, as compared to the use of prescribed preparations containing retinoic acid.

A number of dermatologists agree that prolonged use of retinol or retinaldehyde may have beneficial effects on the skin, similar (but weaker) to that of retinoic acid. The beneficial effect of each preparation depends on many factors such as the active ingredient (retinol, retinaldehyde, or any other retinoid compound), its concentration, the preparation in which it is contained, and the presence of other compounds in the preparation.

Many cosmetic companies produce and market preparations containing retinol, or other retinoids, available without prescription, that can be bought at any retail outlet. The range of preparations is such that the individual customers can choose a preparation to their liking in terms of texture, moisture level, presence of other ingredients, and the way it feels when applied to the skin.

CONCLUSION

Despite the warnings given above—which should be observed—retinoic acid has a beneficial effect. It appears to delay the aging process of the skin, and even reverse it to a certain extent.

18 | α-Hydroxy Acids

Ron Yaniv and Stanley Levy

Contents Overview • Effect of low concentrations of α-hydroxy acids • Effect of moderate concentrations (10% to 50%) of α-hydroxy acid on sun-damaged skin • High concentrations of α-hydroxy acid for superficial chemical peeling • Guidelines for use • Possible side effects • Summary

OVERVIEW

α-hydroxy acids are a group of compounds derived from various plant sources:

- **glycolic acid**, derived from sugar cane,
- **malic acid**, derived from apples,
- **tartaric acid**, derived from grapes, and
- **citric acid**, derived from lemons.

Lactic acid also belongs to this group but is derived from sour milk. Because most of these acids are of plant origin, they are also known as "fruit acids" or "natural acids." However, most of the α-hydroxy acids used in cosmetics are manufactured in laboratories by industrial methods.

α-hydroxy acids preparations may have a beneficial role to play in the skin aging processes—particularly in the aging processes related to excessive sun exposure.

The first reports of their use go back a long way. Cleopatra was said to have bathed in milk, which contains lactic acid (although, to the best of our knowledge, she did not document its effect scientifically!). Van Scott and his colleagues reintroduced the use of these substances in the 1980s. They recognized the beneficial effects of α-hydroxy acids and published scientific articles on the subject.

Of the α-hydroxy acids, glycolic acid is the most widely used. Nevertheless, some manufacturers produce α-hydroxy products based on lactic acid, citric acid, and other acids, or combinations of these with glycolic acid. α-hydroxy acids are used in a wide range of preparations, such as:

- creams,
- liquid emulsions,
- ointments,
- gels, and
- cleansing agents.

In general, α-hydroxy acids are less efficient when incorporated in cleansing agents than when included in other cosmetic preparations since, in the former case, they will be in contact with the skin for a short time only.

The higher the concentration of the α-hydroxy acid, the more marked its effects on the skin. Another parameter determining the potency of the preparation is its level of acidity. When the pH of the preparation is lower, its effect on the skin is stronger. The preparations can therefore be divided into three groups on the basis of their concentrations of α-hydroxy acid:

- **Low concentrations (up to 10%):** The concentration of α-hydroxy acid in preparations that may be sold freely, without a physician's supervision, varies from country to country and within countries, in accordance with the regulations of the local licensing authorities. Higher concentration α-hydroxy acid products may be found in aestheticians' or physicians' offices.

- **Concentrations of 10% to 50%:** These preparations, which require a physician's supervision, are used for a very superficial chemical peeling of the skin. They are usually used in a series of treatments; the treatment is repeated every few days.
- **Concentrations of 50% to 70%:** α-hydroxy acids in these concentrations are used by physicians to achieve superficial chemical peeling of the skin.

In general, the effect of α-hydroxy acids depends mainly on their concentration, the length of time they are in contact with the skin, and the frequency of application. As stated above, the higher the concentration, the more effective the treatment, but then there is more likelihood of skin irritation and undesirable side effects.

EFFECT OF LOW CONCENTRATIONS OF α-HYDROXY ACIDS

At low concentrations (up to 10%), glycolic acid weakens the bonds between the degenerating and dead cells of the outer layers of the skin, thus weakening their adhesion to each other. Hence, the keratinous layer cannot build up, and the new cells coming up from below can replace more easily the cells that peel away. The replacement of the dry, damaged keratinous layer by a new, thinner keratinous layer gives the skin a smooth, younger appearance.

Glycolic acid acts as a humectant, that is, it absorbs water. Thus, it functions as a moisturizer, resulting in swelling of the skin, with the consequent diminution of fine wrinkles; dry, rough skin becomes smoother and softer. Therefore, the immediate improvement in the appearance of dry skin after applying an α-hydroxy acid is mostly attributed to the improvement in the skin's moisture content.

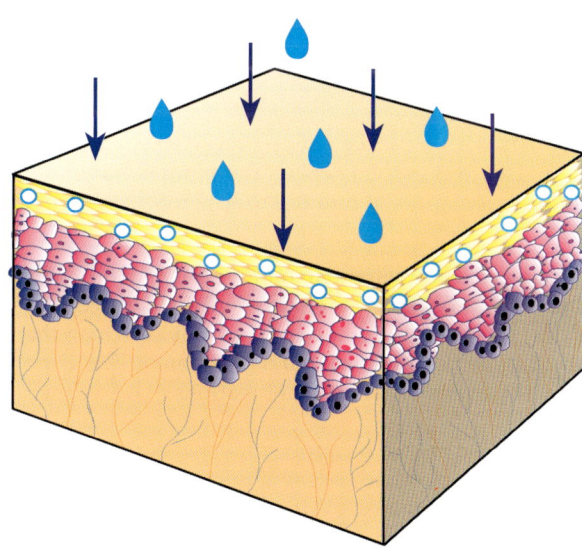

α-hydroxy acid (shown as clear circles) acts as a water-absorbing agent in the keratinous layer.

Note that the effect of α-hydroxy acids as moisturizing agents is more prolonged than that of the standard moisturizing agents. The effect of the latter lasts for a few hours, while the beneficial effects of α-hydroxy acids may even last for several days after discontinuing treatment.

Some α-hydroxy acids have anti-inflammatory properties by virtue of being antioxidants, that is, they may prevent possible damage from oxygen-free radicals.

Preliminary articles have appeared in the medical literature confirming that, even at relatively low concentrations, the daily application of α-hydroxy acids has a beneficial effect on sun-damaged skin. α-hydroxy acids will lighten dark, hyperpigmented blotches on the skin. There is also improvement and a decrease in the appearance of fine skin wrinkles. Preparations of α-hydroxy acids in low concentrations have a beneficial effect on acne (see chapter 9).

EFFECT OF MODERATE CONCENTRATIONS (10% TO 50%) OF α-HYDROXY ACID ON SUN-DAMAGED SKIN

Effect on the Epidermis
After applying 25% glycolic acid daily for several months to sun-damaged skin, microscopic examination of the skin shows that the epidermis becomes somewhat thicker, with improvements in the texture and general structure. The cells appear more uniform and orderly. The skin appears smoother, with less wrinkles. Since most skin wrinkles appear with increasing age and are the result of prolonged exposure to the sun, related to the accumulation of melanin pigment in the epidermal cells, the renewal and organization of the cell turnover in the epidermis lessens the number of wrinkles and improve the skin's appearance. Indeed, many preparations used for bleaching areas of skin contain α-hydroxy acids together with other active ingredients.

Effect on the Dermis
Researchers have formed the impression that constant use of α-hydroxy acids in moderately high concentrations has a beneficial effect on the elastic fibers in the skin, and also results in an increase in the amount of collagen fibers in the skin. Some researchers believe that α-hydroxy acid actually penetrates into the dermis and encourages the formation of new collagen fibers.

The Minipeel Method

In the United States, cosmeticians use products with a concentration of α-hydroxy acids of up to 30% for very superficial skin peeling. This technique is called the minipeel method. The preparation is applied to the face and neck for up to 30 minutes, once or twice a week. There are several crucial points in using this treatment:

- It is essential that the face be thoroughly cleansed beforehand to remove traces of oil, dead cells, and dirt. If this is not done, the acid will not penetrate the skin evenly and effectively, but will be absorbed by the oily layer and by the dirt on the skin. The way in which the cleansing is performed has a significant effect on the final result of the treatment. There are ready-made commercial preparations on the market that are combinations of α-hydroxy acids and cleansing agents.
- Peeling requires that a thin, **even** layer of the substance be applied.
- The preparation must be washed off the face at the time specified in the instructions: **it must not be left on the skin for longer than the specified period**. It should be rinsed off with water or a weak solution of sodium bicarbonate (baking soda).

Note: There is a certain risk of burning the patient's skin using the minipeel method. Other things can also go wrong, whether related to faulty manufacture of the preparation, or to the individual sensitivity of the patient to one of its ingredients.

In most cases, using moderate concentrations (up to 50%) of α-hydroxy acid for facial treatments or "peeling" improves the skin texture. However, the reaction to these treatments, and the degree of improvement achieved, may vary considerably from one person to another (even when using identical concentrations of the active substance). Remember that treatment with 50% glycolic acid is safe if performed by an experienced physician. It is therefore logical to start treatment with this substance first, since, although other products (such as those containing a higher concentration of α-hydroxy acid, or other products used for deeper peeling of the skin) may be more effective, they have more side effects.

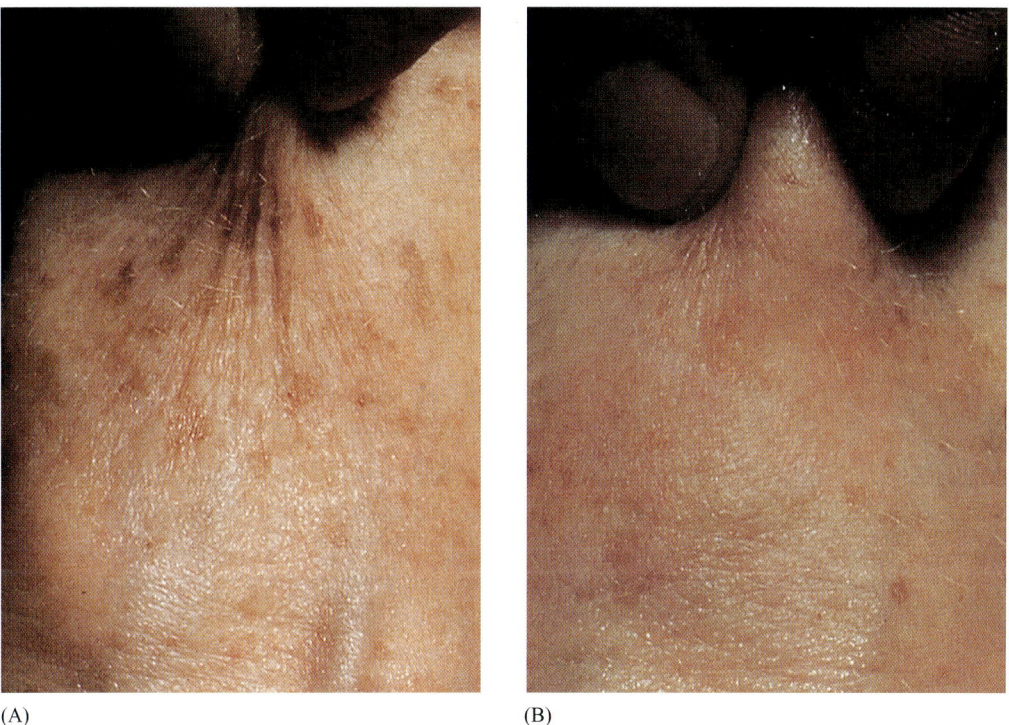

(**A**) Right forearm untreated. (**B**) Left forearm of same patient following six months of treatment with α-hydroxy acids (25%). The treated skin is plumper than that of the right forearm, less wrinkled, and with even pigmentation.

HIGH CONCENTRATIONS OF α-HYDROXY ACID FOR SUPERFICIAL CHEMICAL PEELING

Higher concentrations of α-hydroxy acid have a raised acidity level and can burn the skin. Therefore, any use of high concentrations of α-hydroxy acids requires medical supervision. These highly concentrated solutions (50–70%) are used by physicians to achieve superficial chemical peeling of the skin. Chemical peeling of the skin in fact involves "dissolving" the outer layer of the epidermis. The idea is that after removing this outer layer, new, younger-looking, healthy skin will grow out to take its place. The effect of the high-concentration preparations depends on the length of time the substance is in contact with the skin, and on the frequency of its use.

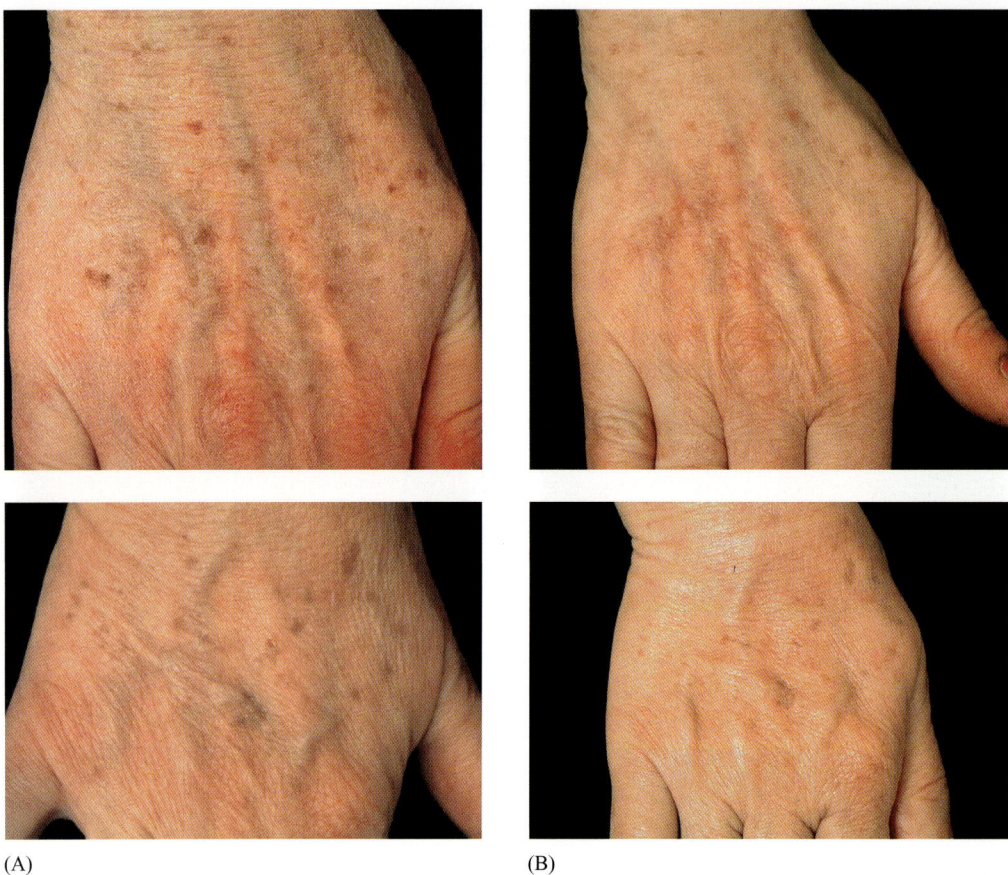

(A) (B)

(**A**) Before treatment. (**B**) Following skin peeling using high concentrations of α-hydroxy acids. The patient was treated with twice-daily applications of glycolic acid 10% lotion and weekly glycolic acid 50% chemical peels for eight weeks.

Epidermis
After repeated treatment by 70% glycolic acid, on several occasions over several months, improvement becomes noticeable in the epidermis. Microscopic examination shows that the epidermis is thicker, while externally the skin looks smoother and slightly thicker, and there are fewer wrinkles.

Dermis
Several research studies on the effects of high concentrations of α-hydroxy acids on the skin have suggested that there is formation of new collagen and elastic fibers deep in the dermis.

The main use for chemical peeling of the skin using high concentrations of glycolic acid is, as we have stated, for treating sun-damaged skin. In addition, this treatment affords an extra benefit in that it lightens hyperpigmented (dark) blotches on the skin.

GUIDELINES FOR USE

Start with Low Concentrations
The standard recommended technique is to start with a daily application of an α-hydroxy compound with a low concentration of acid (3% to 4%) to the skin of the face and neck. After a few days it can be applied twice daily, provided that no skin irritation has appeared. Following several weeks of this treatment (again provided that there are no unwanted side effects), higher concentrations—up to 10%—may be used. Individuals known to have sensitive skin should

undergo a skin test of a small area of unexposed skin before using a preparation containing an α-hydroxy acid on the entire face. Individuals with particularly sensitive skin may begin using α-hydroxy acid products on alternate days to allow their skin to adapt to a more aggressive skin care regimen. Using α-hydroxy acids with other aggressive treatments, such as exfoliating scrubs or retinoic acid, can also increase skin sensitivity.

Sometimes a dermatologist will start treatment in his/her clinic using high concentrations, and then later revert to home treatment with lower concentrations. Although α-hydroxy compounds in which the concentration of the acid exceeds 10% may only be prescribed by a physician, the exact concentration of α-hydroxy acid in preparations that may be sold without a physician's supervision varies from country to country, and within countries, depending on the regulations of the local licensing authorities.

Prevention of Sun Exposure

There are reports in the medical literature showing that prolonged use of α-hydroxy acid can sensitize the skin to ultraviolet radiation. α-Hydroxy acid removes the top dead layers of the skin, allowing ultraviolet radiation to more easily penetrate into the underlying living skin. Therefore, patients being treated with α-hydroxy acid should avoid excessive exposure to sunlight to prevent further skin damage. Patients being treated with these preparations should use a sunscreen with a protective factor appropriate to their degree of sun exposure. Even if the α-hydroxy compound is applied in the evening or at night, the patient should still use a sunscreen during the day. In general, it is absurd to use a preparation that prevents and repairs solar skin damage, while at the same time exposing oneself to the sun! For this reason, many preparations containing α-hydroxy acid also contain sunscreens.

In Combination with Retinoic Acid

α-hydroxy compounds can be combined with retinoic acid, whereby the α-hydroxy compound is applied during the day and the retinoic acid at night. Some researchers feel that this combination enhances the effect of both ingredients, and may increase anti-aging effects.

In Combination with Other Procedures

The use of α-hydroxy acid products or peels may be used in combination with other procedures including other kinds of peels, nonablative lasers, and microdermabrasions. Using microdermabrasion first has been shown to increase the effects of glycolic acid peels. Obviously, there is an increased risk of irritation and more serious side effects with combining procedures. Use of these combinations should only be undertaken with a physician's supervision.

Bleaching Hyperpigmented Lesions

α-Hydroxy compounds can be combined with other substances in the treatment of hyperpigmented skin lesions. This is discussed in more detail in chapter 20 on bleaching.

Matching the Preparation to the Patient's Skin Type

A wide range of α-hydroxy compounds may suit a variety of skin types. The product used should be appropriate for the patient's skin type. For example, for a patient with relatively dry facial skin, an oilier preparation such as a cream or richer lotion should be selected, while for a patient with an oily skin, a gel-based preparation is to be preferred.

Note: Hundreds of companies manufacture α-hydroxy preparations, with concentrations ranging from 1% to 30%. It must be stressed that the efficacy of an α-hydroxy compound depends on how it was prepared, and the constitution of the vehicle in which the acid is dissolved. A glycolic acid cream made by a neighborhood pharmacist or by a local manufacturing plant may be less effective than one produced by a manufacturer with extensive experience in the manufacture of α-hydroxy compounds. Therefore, in general, it is preferable to use products of reputable manufacturers, experienced in the manufacture of α-hydroxy compounds.

POSSIBLE SIDE EFFECTS

Low Concentrations of α-Hydroxy Acids

Transient stinging after applying α-hydroxy acids is quite common and usually disappears with repeated applications. However, persistent stinging, itching, or visible redness is a sign of more significant irritation, and usually means that there is excessive sensitivity to one of the components of the product (which can happen with any medical cosmetic product). In that case, one should discontinue applying the preparation. The FDA 1999 instructions regarding α-hydroxy acids state that even mild irritation is a sign that the product is causing damage. Using another α-hydroxy acid is not recommended without first consulting a dermatologist.

Moderate or High Concentrations of α-Hydroxy Acids

The side effects can vary in severity—slight irritation will be manifested by redness and stinging. Severe cases associated with higher concentrations may be manifested by the appearance of blistering and painful burns. In these cases, a dermatologist should be consulted.

Restrictions on the Use of α-Hydroxy Acids in the United States

The concentration of α-hydroxy acid that may be sold freely, without a doctor's prescription, varies, depending on the local licensing authority. In the United States, the Cosmetic Ingredient Review Panel (the cosmetics industry's self-regulatory body for examining the safety of cosmetic ingredients) determined in 1997 that α-hydroxy acids are safe to use in cosmetic preparations in concentrations up to 10%, provided that the pH of the preparation is not less than 3.5. This is because the more acidic the preparation (the lower the pH), the higher the absorption of the α-hydroxy acid into the skin.

In the United States, preparations containing up to 30% α-hydroxy acid are permitted for use by trained cosmetologists, on condition that the substance is applied to the skin for only brief periods of time and is then immediately rinsed off. However, in recent years, there have been reports of side effects from products containing α-hydroxy acid. Such reports are more common in cases where the concentration of the α-hydroxy acid in the preparation is moderately high, up to 30%—a concentration that, in the United States, may only be used by trained cosmetologists.

Use of α-Hydroxy Acids on Dark-Skinned Patients

The use of α-hydroxy preparations on people of Asiatic origin and dark-skinned people in general, requires particular care (compared with their use in Caucasians). In these people, there is an increased tendency to side effects such as skin irritation, as well as the appearance of dark (pigmented) skin blotches in the treated areas (postinflammatory pigmentation). These effects are extremely uncommon following the use of cosmetic preparations sold without a prescription, in which there is a low concentration of the active ingredient. On the other hand, in those preparations used by physicians for peeling, and in which there is a higher concentration of glycolic acid (more than 20%), these effects are more common.

In spite of all the above, glycolic acid is considered a very safe substance for achieving skin peeling in dark-skinned people.

SUMMARY

α-Hydroxy compounds have a beneficial effect on sun-damaged skin. The substances shown to have the greatest benefit in clinical studies in lessening the effects of aging on the skin are α-hydroxy acids and retinoic acid.

19 | β-Hydroxy and Polyhydroxy Acids

Stanley Levy, Avi Shai, and Howard I. Maibach

Contents Overview • Beneficial effects • Adverse effects • Precautions • Other dermatological uses • Polyhydroxy acids • Summary

OVERVIEW

β-Hydroxy acids are simple organic acids, which resemble α-hydroxy acids in their biochemical structure. They can be found, in varying quantities, in certain plants. In the past, β-hydroxy acids were mainly extracted from willow bark. Nowadays, however, the dermatological and cosmetic industries mainly synthesize β-hydroxy acid in laboratories.

Salicylic acid is the most common β-hydroxy acid used in cosmetics. Other types of β-hydroxy acids are trophic acid, β-hydroxybutanoic acid, and trethocanic acid.

Although β-hydroxy acid is, sometimes, presented as being a recent innovation in skin care products, salicylic acid, the most common form of β-hydroxy acid, is actually a traditional compound, which has been used in dermatology for many years.

BENEFICIAL EFFECTS

β-Hydroxy acids are lipid-soluble compounds. This enables them to penetrate deeper into oily skin than α-hydroxy acids, which are water-soluble only. Due to their lipid solubility, β-hydroxy acids can infiltrate deep into skin pores containing sebum and remove excess material that is blocking the outlet of sebaceous glands and hair follicles.

Hence, β-hydroxy acids and their main representative, salicylic acid, are keratolytic, meaning they dissolve and eliminate/remove *keratin*, a protein found in the outermost layer of the skin. As such, β-hydroxy acids can break up the dead top skin cells in thickened skin and loosen cell adhesion in the upper epidermis. Salicylic acid has been used for many years in the treatment of acne, with the objective to remove keratin that occludes the skin pores.

In the cosmetic industry, β-hydroxy acids are used as exfoliants. They dissolve and "unstick" the cells of the upper skin layers, enabling the dead cells to shed themselves from the skin's surface. This causes the young cells in the epidermis to continuously advance upward without being blocked by layers of closely packed cells.

For chemical peeling, salicylic acid can be used alone, in concentrations of up to 30%. It may also be combined with α-hydroxy acids. β-Hydroxy acids are considered to improve the quality of skin texture and reduce fine wrinkling. Following treatment, the skin becomes softer and smoother.

Lower concentrations of β-hydroxy acid, in the form of preparations containing salicylic acid for use on a regular daily basis, can remove dirt and excess oil from the skin's surface but are not expected to achieve the same effect as peeling procedures. Preparations containing salicylic acid are useful for acne patients, since salicylic acid has a prolonged keratolytic effect within skin pores. It can also have an anti-inflammatory effect on acne lesions.

ADVERSE EFFECTS

Skin Irritation

β-Hydroxy acid may induce skin irritation, depending on the concentration used. This can manifest as redness, itching, stinging and, if severe, as burning. On the other hand, since salicylic acid is related chemically to acetylsalicylic acid, namely Aspirin®, it has some anti-inflammatory effect, which may lessen the degree of irritation.

Sun Sensitivity

β-Hydroxy acids are known to increase sun sensitivity. By exfoliating and reducing the thickness of the stratum corneum, the sun can more readily penetrate the skin. For those using preparations containing salicylic acid, it is advisable to take appropriate sun protection measures, including regular application of sunscreens. Some β-hydroxy preparations contain sunscreens as well.

PRECAUTIONS

The accepted precautions of using β-hydroxy acid-containing preparations, as suggested by the FDA, are as follows:

- Any product containing β-hydroxy acids should be tested on a small area of the skin prior to its use on larger areas.
- Should a skin irritation develop, treatment should be discontinued and a physician consulted.
- Products containing β-hydroxy acids should not be applied on the skin of children.
- Sun protection measures should be taken.

> Additional Data
>
> β-Hydroxy acids exert maximal beneficial effect in concentrations of 1% to 2% with a pH of 3 to 4. In most cases, data as to the accurate pH of cosmetic products are not mentioned on the label. It is possible to examine the pH of a product with a test strip. In addition, it is advisable to purchase such products from cosmetic/pharmaceutical companies of repute.

OTHER DERMATOLOGICAL USES

Salicylic acid is currently used in a variety of dermatological problems due to its keratolytic effect. It can be used in the treatment of viral warts and corns, as well as dandruff and scaly skin.

As stated above, salicylic acid in a concentration of 2% is a common over-the-counter product for mild acne. It dissolves keratin and sebum that block the outlets of the pores, preventing the development of comedones and may reduce the degree of inflammation in the lesions.

POLYHYDROXY ACIDS

The polyhydroxy acid group includes compounds such as lactobionic acid, galactose, and gluconolactone. Polyhydroxy acids are water-soluble compounds, which are similar in their biochemical structure to α-hydroxy acids. They function similarly, and due to their water absorbing capacity they can be used as humectants, increasing the moisture level of the skin. Some polyhydroxy acids, such as gluconolactone, have antioxidant properties as well. In the cosmetics industry, they are manufactured as mild exfoliants. They have a much higher molecular weight compared to α-hydroxy acids and, therefore, take longer to penetrate the epidermis and dermis, which reduces the potential for irritation. This feature makes polyhydroxy acids suitable for achieving mild exfoliation in people with sensitive skin, and in those affected by various skin problems such as atopic dermatitis or rosacea.

In view of the above, some practitioners advocate the use of polyhydroxy acids as an alternative to α-hydroxy acids, being able to achieve similar effects with less irritation in individuals with more sensitive skin. These compounds also provide additional moisturizing benefits.

SUMMARY

β-Hydroxy acids are mainly used as exfoliants. As lipid-soluble materials, β-hydroxy acids may be particularly helpful in acne-prone individuals for reducing clogged pores and diminishing areas of excessive skin pigmentation.

As with α-hydroxy acids, they may be available in lower concentrations in skin care products or in higher concentrations (up to 30%) for skin peels. Polyhydroxy acids take longer to penetrate into the skin, in contrast to α-hydroxy acids, and may be used as relatively mild exfoliants.

20 | Bleaching and Bleaching Preparations
Avi Shai, Robert Baran, and Howard I. Maibach

Contents Overview • Skin color and melanin • Which skin lesions are bleaching preparations used for? • General remarks regarding bleaching preparations • Types of bleaching preparations • Other preparations used for bleaching hyperpigmented blotches • Other forms of treatment that can be performed by a physician • Summary

OVERVIEW

Bleaching is used to treat patches of unusually dark skin such as freckles, sun spots, scarring lesions that result from hormonal conditions, and more. The types of bleaching substances are many and varied. In this chapter, we examine the different types of bleaching substances and the types of lesions for which they are appropriate. The first section, however, provides background information on what constitutes skin color and how irregularities can occur.

SKIN COLOR AND MELANIN

Skin color is determined by several factors, the main ones being the following:

- **thickness** of the skin,
- **blood vessels** in the skin, their density and the extent to which they are dilated (the more closely packed and the more dilated the blood vessels are, the redder the skin looks),
- amount of **oxygen in the blood:** a high level of oxygen in the blood makes the skin bright red, while a low level of oxygen gives the skin a bluish coloration,
- presence of **pigments** that may alter skin color, for example, carotene, a substance with a similar chemical structure to vitamin A, gives the skin a yellow tinge. A person who eats an excessive amount of carrots (which contain carotene) will develop a yellowish skin color typical of carotene accumulation, and
- level of **melanin** in the skin.

Of all the above factors, the most significant is melanin, which is produced by special cells in the skin, called **melanocytes**. The amount of melanin produced depends on

- ethnicity (dark-skinned people produce more melanin),
- genetic factors (heredity),
- hormonal factors, and
- exposure to the sun.

Tanning

The production of melanin during exposure to the sun is manifested by **tanning**. To some extent, tanning is a protective mechanism, since melanin provides the skin with natural protection against solar damage. When its level in the skin rises, there is better protection from the sun rays. However, the protection provided to the skin by melanin is inadequate, particularly for fair-skinned people, and repeated exposure to the sun will lead to damage. Some damage appears in the form of dark areas on the skin, of varying shades of brown. (See chapter 10, "Sun and the Skin," for further details).

Some skin problems appear in the form of dark blotches and lesions on the skin, or as uneven distribution of color throughout the skin. The main reason for these problems is the abnormal and nonuniform distribution of melanin in the skin. A **hypopigmented** lesion is an area of skin in which the amount of melanin is reduced, while a **hyperpigmented** lesion is an area of skin in which the amount of melanin is increased. This chapter discusses problems of hyperpigmentation and methods of bleaching them.

Note: This chapter is included because dark, hyperpigmented lesions are common. The reader should be familiar with the range of treatments available. However, the treatment of dark (hyperpigmented) skin blotches and lesions must only be performed by a physician. Sometimes a hyperpigmented lesion is actually a cancer of the skin. Obviously, the treatment then is not merely to bleach the lesion; such a lesion should be removed and examined microscopically. In any case of a dark lesion, the possibility of melanoma should only be ruled out by a physician. Many preparations for bleaching skin lesions exist. It is important that the appropriate and specific preparation be used for each patient according to his/her medical history.

WHICH SKIN LESIONS ARE BLEACHING PREPARATIONS USED FOR?

Freckles

Freckles are those familiar pale-brown spots, usually found in light-skinned people with light hair, or in redheads. They are generally small—approximately 5 mm in diameter. Freckles appear in early childhood, between the ages of two and four years. They commonly occur in areas of skin exposed to the sun: the face (mainly on the nose), the shoulders, and the upper back. In the summer, freckles tend to become darker, while in the winter they tend to become smaller and lighter and may almost disappear.

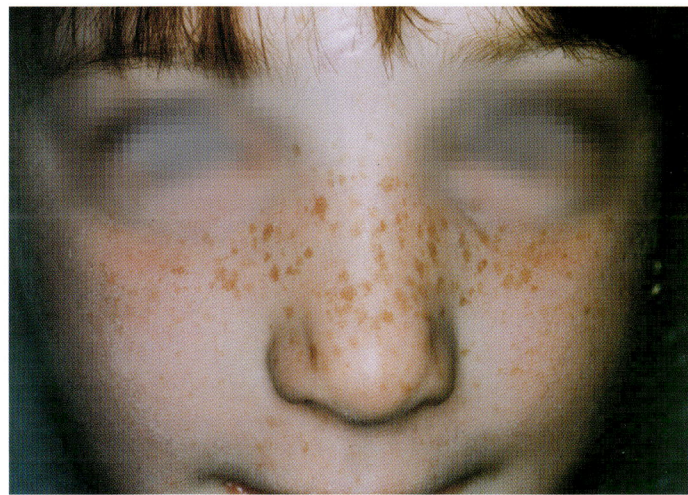

Freckles.

The way to prevent freckles is to avoid excessive exposure to the sun. Some bleaching preparations can bleach freckles to some extent, but these preparations are only partially effective and will not necessarily make the freckles disappear completely.

Sun Spots

The correct scientific name for "sun spots" is **solar lentigines**. Some people call them "liver spots," or "old-age spots," unjustifiably, since the main cause of these lesions is repeated exposure to the sun (and so they appear on exposed areas of the body: the face, the backs of the hands, the upper chest, and the sides of the arms). They are dark spots, ranging from brown to brownish-black. They are usually round or oval, but can be other shapes. Sun spots usually start to appear after the age of 40. They vary in size from a few millimeters to one centimeter. Sometimes, a few spots coalesce, forming a larger lesion. This process usually occurs in skin that has been severely damaged as a result of prolonged exposure to the sun over a number of years. Sun spots are discussed further in chapters 8 and 10, and their treatment is discussed again at the end of this chapter.

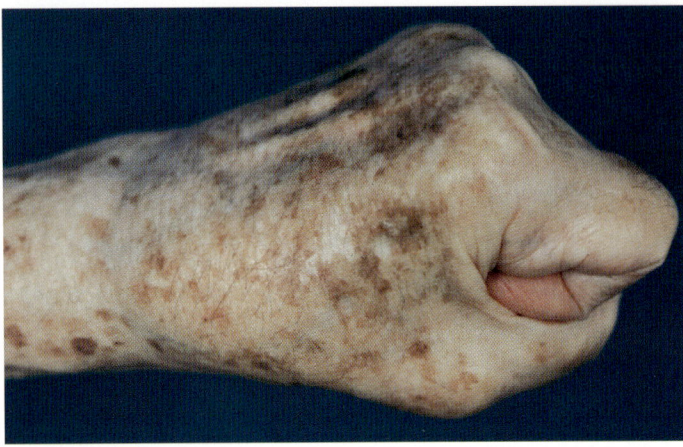

Sun spots on the back of the hand.

Usually, sun spots pose no danger to health but are an aesthetic nuisance that most people would prefer to avoid. Minimizing sun exposure will prevent the occurrence of sun spots or at least diminish the extent of the problem.

Melasma (Chloasma, "Pregnancy Mask")

Melasma is a unique pattern of pigment distribution on the face. It appears mainly in pregnant women, and is often called a "pregnancy mask." In general, there is some accentuation of relatively dark areas of the skin during pregnancy. In its mild form, this phenomenon appears as a darkening of the areola (the area around the nipples). In its more severe form, with involvement of the face, it is called melasma (or chloasma).

Melasma is characterized by the appearance of light to dark brown areas of skin on the face, usually symmetrically distributed. It usually occurs on the upper lip, forehead, and chin. It appears as a result of a hormonal process that is not yet understood.

Although melasma appears mainly during pregnancy, it can also occur in women following the use of contraceptives, or certain other hormonal preparations. Sometimes melasma becomes more prominent before the menstrual period. In many women, it appears for no apparent reason.

When melasma is related to pregnancy, the lesions usually become lighter in the months following the pregnancy.

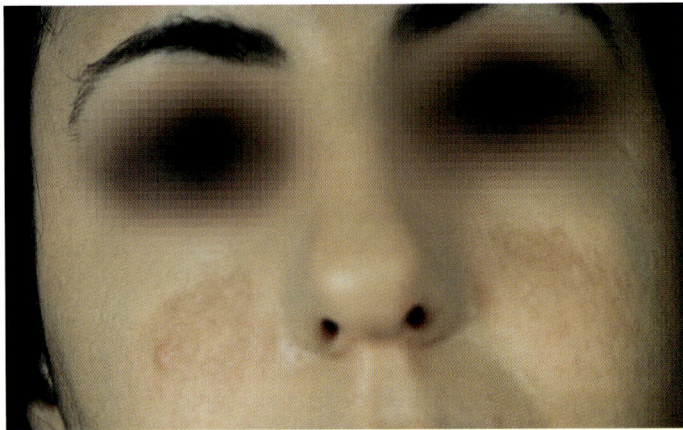

Melasma.

Note: Before using bleaching preparations for melasma, there are two essential steps to be taken:

- minimize sun exposure, and
- consult a dermatologist regarding certain hormonal or other medications that can cause or aggravate the melasma.

Postinflammatory Pigmented Lesions

Hyperpigmented areas of skin may appear following some types of skin inflammation, such as:

- acne,
- contact dermatitis, and
- trauma or burns to the skin.

In these cases, treatment with a bleaching agent is of limited value, since the pigment has "sunk" into the deeper layers of the skin. The earlier the treatment is started following the initial affliction to the skin, the better the chances are for improvement.

> **Berloque Dermatitis**
>
> A unique form of pigmentation of the skin is seen in the skin inflammation known as **berloque dermatitis**. The pigmented area is irregular in shape; the common sites of occurrence are on the sides of the neck, behind the ears, and on the cheeks. The problem occurs as a result of the use of perfumes and aftershave lotion. These preparations contain substances called **furocoumarins**. The application of these compounds, combined with exposure to the sun, results in the pigmented areas of berloque dermatitis. In this condition, skin lesions appear as dark-toned irregular blotches. These compounds do not cause any damage if the skin is not exposed to the sun.

GENERAL REMARKS REGARDING BLEACHING PREPARATIONS

Most cosmetic problems leading to hyperpigmentation are related to sun exposure. Therefore, when using bleaching preparations, the sun should be avoided as much as possible. If it is impossible to totally prevent exposure to the sun, it is worthwhile using a sunscreen when outdoors (some bleaching preparations already incorporate a sunscreen). In many cases, dermatologists advise using the bleaching agents nightly, while applying sunscreens on the affected areas of skin during the day.

When starting the use of any bleaching preparation, it should be applied to a small area of the hyperpigmented area. If no redness and/or irritation occurs thereafter say, up to 24 hours, the preparation may be applied onto the whole affected area.

Bleaching preparations are meant to be applied only to the hyperpigmented areas of the skin. There is obviously no point in bleaching the normal skin adjacent to the hyperpigmented area. If the distribution of the hyperpigmented blotches is such that it is impossible to apply the preparation without some of it getting onto the normal skin, a dermatologist should be consulted. The dermatologist may be able to suggest a more effective form of treatment, aimed only at the pigmented areas (see below).

It could take months before any improvement in the skin can be discerned. The efficacy of a bleaching preparation and its rapidity of action depends on the nature of the active ingredients it contains, and the type of lesion being treated.

More than one bleaching agent can be used for any given lesion. For example, hyperpigmented blotches may be treated with two different preparations—one to be used in the morning, and a different one for nighttime. The rationale of this approach is that different preparations exert their bleaching effect by different mechanisms. In addition, this approach provides a complementary treatment in cases where one of the preparations (such as retinoic acid) cannot be used during daylight. Furthermore, a mixture of preparations containing more than one active ingredient may be used. A common combination used by dermatologists, for example, is composed of **hydroquinone and retinoic acid**.

Bleaching agents should not be used on areas of skin that have been sunburnt. They should not be used on skin which is dry, irritated, or inflamed. One should wait until such conditions have normalized before using any kind of a bleaching preparation. It is advisable that all these treatments, including those which do not necessarily require a prescription, be performed only under a physician's instructions.

TYPES OF BLEACHING PREPARATIONS

Hydroquinone

Hydroquinone is a well-accepted agent for bleaching hyperpigmented lesions. It slows down and prevents the production of melanin in the skin. Commercial products containing hydroquinone are available in the United States in concentrations of up to 4%. In concentrations up to 2%, it can be purchased over-the-counter. At the moment, this policy is under review by the FDA. Products based on hydroquinone in concentrations of 4% or more can only be purchased with a doctor's prescription. In some cases, doctors may prescribe preparations containing up to 10% hydroquinone, and sometimes more. However, at concentrations above 5%, there is an increased risk of skin irritation, manifested by reddening and itching of the skin and a burning sensation.

In countries of the European Union, hydroquinone is no longer permitted to be purchased over-the-counter. It is available on prescription only.

Mode of Use

The preparation should be applied twice a day—in the morning and before retiring to bed. The hydroquinone may be combined with a sunscreen agent. Some physicians advise applying hydroquinone before bedtime and using a sunscreen during the day. After the skin has been cleaned and dried out, a thin film of the preparation should be applied.

The preparation may be based on hydroquinone alone, or on a combination of hydroquinone and other bleaching agents or with corticosteroid compounds.

In melasma, concentrations of hydroquinone up to 10% may be used. It would be advisable to keep on with a maintenance treatment once weekly, for approximately two years after the melasma has faded.

Efficacy

Following at least several weeks of treatment, one can usually discern some bleaching of the lesions. The use of hydroquinone-based preparations results in an improvement for 70% to 80% of patients. After four to five months of its use, further improvement is not expected to occur. It is advisable to discontinue the use of hydroquinone if no improvement has been noted following this time. Once the affected skin has faded to the desired shade, the preparation should be discontinued, but sunscreen still applied. In some cases, the bleaching effect may be only temporary, and after some time without treatment, the skin may darken again to its original shade. In this case, the following options should be considered by the physician:

- the use of a preparation with a higher concentration of hydroquinone, or
- combining hydroquinone with other bleaching agents (this is usually the preferred option).

Adverse Effects and Precautions

Hydroquinone may tint the nails orange. Contact with the nails should be avoided while using hydroquinone.

Not commonly, one may notice irritation of the skin following the use of hydroquinone, with itching and redness. In such cases, the treatment should be discontinued and a physician consulted.

Hydroquinone should neither be used by pregnant women nor by women who could become pregnant during treatment. It is also advisable to avoid its use in breast-feeding women.

Ochronosis

Ochronosis is a relatively rare adverse effect of hydroquinone. It is mainly described in dark-skinned people who have been using high concentrations of hydroquinone for some years, but it has also been documented following its use in low concentrations. Ochronosis is manifested by an increasing darkening of the skin areas that have been treated by a hydroquinone preparation.

> Examples of Preparations Containing Hydroquinone, in Various Countries
> - Alphaquin HP®
> - Eldopaque®
> - Eldoquin®
> - Esomed®
> - Esoterica®
> - Melanex®
> - Lustra®
> - Melpaque®
> - Viquin Forte®

Kligman Formula

Kligman formula is a well-known preparation that combines certain compounds intended to bleach pigmented lesions. The original formula contains 5% hydroquinone, 0.1% retinoic acid, and 0.1% dexamethasone in an ointment base.

> **Hydroquinone Monobenzyl Ether (HMBE)**
>
> Hydroquinone monobenzyl ether (HMBE) is chemically similar to hydroquinone, but when applied to the skin, the effect cannot be controlled. For example, the bleaching may occur in areas away from where it was applied, and the bleaching effect can continue for several months or more after the patient has stopped using the products. **Therefore, this agent is not to be used for bleaching dark, hyperpigmented skin lesions.**
>
> The only use for HMBE is in the disease known as **vitiligo**, where the condition is widespread over large areas of skin. In vitiligo, hypopigmented white blotches appear on the skin for reasons that are not clear. In vitiligo, there is a defect in the function of the immunological system that interferes with the formation of skin pigment. Since the white blotches in vitiligo cannot be darkened, the only way to achieve a more or less uniform skin color is to bleach unaffected (normal) areas of skin using HMBE. The entire skin becomes hypopigmented, becoming all the same color. Obviously, this treatment requires close medical supervision.

Retinoic Acid

The effect of retinoic acid on aging of the skin and on acne lesions has been described and explained in chapters 8, 9, and 17. This substance, alone or combined with other products, has some effect on bleaching dark, hyperpigmented skin blotches. Preparations based on retinoic acid are available (by prescription only) in concentrations of 0.025%, 0.05%, and 0.1%.

> Examples of Preparations Containing Retinoic Acid, in Various Countries
> - Airol®
> - Avita®
> - Locacid®
> - Renova®
> - Retin-A®
> - Retisol-A®
> - Vesanoid®

Azelaic Acid

Azelaic acid is said to inhibit the production of melanin in the skin; it can therefore be considered for bleaching hyperpigmented skin lesions. Preparations containing azelaic acid are usually available in concentrations up to 20% in various countries, and are applied twice daily for several months. There are conflicting reports as to its efficacy in melasma compared with hydroquinone. This compound is also used for treating acne. It may only be prescribed by a physician.

α-Hydroxy Acid

α-Hydroxy acid has some effect on bleaching skin and bleaching hyperpigmented skin lesions. In the past, skin-bleaching properties were attributed to extracts of certain fruits and vegetables (particularly cucumbers, lemons, and strawberries). If indeed there is some bleaching of dark skin following the use of fruit and vegetable extracts, it may be due to the presence of α-hydroxy acids in these extracts.

Combining α-hydroxy acids with other bleaching agents may be considered. It has been shown that the addition of glycolic acid, an α-hydroxy acid derived from sugar cane, may increase the depth of penetration of hydroquinone into the skin. α-Hydroxy acids are dealt with in more detail in chapter 18.

Glabridin

Two decades ago, scientists in Japan identified a certain chemical constituent in liquorice extracts as being an efficient bleaching agent. Since then, **glabridin** has been used in various bleaching preparations. Preparations containing glabridin are considered to be cosmetics and do not require a physician's prescription.

Kojic Acid

Kojic acid is a substance derived from yeast and prevents the production of melanin in the skin. It was originally developed by the Japanese cosmetics industry and subsequently appeared in other parts of the world.

OTHER PREPARATIONS USED FOR BLEACHING HYPERPIGMENTED BLOTCHES

Additional compounds for bleaching of dark skin blotches have recently emerged from the cosmetic industry, but because these are relatively new, it is still difficult to assess their efficacy. It can be assumed that those found to be effective will, in time, join the list of preparations available today.

New compounds used as bleaching agents are extracted from various plants, such as *Catharanthus roseus*, *Chamomilla recutita*, *Theaceae* (green tea), and soy. **Arbutin** is another bleaching compound extracted from *Arctostaphylos uva orsi* (bearberry). In addition, certain derivates of vitamin C have been shown to lighten pigmented areas. Hence, vitamin C can be found in certain bleaching preparations.

Two other compounds that have been introduced recently are **boldine diacetyl**, extracted from the bark of Chilean boldo tree, and **phenylalanine undecylenoyl**. Further research studies are required to assess their efficacy as compared to standard skin-lightening agents and the anticipated outcome of various combinations.

Decades ago, the accepted treatment for bleaching skin lesions included products containing mercury salts. Their use is now prohibited because of their potential adverse effects—these substances are highly toxic. Hydrogen peroxide can also bleach melanin by oxidizing it, but it is not usually used for the bleaching of skin, since it may cause skin irritation. The main use of hydrogen peroxide is for bleaching hair.

OTHER FORMS OF TREATMENT THAT CAN BE PERFORMED BY A PHYSICIAN

Dermatologists may use other chemical and physical treatments. These treatments may, in many cases, be more effective than the treatments described hitherto, depending on the nature of the skin problem. Of the many treatments in use are:

- freezing using liquid nitrogen,
- laser (or light) treatment,
- local peeling with trichloroacetic acid, and
- local peeling with α-hydroxy acids.

The dermatologist decides which particular form of treatment to use for which lesion and hyperpigmented area, depending on the type of skin problem and the medical background of the patient. Take, for example, sun spots, as described earlier in the chapter (see picture on page 160). Because of the distribution of these small, isolated spots on the back of the hand, on a background of large areas of normal skin, the treatment of choice would seem to be to treat each pigmented spot separately by one of the four possibilities mentioned above. These treatments are often preferable to the long-term application of skin-bleaching substances to the back of the hand which, in fact, is mostly made up of normal-colored skin.

Note: Many dermatologists prefer to avoid spraying and freezing pigmented spots by liquid nitrogen in the case of "solar lentigines." Although it may benefit many patients, in some cases, the lesion may later on regain its dark color, making it unresponsive to any bleaching treatments thereafter.

Skin-peeling treatments may also be effective in the treatment of dark blotches. The degree of improvement depends mainly on the depth of the peeling, the peeling preparation used, the type of skin lesion, and the extent of its pigmentation. Chemical peeling of skin is discussed in detail in chapter 24.

SUMMARY

Dark lesions of the skin are known in medical terminology as hyperpigmented lesions, and may include freckles, sun spots, the pregnancy mask, and other lesions. Various substances are used in the treatment of hyperpigmented skin lesions: hydroquinone, retinoic acid, α-hydroxy acids, liquorice extract (glabridin), and kojic acid among others. Each substance can be used separately or can be combined with other substances, for example, with one being used in the morning and another in the evening.

Whenever hyperpigmented lesions appear on the skin, the patient must minimize exposure to the sun and consult a dermatologist.

21 | Astringents
Avi Shai, Robert Baran, and Howard I. Maibach

Contents Astringents and their use • Composition of astringents • Comments

ASTRINGENTS AND THEIR USE

Astringents are used to give the skin a taut, cool, refreshing feeling, to temporarily constrict the skin pores and to remove the outer layer of oil from the skin. Astringents have other names in the cosmetics industry. They are also called, for example, "skin tonics," or "skin toners." They usually come as solutions, although some are in the form of gels.

Astringents are applied following skin cleansing. The commonest form of astringent, as a cosmetic, is in aftershave products.

Note: Not all the claims made about astringents have been tested scientifically. The question of how beneficial they really are for the skin is unanswered. We assume that their benefit to the skin varies depending on the nature of the specific product and the type of skin it is used upon.

COMPOSITION OF ASTRINGENTS

Astringents are solutions containing a mixture of **alcohol** and **water** in various proportions. Astringents for use on dry skin should contain minimal concentrations of alcohol (which tends to dry out the skin). For very dry skin, astringent-containing moisturizers should be used. On the other hand, astringents for use on oily skin have a higher concentration of alcohol.

Astringents usually contain **aluminum** or **zinc salts**, which are said to constrict the pores. This effect has not been tested scientifically. Should it be correct, there may well be some advantage to constricting the pores following cleansing of the face, in order to prevent the entry of dirt, particles of soot and dust into the pores.

Astringent solutions generally contain substances that cool and refresh, such as **menthol** or **camphor**. These substances have some kind of a "medical" fragrance about them. Alcohol also gives a feeling of coolness because of its rapid evaporation from the skin. The solutions may also contain **dyes** and **fragrances.**

Sometimes **"exotic" ingredients**, derived from plants, that give the skin a taut, fresh, and cool feeling, may be included. Witch hazel extract, for example, is derived from the leaves of the *Hamamelis virginiana* tree, found in North America. This extract has anti-inflammatory properties. Because of its reputed astringent properties, it is a common ingredient in astringents and aftershave preparations. Other plants whose extracts are said to have astringent effects include species of oak (*Quercus*), where an extract is produced from its bark, or *Tilia*, where the extract is derived from the flowers.

COMMENTS

The use of astringents following cleansing of the face once had an additional purpose—they helped to remove soap remnants left on the skin. Nowadays, with the increasing use of modern soaps ("soapless" soaps), rinsing the face with water is usually sufficient to remove any residual soap completely, so that this function of the astringent is unnecessary.

Aftershave preparations are made of the same substances as are astringents; they also contain water and alcohol. The assumption is that even the low concentration of alcohol present in an aftershave has some antiseptic effect, which is helpful in dealing with tiny cuts or abrasions in the skin (some of them not even visible or felt) that occur during shaving. Again here, zinc or aluminum salts in the product are said to constrict the skin pores that were dilated following rinsing of the face with warm water. Aftershave lotions give a feeling of freshness and coolness—usually due to the addition of menthol. With regard to aftershave preparations, the only real difference between the various brands is the unique scent of each one. The practical value of astringents is controversial. It has not yet been shown in the medical literature that they indeed have any beneficial effect.

22 | Preparations Used in Dermatology
Marcelo H. Grunwald

Contents Overview • Antibiotics • Antifungal agents • Antiseptics • Preparations containing corticosteroids

Note: This chapter provides information about commonly used preparations. It is not intended that anyone unauthorized should treat him/herself or anybody else on the basis of the information in this chapter. In any case of skin disease, a physician should be consulted.

OVERVIEW

In the average family medicine cabinet, one can usually find remnants of various substances widely used in dermatology. Too often, people try to treat skin lesions with these preparations without appropriate knowledge. Treatment with an incorrect preparation may aggravate the skin problem. It may even make it difficult for the physician to arrive at an appropriate diagnosis and treat the patient correctly. For example, using a cream containing a corticosteroid to treat a skin lesion that is caused by a fungus will mask and alter its clinical appearance so that even an experienced physician may not be able to diagnose the problem correctly. In this chapter, we limit our discussion to those agents that are the most widely used, such as preparations containing:

- antibiotics,
- antifungal agents,
- antiseptics, and
- corticosteroids.

These types of substances are familiar to most of us. They also happen to be the substances that are statistically the most misused ones.

ANTIBIOTICS

Antibiotics are active against bacteria. These medications can kill bacteria or inhibit their growth. Traditionally, antibiotics are produced from various bacteria or certain fungi (moulds). However, nowadays, the term "antibiotics" also includes synthetically manufactured antibacterial agents such as *sulfonamides* and *quinolones*.

Antibiotics work in various ways. Commonly, their activity is accomplished by damaging and breaking the cell walls of the bacteria; these are given orally (tablets, capsules, syrups), injected into a muscle, or given intravenously (infused into a vein).

Antibiotics for use on the skin are usually in the form of solutions, creams, or ointments. They are used for skin lesions infected by bacteria. The following are some examples of antibiotic agents for application to the skin:

bacitracin	fusidic acid	neomycin
chloramphenicol	gentamicin	oxytetracycline
chlortetracycline	mupirocin	tetracycline

For antibiotics used in the treatment of acne, see chapter 9.

ANTIFUNGAL AGENTS

The substances listed here are for the treatment of skin infections caused by fungi. The most common mode of action of these antifungal agents is to interfere with the production of substances that the fungus needs to build its cell walls. As a result, the cell walls develop "holes" which stop the growth of the fungus and eventually leads to its death. Antifungal agents are divided into several groups, depending on their chemical composition:

- Substances made up of compounds from the **imidazole group:**

  bifonazole   isoconazole
  clotrimazole ketoconazole
  econazole   miconazole

- Substances in which the active ingredient is **ciclopiroxolamine**
- Other agents:

  nystatin   tolnaftate
  terbinafine zinc undecylenate

These antifungal agents may be applied in the form of a solution, a cream, a shampoo, a powder, or another form, depending on the region to be treated.

There are combinations of substances that contain corticosteroids or antibiotics in addition to the antifungal agent. These are used in cases where there is both a fungal and a bacterial infection, and the fungal infection has caused severe inflammation of the skin, for which the use of an agent containing a steroid may be advisable.

Certain skin diseases may produce a clinical picture suggestive of a fungal infection. Inappropriate use of antifungal agents on a skin lesion that is not necessarily a fungal infection may aggravate the condition. In spite of the fact that some of the substances listed above can be purchased without a physician's prescription, it is advisable to use them only on a physician's advice.

ANTISEPTICS

Antiseptics are substances that kill or inhibit the growth of bacteria and other microorganisms. They are produced synthetically. The reason we categorize between antibiotics and antiseptics is due to their differing mechanisms of actions. Antibiotics act against bacteria by using a specific mode of action, unique to each class of antibiotics. In contrast, antiseptics are nonselective. They damage any living tissue. The damage may be not limited to the offending bacteria, but may be directed toward human cells as well.

Types of Antiseptics

Antiseptics for Handwashing and Disinfecting the Skin Before Medical Treatment
Antiseptics for handwashing and disinfecting the skin before medical treatment include:

- hexachlorophene,
- chlorhexidine, and
- high-concentration alcohol solutions.

High-concentration alcohol solutions have very effective antiseptic properties. Consequently, alcohol solutions are widely used in cosmetic clinics, medical clinics and hospitals. Alcohol in a concentration of 70% is used to disinfect the skin prior to medical procedures. In addition, medical instruments are disinfected by being soaked in concentrated solutions of alcohol.

Note: Certain cleansing agents in high concentrations can also kill bacteria effectively, for example, quaternary ammonium compounds, which belong to the cationic surfactant group. **Cetrimide**, which belongs to this group, in low concentrations is a component of hair shampoos and in higher concentrations a potent antiseptic used mainly for disinfecting medical instruments.

Antiseptic Agents for Treating Infected Areas of Skin
These antiseptics are used in the form of solutions, in which the active ingredient is present in low concentrations, for example, solutions of **potassium permanganate** or solutions based on **chlorine.** Weak solutions of potassium permanganate are pink/purple in color. They are used

for infected areas of skin, particularly weeping skin, such as an infection on a limb, whereby the limb can be soaked in a potassium permanganate solution for several minutes, two to three times a day.

Another method of treating infected weeping skin is by wetting the area repeatedly. For this, a cotton cloth soaked in the antiseptic solution is placed on the infected area for a few minutes, two or three times a day. Diluted chlorine solutions can also be used for this purpose.

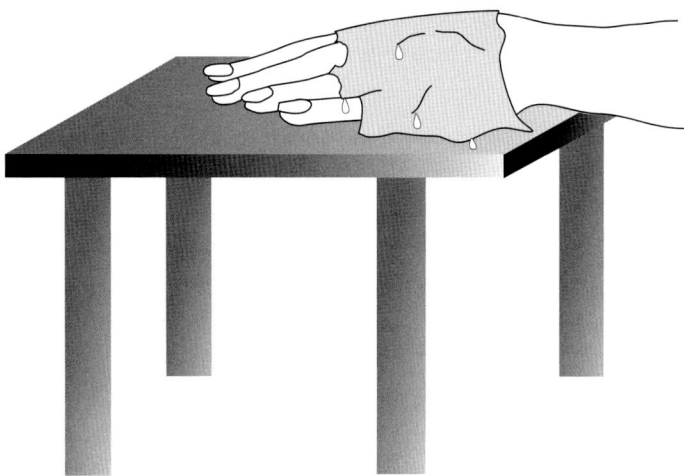

Wetting infected skin with a cotton cloth soaked in a solution of potassium permanganate.

Hydrogen Peroxide

Hydrogen peroxide is a strong antiseptic, which comes as dilute solutions in water. Because hydrogen peroxide itself can damage body tissues, it is not normally used as a disinfectant. Hydrogen peroxide is also used to bleach hair.

Iodine-Based Solutions

It is not clear exactly how iodine kills bacteria and other microorganisms, but it is effective and rapid in its action. It is available in the following forms:

- **Iodoform** is a compound that releases iodine and has a relatively weak antibacterial effect.
- **Povidone iodine** is a mixture of iodine with a polymer that releases the iodine slowly. It is available as a powder, an ointment, or a yellowish-brown lotion. Povidone iodine compounds are used for the treatment of infected areas of skin. In liquid form, they are also used as antiseptic preparations prior to medical procedures. Before use, it is advisable to determine whether the preparation about to be used contains alcohol. If it does, it should not be used on an open wound, since it may cause a severe burning sensation and, to a certain extent, may lead to tissue damage. Povidone iodine compounds that contain alcohol are best reserved for use as antiseptic preparations prior to medical procedures.
- **Tincture of iodine** is based on iodine diluted with alcohol and is used for the same purposes as povidone iodine.

Synthetic Dyes

Synthetic dyes include **gentian violet** and **brilliant green**. These synthetic dyes were formerly used as antibacterial preparations. They have since been replaced by the newer substances already discussed.

PREPARATIONS CONTAINING CORTICOSTEROIDS

Steroids (or **corticosteroids** or **glucocorticoids**) is the general name given to a group of hormones that is produced naturally in the body. Among their many important functions is their anti-inflammatory activity, which is why they are widely used in dermatological preparations for the treatment of various inflammatory disorders of the skin.

Corticosteroids may be given orally, or injected into a muscle or a vein. In addition, corticosteroid preparations can be applied to an affected area of skin. As stated, dermatologists have available a wide range of preparations that contain corticosteroids of varying degrees of potency, which can be selected depending on the intensity of the skin inflammation.

In dermatology, topical corticosteroids are used for allergic skin diseases, as well as non-allergic diseases (e.g., psoriasis). They can also be used in order to alleviate the inflammatory response that accompanies certain medical conditions, such as fungal infections.

What is the Fingertip Unit?

The term "finger tip unit" was coined in the 1990s. It is a practical way to clarify the amount of ointment or cream needed to be applied on a specific skin area. The assumption is that the preparation is applied evenly, in a thin layer, in an amount sufficient to cover the whole area to be treated. Using the accurate amount is highly important for certain medications, particularly with topical steroids.

One finger tip unit is defined as the amount of cream or ointment needed to cover the tip of the index finger, from the skin crease up to the the end of the finger, if the preparation is squeezed out of a tube with a 5-mm diameter opening. The average amount is approximately 0.5 g in adult males and 0.4 g in adult females. In infants of up to one year, the amount is approximately 25% of that of an adult.

The amount of preparation (cream or ointment) needed to be applied varies according to the area of skin surface. For example, for one hand one fingertip unit is required. Face and neck require 2.5 fingertip units. For one arm one should use around three fingertip units.

Topical corticosteroids can produce unwanted side effects, particularly if used for long periods of time. Side effects on the skin include the following:

- The skin may become thin and fragile, the medical term for which is skin **atrophy**.
- Small areas of bleeding within the skin can appear, the medical term for which is **purpura**.
- Acne may appear as a result of prolonged corticosteroid usage called **steroid acne**.
- A network of fine blood vessels may appear on the skin, referred to as **telangiectases** (sometimes called "couperose").
- There may be an increase in the amount of hair in the steroid-treated area, the medical term for which is **hirsutism**.

In addition, prolonged use of corticosteroids reduces the skin's ability to heal wounds. It also makes the skin more susceptible to various kinds of skin infections. Note that when large areas of skin are treated with corticosteroids (especially when a high-potency steroid is used), they may be absorbed through the skin into the blood and, as a result, may have an unwanted systemic effect.

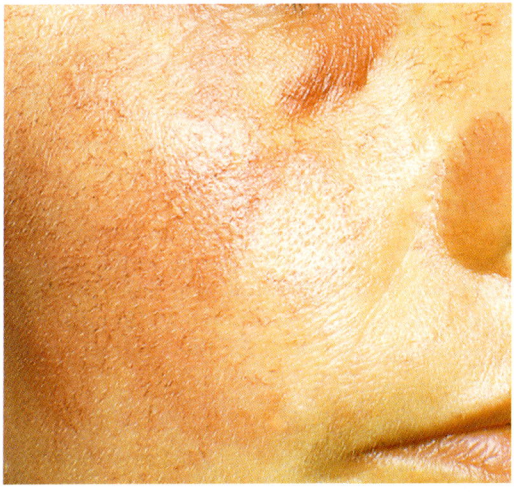

Purpura and telangiectasia following prolonged use of steroidal preparations.

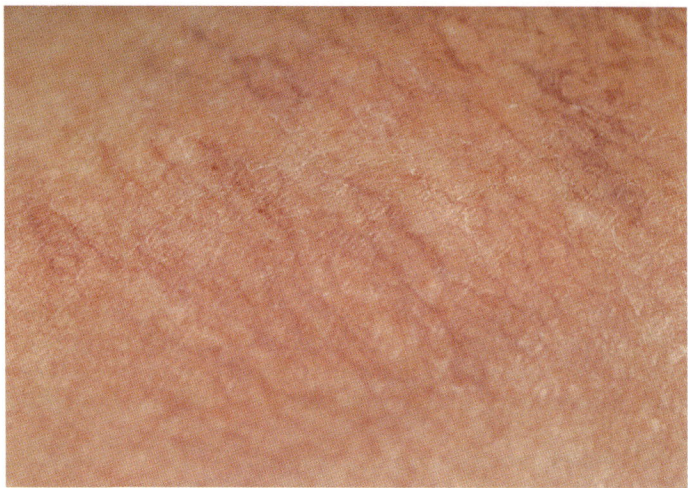

Telangiectasia following prolonged use of steroidal preparations.

> **What is the "Rebound Effect"?**
>
> Skin disorders that have improved with topical corticosteroid therapy may worsen when treatment is discontinued abruptly. This phenomenon in known as the rebound effect. In order to prevent the likelihood of a rebound effect, doctors usually advise patients in whom clinical improvement has occurred, to gradually taper off the frequency of steroid application, rather than to discontinue treatment suddenly. Alternatively, in an advanced stage of therapy, a steroid preparation less potent than those initially applied may be used.

Because of these potential side effects, corticosteroids should not be used indiscriminately or without medical consultation. In many countries, including the United States and the United Kingdom, only preparations that contain a low concentration of hydrocortisone (0.5% to 1%) may be purchased over-the-counter. Other corticosteroid preparations are available by prescription only. The duration of the treatment must be determined by the physician, and steroids must never be used for longer than the recommended period. Furthermore, corticosteroid-containing preparations should not be overused on the face, even with a relatively mild steroid.

As stated earlier, there is a variety of corticosteroid preparations with different strengths. The main factors determining the strength are the type of steroid used, and its concentration. However, there are other factors involved, such as the nature of the preparation itself; thus, for example, an ointment is more potent than a cream containing the same corticosteroid. Similarly, given the same topical corticosteroid, it would be more potent when incorporated into a cream, compared to lotions or solutions.

In the following table, the preparations are divided into seven degrees of potency. Class I includes the "very potent" preparations, while Class VII includes the "mild" preparations. The use of any of these substances, regardless of class, requires a dermatologist's advice. This is especially important in two cases: (1) when they are applied to the face and (2) when treating children (and especially babies), since they are more prone to the adverse effects of corticosteroids. This is highly significant when large areas of skin are treated. In such cases, it is advisable to (1) use a topical corticosteroid of lowest potency; (2) apply the minimal amount of topical preparation; and (3) maintain treatment for the shortest period possible.

	Generic Name	Type of Preparation	Examples of Brand Names
Class I			
	Clobetasol propionate 0.05%	Cream/ointment/lotion	Dermovate
		Cream/ointment/scalp application	Temovate
	Halobetasol propionate 0.05%	Ointment	Ultravate
	Betamethasone dipropionate 0.05%	Ointment	Dicorten
		Ointment	Diprolene
Class II			
	Betamethasone dipropionate 0.05%	Cream	Diprolene
		Ointment/cream	Diprosone
	Fluocinonide 0.05%	Cream	Fluonex
			Lidex
	Halcinonide 0.1%	Cream	Halciderm
		Cream	Halog
		Cream	Halog-E
	Deoximetasone 0.25%	Ointment/cream	Topicort
Class III			
	Betamethasone propionate 0.05%	Lotion/ointment/cream	Diprosone
	Triamcinolone acetonide 0.5%	Cream	Aristocort
	Amcinonide 0.1%	Cream/lotion	Cyclocort
	Fluocinonide 0.05%	Cream	Lidex E
	Diflorasone diacetate 0.05%	Cream	Maxiflor
		Ointment	Florone E
	Mometasone furoate 0.1%	Ointment	Elocon
			Elocom
Class IV			
	Triamcinolone acetonide 0.1%	Ointment	Aristocort
		Cream/lotion	Kenalog
	Mometasone furoate 0.1%	Cream	Elocon
			Elocom
	Fluocinolone acetonide 0.2%	Ointment	Synalar HP
	Desoximetasone 0.05%	Cream	Topicort LP
	Betamethasone valerate 0.1%	Ointment	Betnovate
			Betacorten
Class V			
	Betamethasone valerate 0.1%	Cream/lotion	Betatrex
			Valisone
			Betnovate
			Betacorten
	Betamethasone benzoate 0.025%	Ointment	UtiCort
	Fluticasone propionate 0.1%	Cream	Cutivate
	Fluocinolone acetonide 0.025%	Ointment	Synalar
	Hydrocortisone butirate 0.1%	Ointment	Locoid
Class VI			
	Triamcinolone acetonide 0.1%	Cream	Aristocort
	Triamcinolone acetonide 0.025%	Lotion	Kenalog
	Fluocinolone acetonide 0.01%	Solution	Synalar
	Desonide 0.05%	Cream	Tridesilon
	Betamethasone valerate 0.1%	Lotion	Valisone

(continued)

	Generic Name	Type of Preparation	Examples of Brand Names
Class VII			
	Various preparations containing hydrocortisone in concentrations of 0.25%, 0.5%, or 1%	Cream/lotion/ointment	Alphaderm Anusol HC Bactine HC Caldecort Cetacort Cortaid CortoDome Dermacort Eldecort Hytone Lacticare HC Lanacort Nutracort PeneCort SyneCort TexaCort

This table is reproduced courtesy of Dr Alex Zvulunov.

Classes of topical corticosteroids according to their potencies.

23 | Liposomes
Alex Zvulunov

Contents Background • Structure of cell membranes: phospholipids • What are liposomes? • Basis for the use of liposomes • What substances do liposomes contain? • Are liposomes effective? • Additional possible benefits of liposomes • Conclusion

BACKGROUND

The term **liposome** has become popular in the area of cosmetics. In many cases, a sales person at a cosmetics counter will advise her customers to purchase a certain product claiming that, "it contains liposomes."

To understand what liposomes are, we clarify some basic concepts about how substances penetrate the skin. The main barrier to the passage of substances from the exterior into the epidermis is the keratinous (horny) layer. These outer cells are arranged in compact layers and contain large amounts of horny matter. Liposomes are used in an attempt to create a new method for transferring active products into the epidermis and dermis.

> Penetration of Substances into the Skin
>
> The major factor that determines the penetrating ability of substances into the skin is the **molecule size**. Beyond a certain size, molecules cannot penetrate the skin—only relatively small molecules can do so. For example, collagen, which is present in many cosmetic products, has relatively large molecules that cannot penetrate the skin.
>
> In addition, oily products tend to penetrate the skin more easily than water-based preparations. Substances with better oil solubility can penetrate better into the skin.

STRUCTURE OF CELL MEMBRANES: PHOSPHOLIPIDS

The external membranes of the cells, including skin cells, are made up of phospholipids, polysaccharides, and various proteins. **Phospholipids** are fatty compounds containing phosphorus. They form the cell membrane as a two-layered structure.

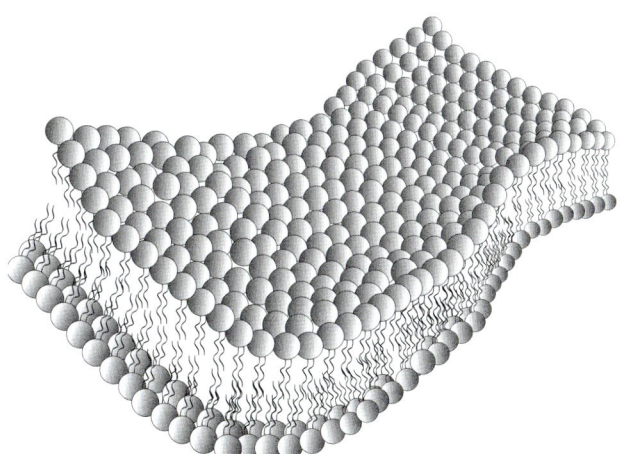

The cell membrane is formed of two layers of phospholipids.

This structural organization prevents the passage of unwanted substances into, or out of, the cell, and allows it to regulate the entry and exit of various substances.

WHAT ARE LIPOSOMES?

Liposomes are spherical vesicles, with a water-filled center. Their diameter is measured in micrometers (microns, i.e., several thousandths of a millimeter). The membranes that form the spherical structure are composed of one or numerous layers.

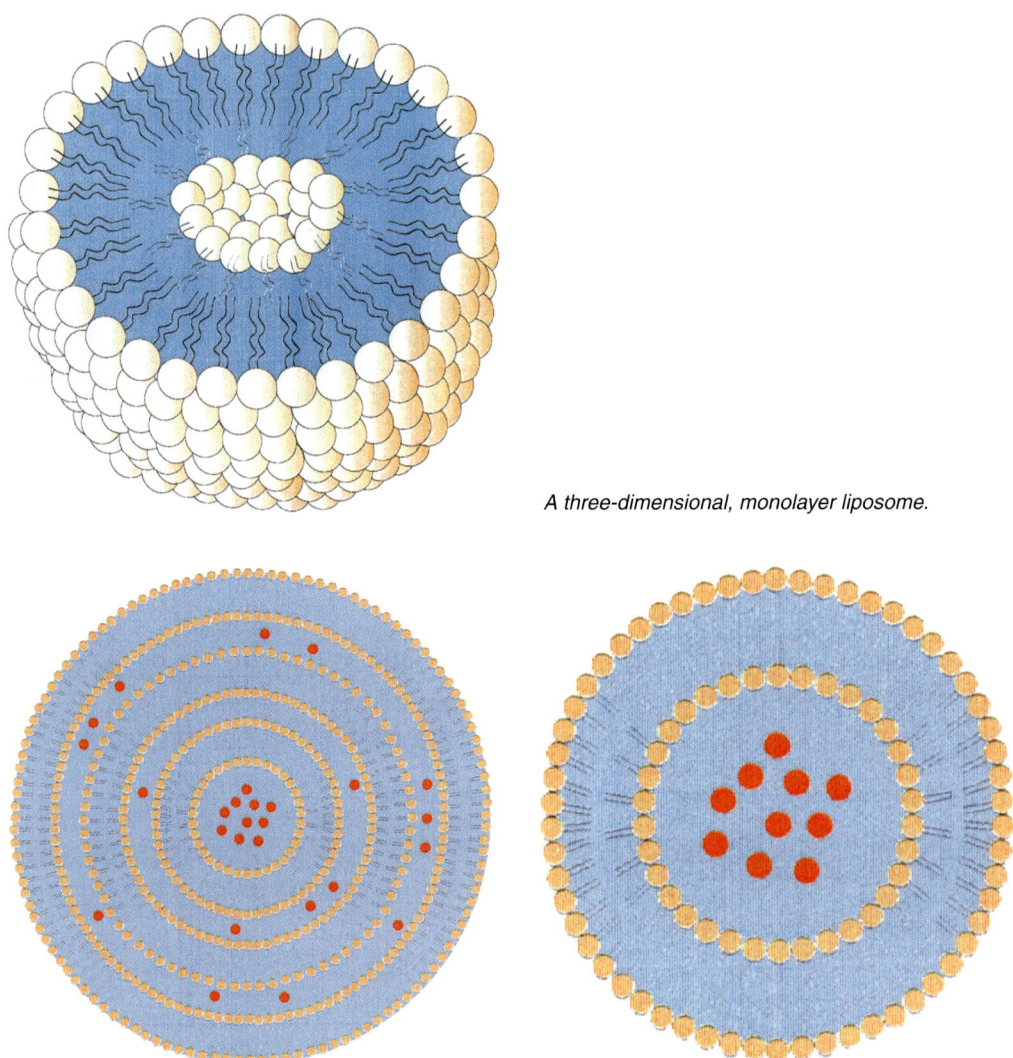

A three-dimensional, monolayer liposome.

*Various medications (marked in red) can be inserted into liposome vesicles. Liposomes can be **unilamellar** (composed of one layer) or **multilamellar** (many-layered).*

BASIS FOR THE USE OF LIPOSOMES

The basic idea of using liposomes derives from the fact that the cell membranes of the body (including the skin, of course) are composed of phospholipids. Therefore, a small spherical liposome itself composed of phospholipids can serve as a carrier for active substances. Substances, such as medications, can be inserted into liposomes. An active product can be inserted to the liposome's core, or it can be anchored to the membrane surface.

In practical terms, it is not yet clear how this transport is achieved. One possible mechanism of transport and delivery would be fusing of the liposome membrane with the cell membrane, thereby allowing penetration into a skin cell. It is not clear whether this hypothetical mechanism is true. Most studies show that liposomes are destroyed on the skin surface or in the outer horny layer. From here active substances can progress deeper into the skin—each substance penetrating according to its individual properties. Other studies raise the possibility that, because of the difficulty encountered in penetrating the horny layer, most of the liposomes enter the skin through the pores.

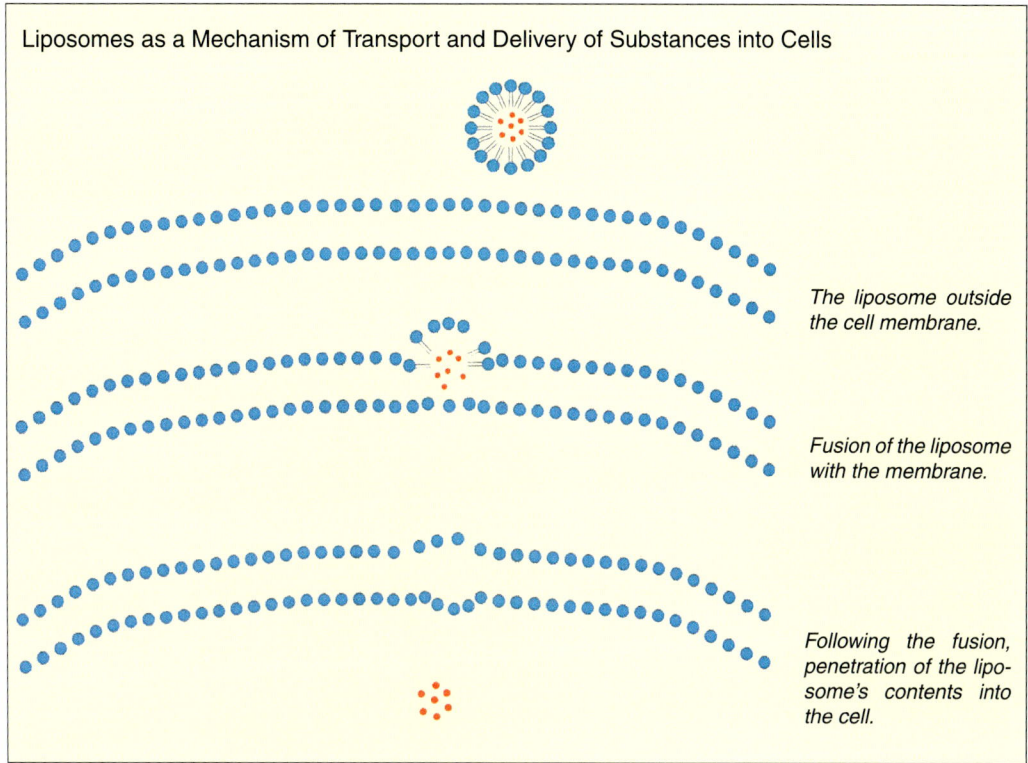

WHAT SUBSTANCES DO LIPOSOMES CONTAIN?

In dermatology, antifungal medications are the main area of use for liposomes. Liposomes are currently also being investigated with regard to their use with antibiotics, corticosteroids, and retinoids.

The cosmetics industries are currently focusing much on liposomes. Whether this is justified has yet to be established. One can reasonably assume that collagen and elastin molecules are too large to penetrate the skin, and their insertion into liposomes is not likely to cause them to shrink. However, substances with smaller molecules may penetrate the skin more efficiently.

The cosmetics industry utilizes liposomes mostly for moisturizers. In addition, products containing various vitamins have been created. However, the value of these, whether or not they are enveloped in liposomes, is controversial.

New Systems: Niosomes

In order to increase the ability to penetrate the skin, niosomes were developed. The full scientific term is **nonionic surfactant vesicles**. They are similar in composition to liposomes, and are spherically structured as well. The vesicle membranes of niosomes are composed of oily compounds of ether or alcohol.

ARE LIPOSOMES EFFECTIVE?

Several studies have examined the efficacy of the liposomal system. An active product enveloped in liposomes was compared with the same product in a regular oil base. Some of the studies proved increased efficacy for the use of liposomes, especially regarding the oral use of certain medications. With regards to the topical use of drugs (i.e., drugs that are to be applied externally to the skin), the issue remains controversial.

Some scientists consider the issue a marketing allure for the cosmetic industry. Others perceive it as a significant turning point in cosmetics and dermatology. The issue is currently under investigation, so a definite conclusion concerning the efficacy of liposomes used in topical preparations cannot yet be established.

Note that the main function of liposomes is to carry active ingredients into the skin. Therefore, the potential beneficial effect of a preparation that contains liposomes is determined mainly by the biological properties of the specific ingredients that are carried by the liposomes.

ADDITIONAL POSSIBLE BENEFITS OF LIPOSOMES

Liposomes, composed of an oily substance, form a thin, oily film on the skin surface. There is a weak occlusive effect and an increase in skin moisture. However, there is no significant advantage when compared with other moisturizers. Contact between skin cells and active substances or topical medications decreases when these are enveloped in liposomes. This may decrease or modify allergic reactions.

CONCLUSION

Liposomes are not active substances in themselves. They act as a medium for penetration of active products in the skin. Their efficacy for topical preparations has yet to be established.

24 | Chemical Skin Peeling
Josef Shiri

Contents Overview • For which problems is chemical skin peeling used? • Peeling Agents • Depths of chemical peeling • Procedure for chemical skin peeling • Level of pain with chemical skin peeling • Course following chemical skin peeling • Possible complications of chemical skin peeling and their management • Summary

OVERVIEW

Chemical skin peeling is a method of peeling the outer layers of the skin by creating a chemical burn. As the burn heals, a new outer layer of skin forms. The new skin that appears is smoother, pinker, tauter, and has a more uniform texture. After chemical peeling, sun spots (solar lentigines) on the skin become paler. Similarly, wrinkles are smoothed out to a certain extent, and some even disappear completely.

The following paragraphs describe the technique of chemical peeling for information and interest only. Under no circumstances do we suggest that this technique be used for self-treatment. Chemical skin peeling must only be performed by a physician experienced in the technique.

FOR WHICH PROBLEMS IS CHEMICAL SKIN PEELING USED?

Chemical skin peeling is mainly used to treat solar damage in the form of sun spots, to smooth out the skin and to eliminate wrinkles. For fine wrinkles, superficial peeling is sufficient. For deeper wrinkles, such as those found around the mouth and at the corners of the eyes, deeper peeling is needed.

Similarly, skin peeling can improve other abnormalities of pigmentation in the form of dark blotches on the face, such as the "pregnancy mask" (melasma), as well as superficial acne scars.

Superficial and medium depth (see below) skin peeling, although helpful in treating the above-mentioned problems, are ineffective in solving the problem of sagging skin. In contrast, deeper peeling may contract the skin to a certain extent, partially treating the problem of sagging skin. However, this procedure is not able to achieve the same results as a surgical face-lift as performed by a plastic surgeon.

PEELING AGENTS

The following substances are commonly used for chemical skin peeling:

- "dry ice" (carbon dioxide snow);
- Jessner's solution, which contains resorcinol, salicylic acid, and lactic acid;
- α-hydroxy acids (see chap. 18);
- trichloroacetic acid (TCA);
- phenol.

There are also other substances that are used for chemical peeling; moreover, several substances can be mixed in a "combination" product for peeling. Each physician selects an appropriate substance, depending on the depth of peeling to be achieved, the patient's skin type, and the physician's personal experience with that particular product.

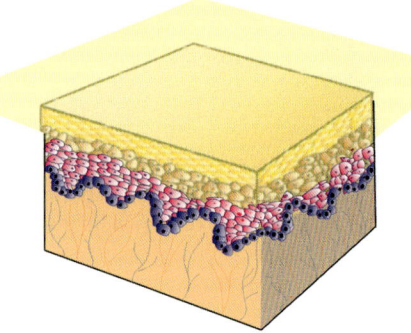
Very superficial peeling—only epidermis.

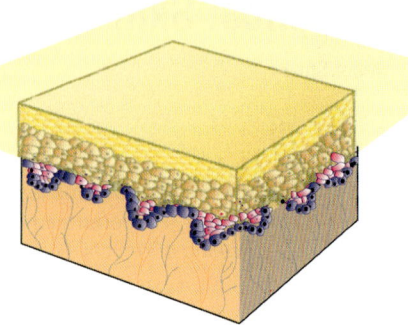
Superficial peeling—epidermis and outer dermis.

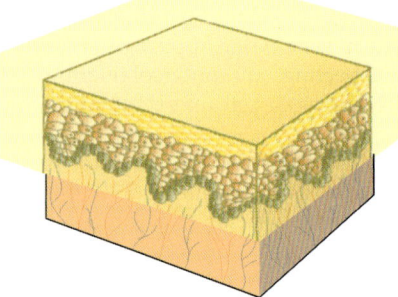
Medium peeling—deeper into the dermis.

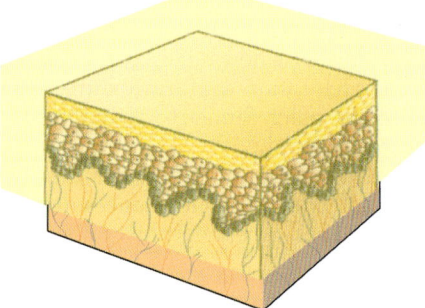
Deep peeling—half the depth of the dermis.

DEPTHS OF CHEMICAL PEELING

Chemical skin peeling can be performed to reach four different depths of penetration, each intended to achieve a different end result. These are as follows:

- **Very superficial peeling,** which involves only the epidermis. There may also be minimal involvement of the dermis.
- **Superficial peeling,** which includes the epidermis and the outermost part of the dermis.
- **Medium peeling,** which reaches the dermis deeper than superficial peeling.
- **Deep peeling,** which reaches deeper into the dermis, to approximately half its depth.

The deeper the peeling, the more significant its influence on the facial skin. With increasing depth of peeling, the possibility of lightening various blotches and erasing relatively deep wrinkles increases substantially. Not infrequently, the procedure of superficial peeling has to be repeated several times until satisfactory results are obtained.

Skin Regeneration Following Chemical Peeling

If the peeling is superficial, the skin will regenerate from cells in the epidermis that replicate, multiply, and produce a new layer of epidermis.

If deeper peeling reaches the dermis—destroying the epidermis in its path—how does the skin regenerate after such a procedure? In these cases, the regeneration is mainly from cells coating the hair follicles, which go down quite deep into the dermis. Although these cells are situated "deep" in the dermis, they are, in fact, epidermal cells. These cells replicate and divide until they cover the entire area that was denuded by the peeling. Within the dermis, new collagen tissue forms, which replaces the collagen destroyed by the chemical treatment.

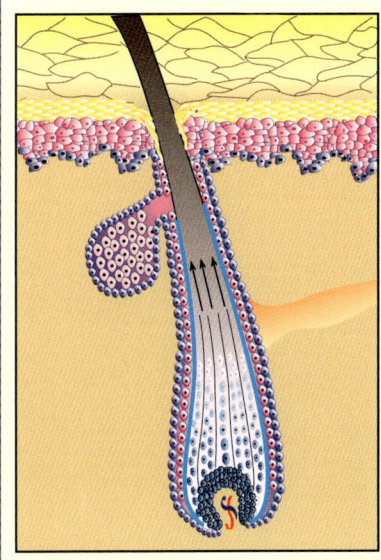

As this illustration shows, even at the depth of the dermis where the hair follicles extend, there are epidermal cells. It is from those cells that new skin regenerates following deep peeling.

The major factors that determine the depth of the burn that results from peeling are:

- the chemical (or mixture of chemicals) used,
- its concentration,
- the length of time of contact with the skin, and
- whether an occlusive dressing is used.

Several other factors include skin thickness and the use of other preliminary treatments before peeling (such as the daily application of retinoic acid for approximately two weeks prior to chemical peeling).

Some Preparations Used in Chemical Skin Peeling

- **Very superficial peeling** may be performed using 10% to 20% trichloroacetic acid, Jessner's solution, or α-hydroxy acids (see chap 18).
- **Superficial peeling** may be performed using 35% trichloroacetic acid or 50% to 70% α-hydroxy acids (see chap. 18).
- **Medium peeling** may be carried out using 35% trichloroacetic acid combined with dry ice or with Jessner's solution.
- **Deep peeling** usually utilizes phenol.

There are many methods of skin peeling apart from those already mentioned. Each physician uses the technique with which he/she feels most comfortable and with which he/she has had the most experience.

PROCEDURE FOR CHEMICAL SKIN PEELING

As an example, we describe the procedure for chemical skin peeling using trichloroacetic acid.

1. **Cleansing**

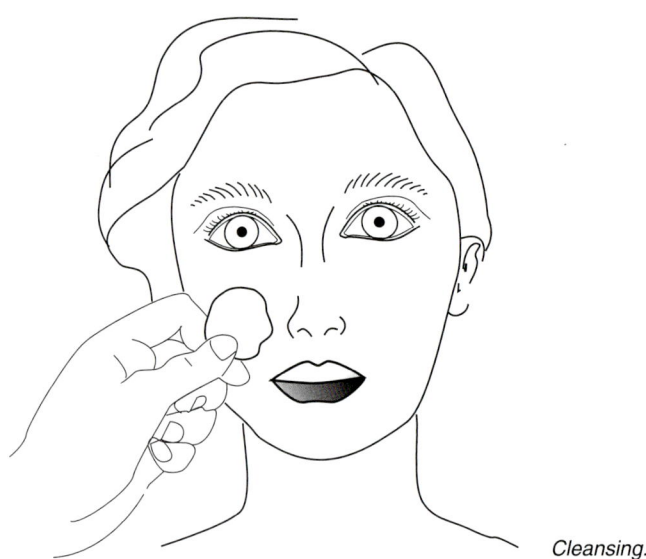

Cleansing.

2. **Applying trichloroacetic acid to the skin using a cotton swab applicator**—Within a short time, the skin develops a gray-white color because of the chemical destruction of the outer layers of the skin, as shown in the illustration.

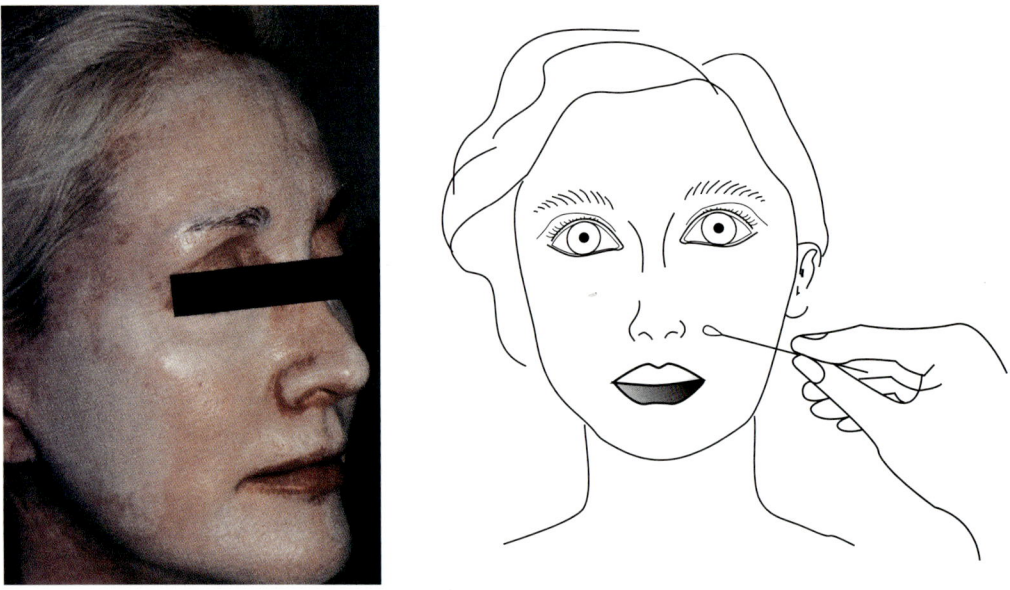

Applying trichloroacetic acid to the skin: following exposure to the trichloroacetic acid, the epidermis changes color.

3. **Rinsing the substance off after two minutes of skin contact**—The patient will feel a certain degree of discomfort, depending on the concentration of the substance.

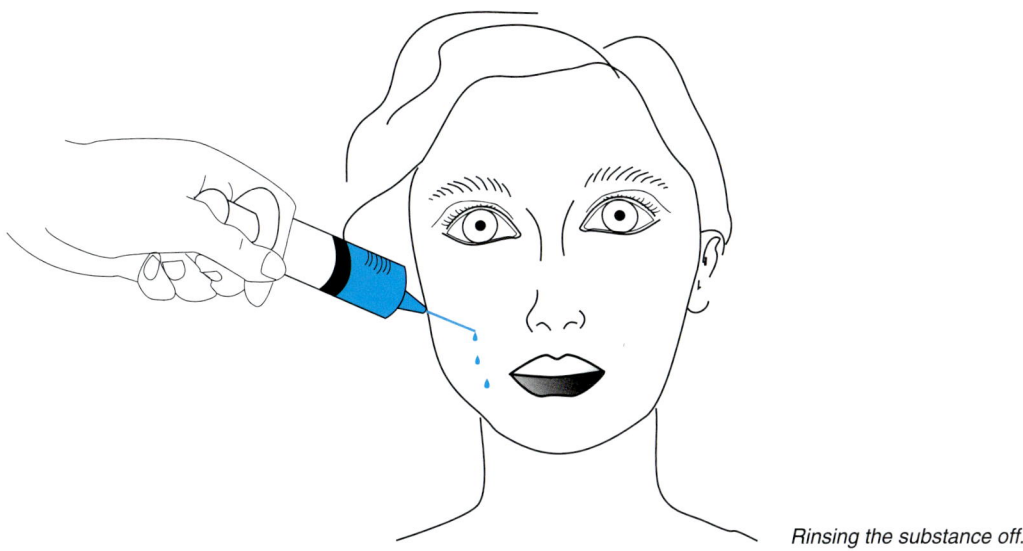

Rinsing the substance off.

4. **Application of an occlusive dressing**—Antibiotic cream may also be applied.

Preparation Prior to Chemical Skin Peeling

Many physicians recommend applying retinoic acid to the face at night for approximately two weeks prior to the skin peeling treatment. This preparatory treatment apparently improves the penetration of the active peeling substance into the skin, and the subsequent healing of the peeled area is quicker and more effective.

Dark-skinned patients should undergo preparation with skin bleaching agents prior to skin peeling. This prevents the appearance of dark pigmented areas of skin following the peeling treatment. One preparation commonly used for this purpose is **Kligman's solution**, which contains hydroquinone, hydrocortisone, and retinoic acid. It must be applied daily for three weeks prior to skin peeling.

A month or so prior to the peeling, a "spot test" should be performed using a small amount of the preparation to be used for the peeling. This test is performed on area of skin that is not readily seen, such as behind the ear. Over the next few weeks, any untoward reaction to the substance (such as inflammation or darkening of the skin) will become obvious, in which case the chemical peeling treatment should not be carried out.

LEVEL OF PAIN WITH CHEMICAL SKIN PEELING

- Superficial skin peeling is associated with a mild burning sensation at the time of the treatment, which in most cases amounts to no more than mild discomfort.
- Medium skin peeling (particularly if carried out with trichloroacetic acid) is associated with bearable pain during the treatment, which subsides quickly thereafter.
- Deep peeling, using phenol, causes severe pain during the treatment and for up to two days afterward. The patient must be given intravenous analgesic medications, or general anesthesia, depending on the physician's and patient's choice.

COURSE FOLLOWING CHEMICAL SKIN PEELING

Superficial Peeling
Superficial peeling, if performed only once, has almost no discernible effect, but if the treatment is repeated several times over a period of months, good results can be achieved. Shortly after the treatment, the skin becomes red, and within two days it develops a brown coloration. The mild burning sensation, which is transient, can be alleviated by applying cold compresses or by directing a flow of cold air from a fan onto the skin. Within three to five days, the superficial layers of the skin start to peel. Healing is almost complete a week after the treatment. Overall, this treatment is simple, the risks are minimal, and healing is quick.

Superficial skin peeling can be repeated at short intervals (every few weeks) in order to achieve a deeper peel with each treatment.

Medium Peeling
Redness of the skin appears approximately an hour after the treatment, and apart from cold compresses or a flow of cool air over the area, usually no further treatment is needed. Later, the face becomes swollen, and five to seven days later, the skin starts to peel. It takes approximately two weeks for healing to occur, at which time new, smooth, delicate skin covers the area. Sun spots are much less obvious, and fine wrinkles become flattened out. The redness of the face lasts for a few weeks and then gradually disappears.

Deep Peeling
Healing following deep peeling is slower than that following superficial or medium peeling. The face becomes more swollen than with medium peeling, and the redness is much more obvious. The swelling and redness last for three to six months. During that period, the patient is unable to tolerate any cosmetics on the face, and they should not be used. Even dyeing the hair can cause severe itching. Deep peeling can help in the elimination of relatively deep wrinkles around the mouth and eyes.

When Should a Physician Avoid Chemical Skin Peeling?

There are several situations in which a discerning physician will choose not to perform chemical skin peeling. Anyone falling into one of the following categories should not have this treatment:

- Patients with a tendency to form excessive scarring.
- Patients with relatively dark skin.*
- Patients who are going to be exposed to the sun following the treatment (because of their occupation or because they are unlikely to follow instructions to avoid exposure).
- Smokers.**
- Patients who are emotionally unstable or have exaggerated, unrealistic expectations of the outcome of treatments.

*In certain cases, these patients may undergo superficial peeling.
**It is preferable for smokers not to undergo chemical skin peeling, as their skin's ability to heal is generally not as good as that of nonsmokers. They also have a higher risk of skin infection following treatment, and wrinkles are more likely to recur.

POSSIBLE COMPLICATIONS OF CHEMICAL SKIN PEELING AND THEIR MANAGEMENT

The complications of skin peeling are usually preventable and treatable, and an experienced physician knows how to avoid them.

Bacterial Infection
The risk of bacterial infection can be minimized if the physician pays careful attention to correct treatment technique and the patient carefully follows the physician's advice following treatment. The more superficial the peeling, the less the likelihood of infection.

Alterations in Skin Pigmentation
Skin color may become either paler or darker. Using concentrations of phenol that are too high can cause pale areas of skin to appear (hypopigmentation). Trichloroacetic acid, on the other hand, usually causes dark areas of pigmentation (hyperpigmentation). To minimize this risk:

- the physician should take care to use the appropriate concentrations of the peeling substance,
- the patient should be advised to avoid exposure to the sun after peeling, and
- in patients with dark skin (who tend to develop hyperpigmentation following peeling), it is advisable to prepare the skin before treatment with skin bleaching agents.

Scarring
The most common reason for the appearance of scars after peeling is infection (viral or bacterial) of skin that was not treated correctly. Meticulous care in taking the appropriate preventative measures, and immediate and effective treatment at the first sign of infection, will significantly decrease the risk of scarring. Less commonly, scars can appear if the concentration of the peeling substance was inadvertently too high. A wise physician will prefer to use a concentration a little less than what is "officially" recommended, in order to provide a safety margin to allow for possible errors in the preparation of the product. For example, using 60% phenol instead of 50% may have drastic effects on the skin.

Herpes Virus Infection in the Peeled Area
It is common practice to prevent this complication by routinely giving the patient antiviral medication orally, starting from the day prior to the treatment until a few days thereafter. The currently accepted treatment is with tablets containing **acyclovir**. Newer preparations for the prevention and treatment of viral infections include **famciclovir** and **valacyclovir**.

Sensitivity to Cold
Marked cold sensitivity of the face can occur following chemical peeling.

Prolonged Redness
Prolonged redness may occur following chemical peeling. It may be accompanied by itchiness and an intolerance to certain cosmetics.

Heart and Kidney Problems
There have been reports of complications involving disturbances of heart rhythm and possible kidney damage following the use of phenol for deep chemical peeling because of its absorption into the bloodstream. Therefore, patients undergoing this treatment may need to be connected to a heart monitor to watch for possible alterations in the heart rhythm. They should also be given intravenous fluids to prevent kidney damage.

Effects of Sunlight
Exposure to sunlight following a peeling procedure can cause changes in skin pigmentation, resulting in the appearance of dark blotches in the new skin that grows back following the peeling. Therefore, the patient should be told to strictly avoid any exposure to sunlight following the treatment. The length of this period of strict avoidance of sunlight will vary, depending on the depth of peeling, and is determined by the physician. However, even after this period of strict, *total* avoidance of sunlight, it is still advisable to avoid sun exposure as much as possible. If it is impossible to totally avoid exposure to the sun, a high-level protective sunscreen should be used when outdoors. The skin that regrows following peeling is particularly delicate and sensitive, and the harmful effects of the sun rays on skin are well known.

Avoidance of Cosmetics
There is intolerance to cosmetic preparations following deep peeling, and the patient should be advised to refrain from applying cosmetics to the face for several weeks or months following chemical peeling, depending on the depth of the peeling.

Note: In older women who have solar damage to the skin, peeling treatment that is "too" effective may not be beneficial. The contrast between smooth facial skin, free of wrinkles, and the deeply wrinkled untreated skin of the neck, with sun spots scattered over it, is not an aesthetically desirable result.

SUMMARY

Chemical skin peeling is a technique whereby the outer layers of the skin are peeled away by means of a chemical burn. The substances used to achieve chemical peeling include dry ice, Jessner's solution, α-hydroxy acids, trichloroacetic acid, phenol, and other substances. Chemical skin peeling is used mainly to lighten dark skin blotches (such as "sun spots") and to smooth out or eradicate wrinkles.

25 | Laser and Light Treatments in Dermatology and Their Cosmetic Applications

Moshe Lapidoth

Contents Overview • Removing tattoos using a laser • Treating blood vessels • Skin peeling using lasers • Further developments • Hair removal using lasers • Laser treatment for sun spots • Intense pulsed light • Final comment

OVERVIEW

The ability of lasers to treat a range of dermatological conditions is based on two basic properties:

- their ability to produce a powerful, focused light beam that destroys precisely the tissue being treated, and
- the ability of the laser beam to home in on a specific target, depending on the color and other characteristics of the target tissue. This color-specific targeting ability significantly reduces damage to surrounding tissues whose color differs from the target tissue.

It follows from the above that there are various types of laser instruments designed to treat skin lesions of various colors: **Ruby lasers** are effective in the treatment of certain skin lesions that have a blue or brown coloration, and **pulsed-dye lasers** can be used to treat lesions that are very vascular (i.e., contain many blood vessels), and are therefore the appropriate instruments for treating fine networks of blood vessels (telangiectases) that appear on the skin or various growths derived from blood vessels in the skin.

Apart from these, there are lasers designed to treat a wide range of skin lesions, including warts, skin tags, scars, and skin tumors of various types. Other uses of lasers, such as in facial skin peeling and hair removal, will be discussed in detail below.

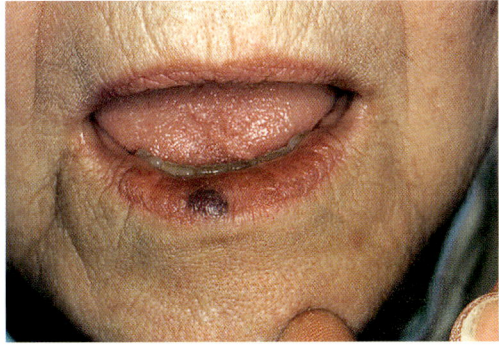 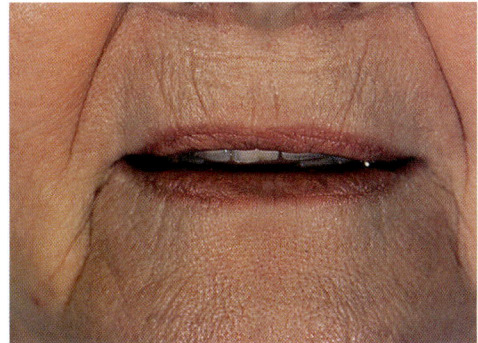

A lesion composed of blood vessels (the medical term is "venous lake") before (left) and after (right) treatment with a laser.

REMOVING TATTOOS USING A LASER

The laser devices used for tattoo removal are the Q-switched Nd:YAG, the Q-S alexandrite, and the ruby laser. Tattoos result from dyes penetrating the skin. The light that these lasers emit is selectively absorbed by the dye, causing it to "burst" into tiny particles. The particles are then engulfed by a special subgroup of white blood cells (macrophages). Since the normal skin in the region does not have the same color as the dye, it does not absorb the laser energy and is, therefore, not damaged. For this method to be effective, the laser used must be selected according to the color(s) of the tattoo. The final result depends mainly on the type of dye used for the tattoo and the skin color of the treated patient. It is usually better in "amateur" tattoos. In more professional tattoos, the beneficial effect may be only partial, if at all. Therefore, in some cases, it would be preferable to remove these kind of tattoos surgically.

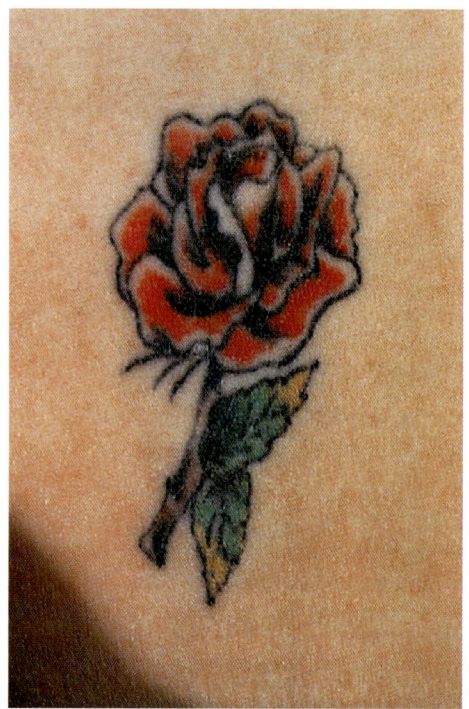 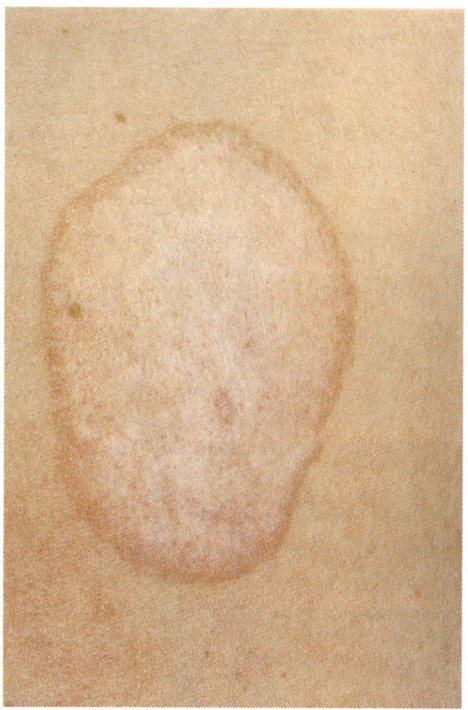

A tattoo, before (left) and after (right) laser treatment.

Professor Rox R. Anderson, United States, a leading figure in the development of highly advanced laser devices, developed an innovative concept of removable tattoos. He suggested the use of minute "balls" containing the specific dye intended for the tattoo. These balls of dye can keep the material contained within them for life. However, if one regrets and would like to erase the tattoo, the balls of dye are easily removed with laser therapy. The laser energy destroys the external coating of the ball, releasing the dye into the skin where it gradually disappears. In this case, one laser treatment would be enough, in contrast to conventional laser treatment for tattoos, which usually requires repeated therapeutic sessions, with no certainty as to the final outcome.

TREATING BLOOD VESSELS

Laser instruments intended for treating blood vessels are the Pulsed Dye Laser, and the Nd:YAG (Yttrium Aluminium Garnet). Intense pulsed light may also be used for this purpose. The treated lesions are usually fine networks of blood vessels (telangiectases) that appear on the skin, or various growths derived from blood vessels in the skin. Laser instruments also enable treating distended (varicose) veins of lower limbs. In some cases, the treatment is combined with other measures, such as electrical energy of radio wave frequency.

SKIN PEELING USING LASERS

The principle behind skin peeling using lasers (also termed "skin resurfacing") is the same as that of chemical skin peeling. In both cases, the aim is to create a superficial burn on the skin of the face, so that as the burn wound heals, new rejuvenated skin appears.

Advances in laser technology have led to the development of laser instruments that can produce extremely short pulses (less than a thousandth of a second). This means that the actual time the beam is in contact with the skin is shorter, thus allowing lasers to be introduced for skin peeling. As a result of these technical advances, the operator can now determine the precise depth in the skin to which the laser beam penetrates, and can therefore achieve exactly the depth of peeling required. The standard laser instruments used in recent years for skin resurfacing are:

- the CO_2 laser, and
- the erbium:YAG laser.

These devices are mainly used for removing acne scars and in the treatment of wrinkles around the eyes and mouth. Deeper wrinkles, resulting from movements of the facial muscles (such as wrinkles on the forehead or between the eyebrows), respond less well.

The beneficial effect of laser skin peeling lasts for a variable amount of time, differing from person to person. The possible adverse side effects of laser skin peeling are similar to those following chemical skin peeling. The main potential problems are redness of the face that may last up to three months following treatment, the development of scars, and changes in the pigmentation (color) of the skin. One has to also bear in mind that the procedure is painful, requiring topical anesthetics.

This mode of laser skin peeling has been considered a relatively safe procedure, provided that the operator is skilled and that the treatment is performed in accordance with accepted medical guidelines.

FURTHER DEVELOPMENTS

Noninvasive Lasers

In the search for novel modes of treatment that may change and improve the structure of collagen, while minimizing the risk of adverse effects, researchers have developed noninvasive technologies, such as infrared lasers and intense pulsed light. These devices are based on a therapeutic concept claiming that new collagen may be produced, with consequent flattening of wrinkles but without external damage to the skin. Four to six therapeutic sessions are required at one-month intervals. They are considered relatively safe, but are less effective than the standard lasers used for skin resurfacing such as the CO_2 laser and the erbium:YAG laser. Most physicians agree that noninvasive lasers may well erase small blood vessels and pigmented lesions, but their effectiveness in treating wrinkles is less optimal.

Fractional Photothermolysis

In order to combine the advantages of invasive and noninvasive lasers, another technique was introduced in 2003. The technique uses a noninvasive laser beam that emits light with a wavelength of 1550 nm. The laser beams are transmitted into the skin via a special lens. The beams do not affect the tissue uniformly but in a partial form, which resembles a very fine net (hence the term "fractional"). The laser beams produce tiny, microscopic thermal wounds. These tiny wounds lead to the development of microscopic "plugs" that advance and are discharged within two weeks onto the skin surface, while being replaced by new tissue. Significant damage to the skin (as seen in standard laser treatment or chemical peeling) is avoided. There is mild redness, similar to sunburn, which is transient and disappears within several days. Several treatment sessions are required in order to obtain a discernable improvement.

Fractional Ablative Skin Resurfacing by Erbium and CO_2 Lasers

This method implements the principle of partial damage to the skin, as already described, to laser instruments such as the CO_2 and erbium lasers. As in the fractional photothermolysis method, the use of the erbium or the CO_2 lasers results in a net-like resurfacing of the skin, with the removal of the epidermis, while the dermis undergoes regulated thermal damage. The adverse effects seem to be milder than those that characterize invasive lasers or chemical skin peeling (most probably due to its partial activity) and include redness, a burning sensation, and discomfort that tends to disappear within several days. These lasers seem to be more effective in skin resurfacing than noninvasive lasers, and they should be considered as a therapeutic option for photoaged skin, wrinkles, and acne scars.

HAIR REMOVAL USING LASERS

The idea of removing hair using laser technology was first published in 1995. Several types of laser devices are used for this purpose: alexandrite, diode, and Nd:YAG. Intense pulsed light may be used for hair removal as well. The type of laser used should be adapted according to the color of the skin and the area to be treated. The principle on which this treatment is based is that there is a difference in color between the hair follicle and the skin; the light energy is absorbed by the dark pigment in the hair follicle causing damage to the follicle, thereby reducing hair growth. The lighter the skin and the darker the hair, the more selectively the laser will affect the follicle and not the surrounding tissue. The main side effects of this treatment are:

- mild discomfort during treatment (usually bearable, but may require local anesthetic),
- local redness, which may last from a few minutes to a few hours, and
- superficial burns, usually resolving without leaving any residual sign.

Note: In view of the above, laser treatment for hair removal in people with dark skin is not desirable because there is insufficient difference between the color of the hair and the color of the skin, which is what the laser treatment requires for it to be effective and safe. In dark-skinned people, laser treatment may cause burns and/or **hypopigmentation**, i.e., lightening of the skin, around the hair follicle. In most cases, however, this phenomenon resolves by itself in time. Similarly, light hair cannot be treated by laser techniques.

> ### Laser Treatment and the Life Cycle of the Treated Hair
>
> The efficiency of laser treatment for hair removal partly depends on which phase the treated hair is in. Lasers are most effective in dealing with hairs that are in the growth phase (anagen phase). On hairs that are in the telogen phase, laser therapy has been considered less effective, since the hair that is about to degenerate is situated some distance from the place in the follicle from where the new hair will grow. (The phases of the life cycle of a hair are described in chapter 30 on the structure of hair.) In practice, however, there is some response to laser treatment even in telogen phase, which is attributed to laser-induced damage to blood vessels in the dermal papillae.
>
>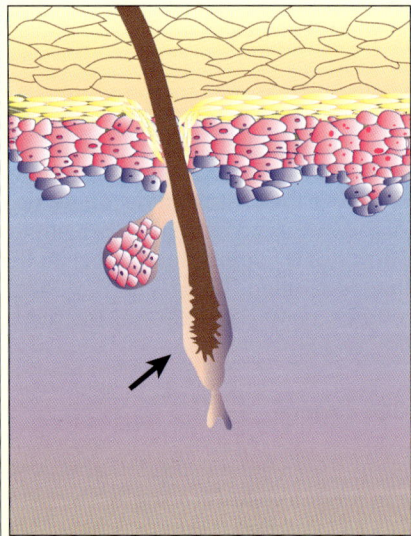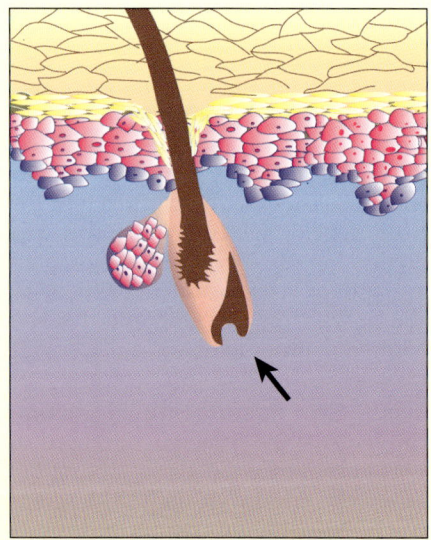
>
> *Telogen hair, about to degenerate.*   *Next stage: the new hair begins to grow from another point (not treated by laser).*

Laser treatment arrests the active growth period of the treated hair for long periods—sometimes for several years. The response varies according to the region of the body being treated, skin type, and the age of patient. For instance, the hair in the armpits, groin, and legs is more responsive to laser treatment than facial hair. Laser treatment is less effective on darker skin. Also, younger individuals usually require more treatment sessions. The response to the treatment may also vary considerably from person to person, for reasons that are not fully understood. However, in most cases, 6 to 12 treatment sessions are usually sufficient. Hair that has not reappeared within a year after treatment is not expected to regrow.

The results obtained to date from many patients are encouraging and justify the continuing use of lasers for hair removal. It should be remembered, however, that laser techniques are constantly being improved upon and further developments can be expected.

> What Is the Appropriate Age to Start Hair Removal with Laser?
>
> The most recommended approach would be to start laser therapy after adolescence. During adolescence, there is an increase in the level of certain hormones that stimulate hair growth in various body regions. This also causes a thickening of the hairs, making them better targets for laser energy. Therefore, laser treatment before adolescence would not be effective enough. In addition, the treatment is painful and could distress the treated children. Moreover, removal of vellous hair in the face in preadolescence can actually cause stimulation of hair growth, aggravating the problem.

LASER TREATMENT FOR SUN SPOTS

The scientific name for sun spots is "solar lentigo" (plural "solar lentigines"). The lasers used to treat sun spots are Q-switched Nd:YAG and ruby lasers. In most cases, the aesthetic outcome is quite good. The number of therapeutic sessions required is between one and three. Note that other options for treating such lesions are available. In any case, using bleaching agents before and after treatment would be desirable.

INTENSE PULSED LIGHT

As mentioned above, a laser instrument produces a powerful, focused light beam, composed of a constant wavelength. In 1993, a new mode of therapy was introduced called intense pulsed light, most commonly known as IPL. It uses a xenon lamp, which emits light for extremely short periods, measured in milliseconds. The light produced by IPL is not composed of a single wavelength, as is the case with laser devices. IPL produces light pulses within the spectrum of 400 to 1200 nm. In order to adapt the IPL device to specific indications, different filters are used, which let through only the segment of light wavelengths required to treat the skin problem.

IPL does not have the specificity of a laser with one, uniform wavelength, and tends to produce more adverse side effects. However, as opposed to laser devices, which are each designed to treat a particular kind of lesion according to the wavelength it emits, each IPL device may be used to treat several types of lesions.

FINAL COMMENT

In spite of all the advantages of laser treatment discussed here, it should be remembered that the laser is not the definitive answer to all skin problems. Medical problems that require laser treatment must be distinguished from those that are best managed by other methods. For example,

- The recommended and accepted treatments for solar keratoses are 5-fluorouracil (5-FU) preparations, imiquimod, and liquid nitrogen. Not necessarily lasers.

- Laser treatment is not the accepted method for treating lesions that may be malignant. In such cases, the lesion should be completely excised, with an appropriate safety margin around it, and sent for microscopic examination. Moles (melanocytic nevi) are definitely not to be treated by laser.
- In some cases, a dermatologist will prefer to perform skin peeling (for removing wrinkles in the skin) using a chemical peeling substance rather than a laser.

The laser should not be thought of as the be-all and end-all for cosmetic treatments. In general, before starting laser treatments, one should consult a dermatologist and examine possible alternatives.

26 | Fillers and Soft Tissue Augmentation
Ines Verner and Christopher Rowland Payne

Contents Overview • History • Indications and patient selection • Soft tissue fillers: biodegradable vs. nonbiodegradable • Biodegradable fillers • Nonbiodegradable fillers • Complications • Summary

OVERVIEW

Loss of facial volume is one of the most important determinants of facial aging.

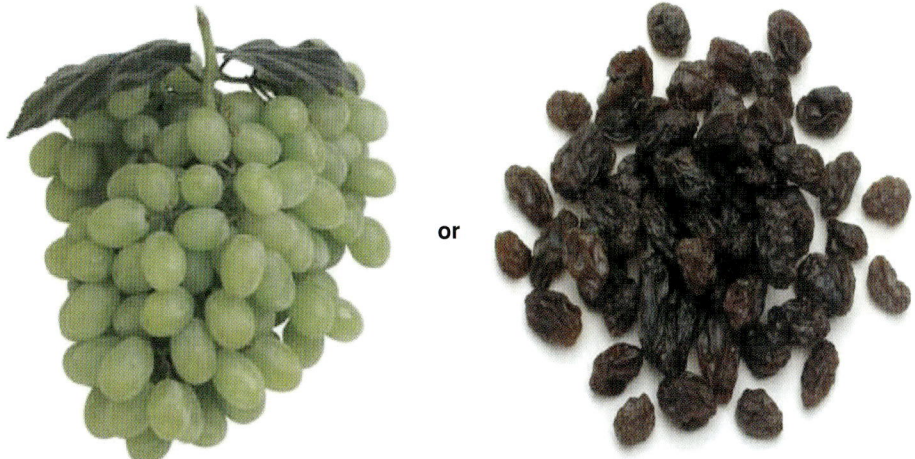

A raisin is a wrinkled grape. A raisin is a grape that has lost volume. A similar principle applies to the loss of volume in subcutaneous tissue.

With age, skin thins and its subcutaneous fat and bony support are gradually lost.

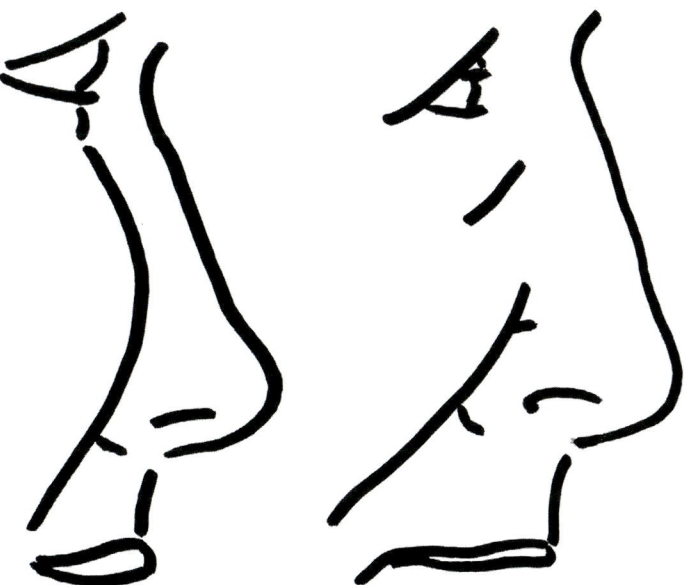

The facial outline of a woman and her grandmother. Note the loss of cheek volume with age.

Facial volume loss can be partially restored by the injection of soft tissue fillers into the subcutaneous tissue skin. With the vast technological developments in the last few decades, many different soft tissue fillers have become available. Soft tissue augmentation has now become one of the most popular noninvasive cosmetic procedures.

Fillers can be divided into biodegradable and nonbiodegradable. Biodegradable fillers, such as hyaluronic acid, are injected and remain, inert, until the body resorbs them. Nonbiodegradable fillers, such as silicone, elicit a granulomatous host response, which ensures a longer lasting effect.

HISTORY

From time immemorial, human beings have sought beauty and tried to slow aging. With the advent of anesthesia and surgery towards the end of the 19th century, more invasive cosmetic procedures became available, including soft tissue fillers. Fat was the first soft tissue filler to be used after trauma and is still widely used today. However, fat transplantation is considered a relatively major procedure, as it necessitates the removal of fatty tissue from another site, and its results may be variable. Towards the end of the 19th century, paraffin oil was used for the restoration of volume and symmetry. However, its use was accompanied by a high incidence of inflammatory granulomatous nodules (*paraffinomas*) with consequent facial distortion and, occasionally, life-threatening paraffin emboli, which passed through the blood stream and obstructed the blood vessels of the lung. Hence, the use of paraffin oil was discontinued.

Liquid silicone gained some popularity in Europe in the 1940s, when thousands of patients were treated with it. Since the 1960s through to the present, excellent, safe and durable results have been reported in the United States and the United Kingdom with silicone, using the serial microdroplet technique. On the other hand, the use of inappropriately large volumes of silicone or impure silicone has been followed by complications, such as neurological dysfunction, blindness, and erysipelas-like inflammatory reactions. These problems have cast an unwarranted cloud of unease over the safe and proper use of serial microdroplet silicone.

Injectable bovine (i.e., from cattle) collagen, for example, Zyderm® collagen implant, was the first biodegradable filler available. The FDA approved it in 1981 for soft tissue augmentation because of its relative safety. The "minimally invasive" nature of the procedure, with no downtime, led to a growing demand for soft tissue augmentation. However, its very short duration in tissue and high incidence of allergic reactions led to the development of other fillers with enhanced longevity and safety, notably, hyaluronic acid. Now there are many different soft tissue fillers, each with its own strengths and drawbacks. The use of fillers has now become commonplace.

INDICATIONS AND PATIENT SELECTION

The development of newer fillers, with many different physical properties, has led to new therapeutic possibilities and thus new indications. While during the 1970s and 1980s, the trend was to fill out wrinkles, nowadays the trend is for the restoration of facial volume and contour. In the past, facial rejuvenation was achieved by pulling up tissue by surgical facelift. Nowadays, fillers are used as a first-line treatment to lift the face before, and often instead of, surgery.

Fillers can be used for many different indications, not only to treat the manifestations of aging but also to treat facial defects and asymmetry due to trauma or disease.

Correction of Changes Due to Aging

The main features of aging in the upper third of the face are loss of the convex projection of the supraorbital ridge with a consequent descent of the eyebrows. Fillers can be used in this area to partially elevate the brows, to treat deep glabellar folds (between the eyebrows), and to treat the wrinkles on the outer side of the eyes (crow's feet).

The main features of aging of the middle third of the face are the appearance of hollows under the eyes and loss of volume in the medial and lateral cheek. By correcting the hollows under the eyes, a tired appearance can be effaced, and the face can gain a smoother

FILLERS AND SOFT TISSUE AUGMENTATION

appearance. Fillers can restore volume loss in the medial and lateral cheeks and can accentuate the cheekbones.

The main features of aging in the lower third of the face are deepening of the nasolabial fold (the fold between the nose and mouth, i.e., the "smile" lines), the appearance of marionette or "drool" lines (lines from the corners of the mouth down towards the sides of the chin), changes in the position and structure of the lips, and jowling of the jaw line. The nasolabial fold is one of the most popular indications for fillers. Filling this fold can give excellent and durable cosmetic results. Treating marionette lines also helps support the sides of the mouth. Fillers can be injected into the angles of the mouth to correct down turning.

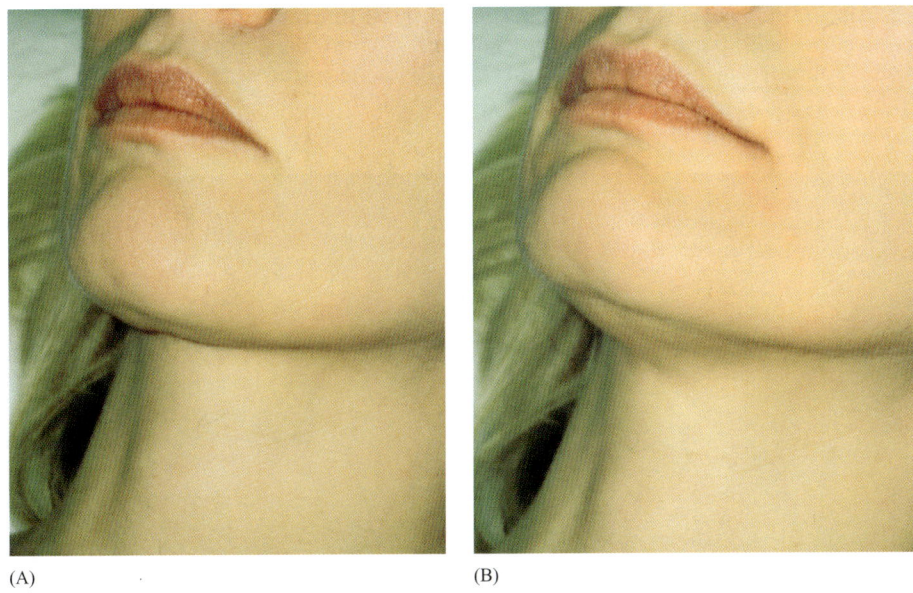

(A) (B)

*Filling the angles of the mouth: Before (**A**) and after (**B**) filler.*

Aging lips become thin and flat, fine radial or crosshatched wrinkles develop on the upper and lower lips and the lipstick may "bleed" out from the vermillion (the red part of the lips) into the surrounding skin. Fillers can be used to efface crosshatched wrinkles of the vermillion and can restore the natural fullness and definition of the lips.

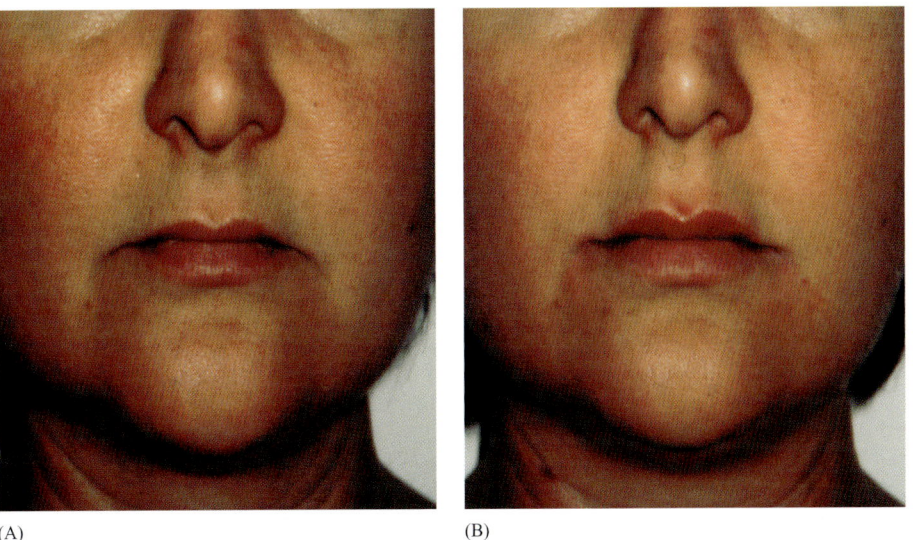

(A) (B)

*Lips before filler. (**B**) Lips after filler. Note the elevation of angles of mouth.*

Aging also leads to loss of jaw line definition with jowling. The corresponding prejowl sulcus (depression) can be filled to redefine the jawline.

Correction of Facial Defects Due to Trauma or Disease

Even though fillers have gained their popularity by facilitating the treatment of aging, they can also be used for the correction of many facial defects, asymmetries, and scars.

In the upper third of the face, forehead asymmetries or depressions can be corrected, such as sunken scars or even tissue loss due to certain skin diseases or trauma. In the mid-face, cheek hollowing due to disease, for example, HIV-related facial lipoatrophy or trauma, may be corrected. Also, minor nasal imperfections, such as nasal tip descent or an overdeep nasal bridge, can be corrected, sparing the need for surgery. A prominent mandible can be made less evident by submucosal filling of the upper lip. Deepened acne scars can be treated by silicone.

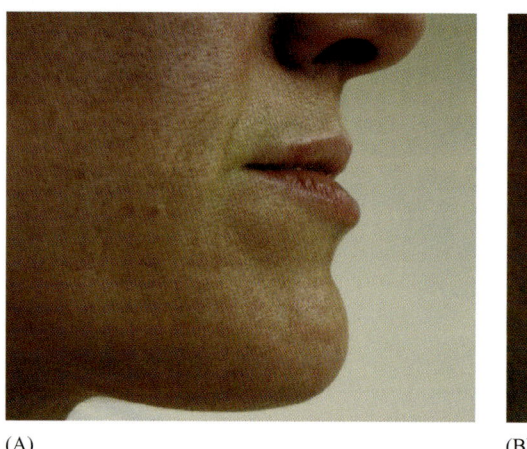
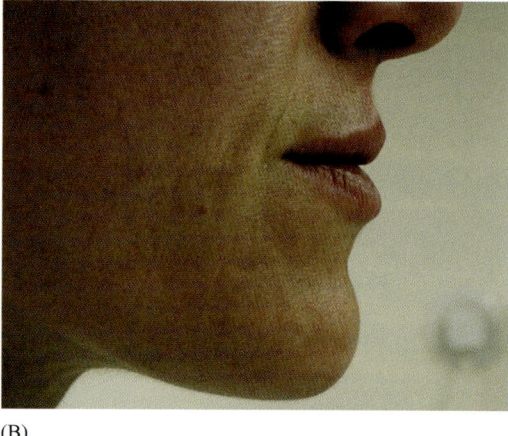

(A) (B)

*Before (**A**) and after (**B**) upper lip submucosal filler treatment.*

In the lower third of the face, lip asymmetries or defects can be corrected. If the chin is too small, chin augmentation can also be achieved by fillers. Cleft lip scars can benefit from silicone.

New fillers with high safety profiles, reasonable longevity, and different physical properties continue to be developed. With these refinements, new indications are being added to the growing list of diseases and defects that can be treated by fillers.

Patient Selection

During the pre-operative consultation, the patient will usually indicate which area of their face they wish to have improved. Patients are often unaware of their asymmetries, wrinkles, nevi, or facial anomalies. It is important that the physician discuss the baseline condition with the patient, while the patient looks in a mirror, so that the patient understands what can and what *cannot* be corrected by fillers. It is very important for the patient to have realistic expectations of the treatment. Patients with severe photoaging and disseminated wrinkles are not good candidates for fillers and should be treated in other ways, for example, ablative resurfacing by a deep chemical peel. Patients with wrinkles that are caused by excessive muscular movement (e.g., deep glabellar furrows) will only get a very transient improvement from the injection of a filler, unless the muscles that cause the wrinkling are also relaxed by botulinum toxin A.

Not all fillers are suitable for all indications and different fillers may be used in the same patient. For example, it may be better not to use the same filler in the cheeks as in the lips. In the cheeks, a large particle filler may provide more and longer lasting volume enhancement, whereas, in the lips, a finer filler may allow more precision of placement and also the use of a finer, more comfortable needle.

SOFT TISSUE FILLERS: BIODEGRADABLE VS. NONBIODEGRADABLE

Soft tissue fillers can be divided into two large groups: biodegradable and nonbiodegradable.

The biodegradable fillers mostly have the advantage of a high safety profile and the disadvantage of a temporary result. The nonbiodegradable fillers, on the other hand, have the advantage of long durability but may harbor a risk of long-lasting problems such as inflammatory nodules or granulomas, or the problem that misplaced injections will not disappear effortlessly in 6 to 12 months. Also, it must be remembered that faces change with aging. What is a good result in a young person may look strange in an older face (e.g., lips that stay large while the face becomes smaller due to the volume loss that goes with aging).

In the past, the longevity of most biodegradable fillers was short (few months) and therefore some preferred the more permanent fillers. Nowadays, some biodegradable fillers have enhanced longevity and remain one to two years in the tissues, providing a longer-term result after injection. The need for permanent fillers, with their attendant risks of permanent problems, is thus gradually lessening. If a problem arises after the injection of a temporary filler (e.g., an inflammatory nodule or if the patient is dissatisfied with the result), the filler will eventually resorb and the problem will resolve.

BIODEGRADABLE FILLERS

Injectable Collagens

Collagens are proteins that form the bulk of the extracellular matrix and comprise 80% of the dry weight of the dermis of human skin. The physiological role of collagen fibers in the skin is to provide tensile properties to the skin. With aging, the amount of collagen in the dermis decreases. This contributes to the development of wrinkles.

The first biodegradable soft tissue filler was bovine collagen, introduced in 1951. It was the first soft tissue filler to receive FDA approval in 1981 (Zyderm I®, followed by Zyderm II® and Zyplast®). Bovine collagen was the most popular US filler until 2003, when Restylane®, an injectable hyaluronic acid filler, also received FDA approval.

Three bovine collagen products are available today: Zyderm I®, with 35 mg/ml collagen; Zyderm II®, with 65 mg/ml collagen; and Zyplast®, with 35 mg/ml cross-linked collagen. Zyderm I® is used for superficial wrinkles, Zyderm II® for intermediate wrinkles, and Zyplast® for deep wrinkles or folds. Although these products are safe and yield good cosmetic results, there are disadvantages of very short longevity (3 to 6 months) and a high level of immunogenity. Three percent of patients are sensitive to bovine collagen, so a skin test is needed prior to injection of this filler. Because of this, new collagen products have been developed.

Some less immunogenic human collagen products have been produced from cadaver skin (Alloderm®, Cymetra®, Cosmoderm®, Cosmoplast®, Dermalogen®), but as these products do not offer sufficient longevity, with results lasting only 3 to 6 months, they are losing popularity.

The most interesting addition to the injectable dermal collagens is Evolence®. This filler is produced from porcine (pig) collagen with the allergenic part of the collagen (telopeptide) removed. Both these features make it less allergenic than bovine collagen, removing the need for an allergy test. Cross-linking (binding multiple molecules together to form large macromolecules that prolong the longevity of the filler) is performed by the "Glymatrix" technology, in which a sugar (ribose) is used. As the sugar is nontoxic, more cross-linking is possible which ensures a slower degradation in tissue and thus greater durability (12 to 18 months). Similar to bovine collagen, this filler has different viscosities: Evolence® (high viscosity) for the deeper folds and wrinkles, and Evolence Breeze® (low viscosity) for moderate to fine wrinkles and for lip augmentation.

Hyaluronic Acid Dermal Fillers

Hyaluronic acid is a linear polysaccharide present in tissues of all vertebrate animals. In the skin, it is the viscous fluid in which the collagen fibers, elastic fibers, and other intercellular structures are embedded. Unlike collagen, its chemical structure is not specific to any particular organism; it is identical in all species. Therefore, in its pure form, it is not immunogenic. With aging, the amount of hyaluronic acid in the skin decreases, which results in reduced volume and reduced intradermal hydration (hyaluronic acid binds water in the skin).

When injected into the skin, native hyaluronic acid will stay for only one to two days, making it a poor candidate for tissue augmentation. To improve the longevity of hyaluronic acid in skin, cross-linking of the hyaluronic acid molecules was developed in the 1980s. In this process, a chemical binds single hyaluronic molecules into large macromolecules, making the hyaluronic acid more resistant to degradation, thereby increasing its durability after injection.

Types of Cross-Linked Hyaluronic Acid

The first cross-linked hyaluronic acid preparation that was widely used for tissue augmentation was Hylaform®. This was produced from roosters' combs and cross-linked with divinyl sulfone. As it lasted only three months in tissue after injection, it lost much of its initial appeal.

The first hyaluronic acid product to receive FDA approval was Restylane® (December 2003). This filler is nonanimal derived and produced by bacterial fermentation followed by cross-linking with butanedioldiglycidyl ether (BDDE). As it is less immunogenic than Zyplast® collagen and gives longer lasting results (6 to 12 months), this filler has rapidly become the new gold standard of soft tissue augmentation. Restylane® is distributed worldwide in different forms: Restylane®, Restylane Fine Lines®, Perlane®, and Restylane SubQ®. All these products contain 20 mg hyaluronic acid per milliliter. The products differ according to the size of the hyaluronic acid particles, the number of gel particles per milliliter, and the intended depth of implantation. The product with the highest number and the smallest size of particles is Restylane Fine Line®. It is the least viscous product of all and is designed to correct fine lines and superficial, easily distensible defects by injection into the upper dermis. Restylane® has fewer and larger gel particles, and therefore higher viscosity. Perlane® has an even lower number of larger particles and is even more viscous than Restylane® and Restylane Fine Line®. It is designed to correct deep folds or wrinkles by injection into the subcutis.

Juvederm® is another widely used hyaluronic acid filler that was approved in Europe in 2001 and received FDA approval in 2006. This filler, like Restylane®, is produced by bacterial fermentation and cross-linked by BDDE. Although many different Juvederm® products are available, all are composed of a homogeneous gel with 24 mg hyaluronic acid per milliliter. The products differ by their degree of cross-linking. The greater the cross-linking, the more viscous the product, and the deeper it should be injected. Thus, the denser products are more suitable for deeper wrinkles and folds, and the less viscous, less cross-linked products are more suitable for more superficial wrinkles.

Many other products containing hyaluronic acid are available in various parts of the world, such as Teosyal®, Surgiderm®, Esthelis®, Puragen®, and many others. Most of them have a good safety profile, good viscoelastic properties, and good durability in tissue. As hyaluronic acid injection is the fastest growing noninvasive cosmetic procedure, new products with improved characteristics are constantly being developed.

Other Biodegradable Fillers

Radiesse® is a biodegradable filler composed of 30% microspheres from calcium hydroxylapatite (CaHA) particles suspended in a carboxymethylcellulose gel carrier. After injection, the carrier gel is gradually absorbed by macrophage phagocytosis and a local fibroblastic response develops around the CaHA particles. These particles are gradually degraded after 12 to 24 months, which is the duration of action of this filler. As a more viscous filler, it is especially suitable for the deeper folds or facial volume replacement and should be injected deep into the dermis or into the subcutaneous tissue. For the same reason, it is not suitable for lip augmentation or for areas with a lot of movement and thin skin, as it may become palpable or visible in these areas. With the right injection technique this filler has an excellent safety profile.

Poly-L-lactic acid (PLLA; Sculptra®) is considered a slowly degradable filler (or a semi-permanent filler), as it may take up to 40 months or even longer to degrade. It works by stimulating the production of new connective tissue. It is mainly suitable for facial volume replacement. The FDA has approved it for the treatment of volume loss in HIV-mediated lipoatrophy. Initially, this filler was marketed in Europe as New Fill®. It lost part of its popularity in Europe because of complications such as subcutaneous nodules and papules. Some researchers state that this was due to wrong dilution or incorrect injection techniques, incorrect injection volumes, or inappropriate sites of injection. Apparently, by using large dilution volumes, by preparing the mixture 12 to 24 hours before treatment, and by injection of this filler into the subcutaneous plane, the risk of complications is relatively low.

NONBIODEGRADABLE FILLERS

Silicone
Liquid silicone is the most controversial of the permanent soft tissue fillers. Its advocates are adamant that when used correctly it is extremely safe and effective. Its adversaries point out that silicone has been associated with massive deformation, and sometimes unresolvable inflammatory nodules (granulomas), even many years following injection.

Liquid silicone is a synthetic polymer of dimethylsiloxane. Its viscosity is a function of its polymerization and is measured in centistokes. Injected deeper into the dermis and/or subcutis, silicone elicits a granulomatous tissue response with collagen formation around the injected silicone, such that tiny collagen capsules develop around each microdroplet. To achieve the desired result, a series of four or five sessions of injections, at four-to-six-week intervals, are needed (the serial microdroplet technique).

Silicone, like hyaluronic acid, can achieve excellent results: silicone can do everything that hyaluronic acid can do; silicone can also do some things that hyaluronic acid cannot do. Silicone can lift depressed scars, which hyaluronic acid cannot do. To do so, tiny microdroplets of silicone are serially injected into the scar. These stimulate the host tissue response that gradually, over the ensuing weeks, lifts the scar. It is not physically possible to inject sufficient volume of an inert filler, such as hyaluronic acid, into a bound down scar to achieve the same effect. Silicone, unlike hyaluronic acid, is long lasting. This is a clear advantage but it also means that silicone is unforgiving and imperfect results, for whatever reason, will also be long lasting. Correct injection technique is critical. It will avoid "silicone lakes" (injection of droplets that are too large) and "beading" (the formation of palpable lumps just under the skin due to too superficial an injection). Silicone fills tissue by inducing a granulomatous host response. As there is variability of intensity of granulomatous response between different people and even variability within the same person over time, great care is needed to avoid overcorrection—hence, the use of four or five injection sessions. Occasionally, unexpectedly severe granulomatous reactions can occur (in perhaps 1 in 1000 patients). In the hands of an inexperienced practitioner, the frequency of such events is probably higher. These reactions may even happen many years after injection of silicone and without any obvious precipitating event (e.g., infection). At least some of these cases may be due to the later development of certain diseases such as sarcoidosis.

Artefill® and Artecoll®
Artefill® is composed of 20% homogenous polymethylmetacrylate (PMMA) microspheres evenly suspended in 3.5% bovine collagen and 0.3% lidocaine. It is more highly purified than Artecoll®, a similar product that has been used in Europe for many years. One to three months after injection, the bovine collagens are completely resorbed and replaced by newly formed human collagen that individually encapsulates the permanent PMMA microspheres. Patients must be skin tested for allergy to the bovine collagen component just as with the other bovine collagen products. Even though inflammatory nodules are very rare after injection of this filler (incidence <0.02%), they may be very long lasting and resistant to treatment. Artecoll® has therefore fallen from favor.

Polyacrylamide Gels
Aquamid® is composed of 2.5% polyacrilamide gel in water. Bio-Alcamid® is composed of 4% cross-linked polyacrylamide with polyalkylimide. These two gels are very slowly resorbed by the body over many years. They either dissipate (like Aquamid®) or are kept in place (like

Bio-Alcamid®) by a fibrous capsule. When injected in large quantities, these gels have a relatively high incidence of complications.

Complications

The use of fillers is growing rapidly due to their effectiveness, versatility, high safety profile, and the absence of any social stigma surrounding their use. However, adverse events and complications do sometimes occur.

Injection site reactions are the most common adverse events. These include pain, swelling, redness, bruising, itching, and tenderness. These reactions (mostly mild) may occur to some extent after any filler injection and mostly subside in less than seven days. No treatment is necessary. Rarely, some temporary fillers (notably hyaluronic acid products when used subcutaneously) have been associated with the appearance of delayed red, painful, swollen lumps at the sites of injection. In most of these cases, an oral antibiotic will solve the problem, indicating that imperfect aseptic technique may be the cause of this subacute cellulitis. Injections in the subcutaneous plane require the strictest possible aseptic technique to avoid this.

Over correction or too superficial placement of a filler may lead to visible lumps under the skin. This problem is mainly seen in areas of thin skin with a lot of movement, such as around the lips or the eyes or in the nasolabial grooves. These lumps may be treated either by firm compression between finger and thumb, by aspiration or, in superficial cases, by puncture incision expression (this last method is particularly useful when blueish beading is apparent, notably in the nasolabial grooves, after too superficial dermal injection of filler). Injection of hyaluronidase (an enzyme that breaks up hyaluronic acid) may be used when the problem arises after the injection of a hyaluronic acid product. When a temporary biodegradable filler is used, any unwanted lumps are usually temporary and treatable.

Persistent inflammatory nodules (granulomatous foreign body reaction) have been reported after injection of most fillers and can be resolved by serial intralesional steroid injections. With the more inert fillers, these "sensitivity" granulomatous reactions are very rare: these nodules were quite common with the older types of bovine collagen having an incidence of 1.3%; Nowadays, with the newer porcine collagens (e.g., Evolence®) and with the hyaluronic acid products, these reactions are very rare. When inflammatory nodules occur after the injection of a permanent (e.g., silicone) or semi-permanent (e.g., PLLA) filler they may, in some cases, be long lasting and more difficult to manage.

SUMMARY

The use of soft tissue fillers is increasing rapidly. This is due, in part, to the development of fillers with better longevity and higher safety profiles. Currently there are different fillers for different indications. Any former social pressure against fillers has been replaced by a peer pressure that encourages their use.

Even though the complication rate of most fillers is low, it is usually preferable to begin by using temporary soft tissue fillers, as any (rare) complications will be resolved spontaneously in due course.

27 | Cosmetic Use of Botulinum Toxin

Ines Verner and Christopher Rowland Payne

Contents Overview • History • Dynamic wrinkles • Patient selection • Indications • The procedure • When not to use botulinum toxin • Botulinum toxin for the upper face • Complications • Summary

OVERVIEW

Botulinum toxin (BTX) is a neurotoxin that is used in the treatment of dynamic wrinkles and facial rejuvenation. When injected in small quantities, it temporarily reduces the power of the target muscles, thereby reducing or effacing the wrinkles associated with those muscles for a period of four to six months. Since its first cosmetic use some 16 years ago, BTX has revolutionized aesthetic medicine. BTX injection has since become the most commonly performed noninvasive cosmetic procedure in the world.

HISTORY

BTX is naturally produced by the bacterium *Clostridium botulinum*. Over 100 years ago, it was discovered to be the cause of food poisoning-induced muscle paralysis (botulism). The first serotype, BTX-A, was isolated for the US Army by Edward Shanz in 1946. Three years later, in 1949, its mechanism of action was discovered. Seven distinct serotypes (BTX-A,B,C,D,E,F,G), each produced by different strains of *C. botulinum*, have been identified so far.

During the last three decades, BTX has been used for certain neuromuscular disorders, such as involuntary muscle spasm and strabismus ("cross-eyes").

The first observation that BTX might be helpful in treating wrinkles was made by Dr. Jean Carruthers, a Canadian ophthalmologist from Vancouver. She noted that many patients she treated with BTX for ocular indications also showed a reduction in dynamic wrinkles.

The first report of the cosmetic use of BTX and its effectiveness in reducing dynamic wrinkles in the glabellar region (i.e., the area between the eyebrows, above the root of the nose) was published in 1992 by Jean Carruthers and her dermatologist husband, Alastair Carruthers. This was followed by numerous publications that confirmed the impressive efficacy and safety of BTX-A and led to its FDA approval for treating facial wrinkles in 2002. Since then, its use has rapidly expanded to include many other cosmetic and medical indications. BTX injection has gained tremendous popularity. In recent years, it has also been used to treat migraine and hyperhidrosis (excess sweating).

BTX: Mode of Action

BTX exerts its effect at the neuromuscular junction where it blocks the release of the neurotransmitter, acetylcholine. Acetylcholine is the messenger substance, released by the stimulated nerve ending, which activates the muscle and leads to muscle contraction. Blocking its release stops muscle movement. The release of acetylcholine is triggered by the action of membrane proteins located in the terminal nerve endings. BTX blocks the release of acetylcholine from the nerve endings by binding to these specific proteins. Each of the BTX serotypes cleaves to a different membrane protein, thus exerting a different clinical effect. Only five serotypes affect the human nervous system, BTX-A,B,E,F,G, and only two of these are available as medicines, BTX-A and BTX-B.

The clinical effect of BTX-A begins to be apparent after 48 hours, reaches its maximum after one to two weeks, and lasts for four to six months. Its action decreases slowly over time as collateral sprouting of new nerve endings occurs. This begins four weeks after treatment. Later, the damaged nerve endings regenerate and regain their function. The new collateral sprouts then retract and disappear.

DYNAMIC WRINKLES

Dynamic wrinkles and expression lines gradually develop over the years due to repeated contraction of the facial muscles. These can be treated by BTX.

While other muscles in the body are attached to the bones, the muscles of the face are attached to the skin. Each facial muscle contraction causes puckering of the skin. Repeated puckering leads to wrinkling, which is always perpendicular to the underlying muscle.

In the young, these lines can be discerned only in animation. Thus, horizontal lines on the forehead can be seen when the eyebrows are elevated, only to disappear when the muscles relax and the eyebrows return to their original position. With aging, these dynamic wrinkles evolve into resting wrinkles that become permanent and gradually deepen.

PATIENT SELECTION

"Dynamic" wrinkles need to be distinguished from "fine" wrinkles of the skin associated with chronological aging and photoaging. Fine wrinkling is due to the gradual degeneration of elastin and collagen fibers in the skin. It is not directly influenced by muscular activity and, therefore, cannot be expected to improve with BTX injections. So, for the treatment to be successful, appropriate patient selection is crucial. It is important to select patients in whom the negative facial signs are caused by an underlying muscle pull. Patients with advanced or severe photoaging, who have many wrinkles at rest, are not good candidates.

INDICATIONS

The common indications for BTX-A lie in the upper face and include glabellar lines (the vertical lines between the eyebrows), forehead wrinkles, and crow's feet (wrinkles at the outer edges of the eyes). Less common indications are in the mid and lower face and include lip wrinkles, marionette lines, cobblestoning of the chin, and facial asymmetries. During the past few years, many indications have been added, and BTX is used more and more for facial rejuvenation.

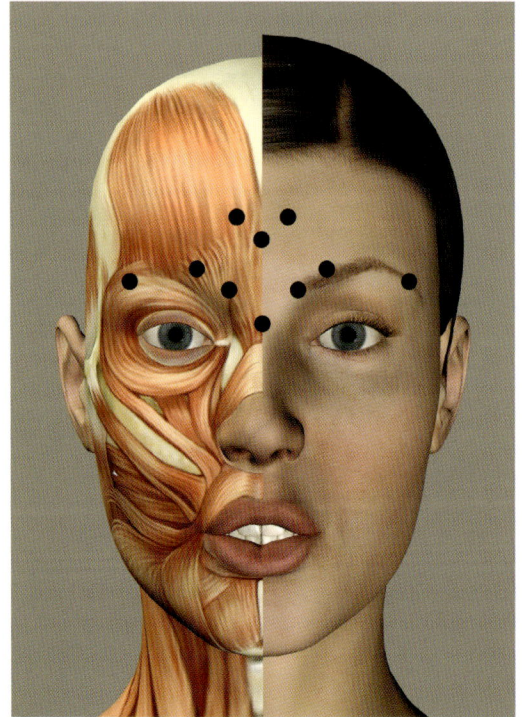

Injection points for the glabellar area and forehead in a female patient.

COSMETIC USE OF BOTULINUM TOXIN

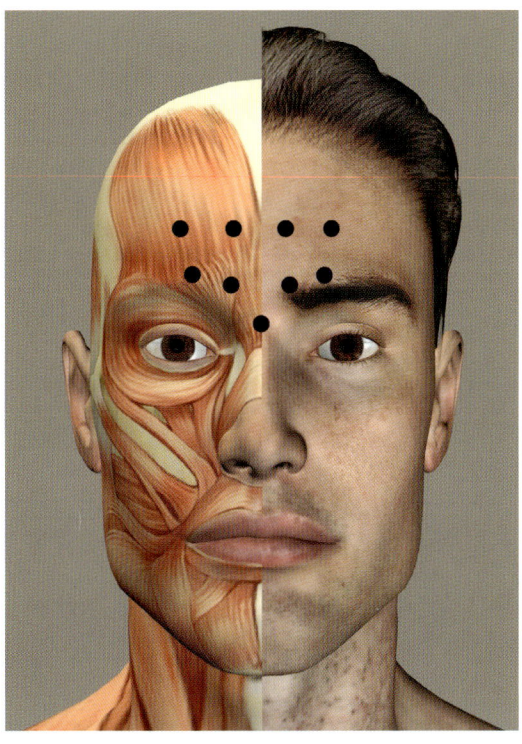

Injection points for the glabellar area and forehead in a male patient.

BTX Products

Up to now, BTX-A, being the most potent of the serotypes, is the principal serotype used in aesthetic medicine on humans. BTX-B has a shorter duration of action and is associated with more adverse effects. Several BTX-A products (Botox®/Vistabel®, Dysport®, Xeomin®, Neuronox®) and one BTX-B product (Myobloc®/NeuroBloc®) are commercially available. Botox® (Allergan Inc.) and Dysport® (Ipsen Inc.) share the majority of the aesthetics market. The main difference between these two products is the amount of human serum albumin (HSA) and BTX in each product. Botox® contains 500 μm of HSA and 100 Botox units per vial, whereas Dysport® contains 125 μm HSA per vial and 500 Dysport® units. The conversion ratio of Botox® units to Dysport® units is estimated to be somewhere between 1:3 and 1:4 and so, when stating doses, it is essential to specify the brand name.

Several companies are working on new BTX preparations and some new products such as Puretox® (Mentor) and Linurase® (Prollenium & Merz NT 201) are on the way. Other BTX-A preparations such as Neuronox® and CBTX® are being manufactured in Asia. Randomized controlled clinical trials in specific aesthetic indications are needed to compare these newer preparations to the older ones.

Storage and Dilutions

Botox® and Dysport® must be stored in the refrigerator. Other types of BTX-A preparations, such as Xeomin®, can be stored at room temperature.

All BTX-A preparations have to be diluted with saline, the amount chosen varies between practitioners and depends upon the concentration desired. Mostly, a 2-ml dilution is used for 100 Botox® units or a 2.5-ml dilution for 500 Dysport® units. It seems that a lower volume (higher concentration) keeps the effect more localized and that a greater volume (lower concentration) allows greater diffusion of the toxin, meaning fewer injections but also a higher risk of undesired effects.

THE PROCEDURE

BTX is injected in very small quantities through a very fine needle, either into the muscle or just under or into the skin. Usually, the patient is asked to make certain facial expressions so that the muscle pull becomes visible under the skin. The BTX-A is then injected after the patient relaxes the target muscles.

As fine needles are chosen, the pain sensation from the needle prick is mild and may be reduced further by the application of anesthetic cream beforehand.

The clinical effect of BTX begins to be apparent at 48 hours, reaches its maximum after one to two weeks and lasts for four to six months. The treatment should then be repeated to maintain the desired result.

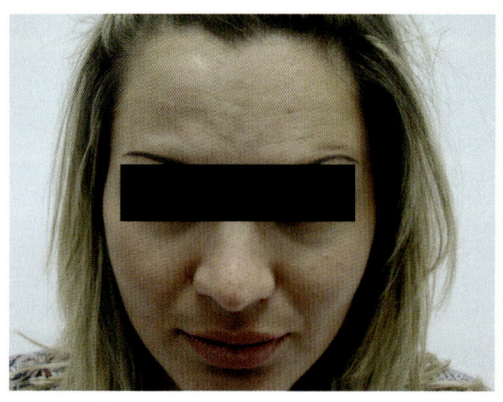
(A)

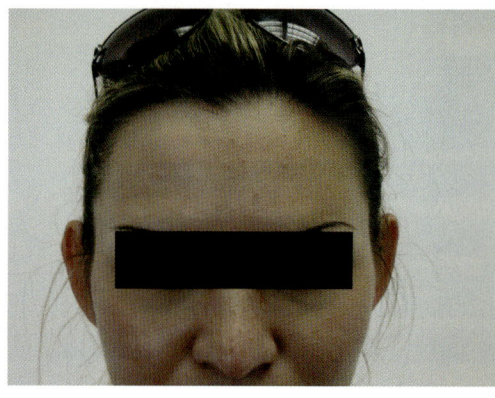
(B)

BTX-A for forehead before (**A**) and two weeks thereafter (**B**).

CONSIDERATIONS

Because muscular anatomy and physiology differ in each patient, treatment must be individualized. The patient needs to know that the effect is temporary and that further treatment will be necessary after three to six months.

Many fear the "frozen" look that was seen in the past with higher BTX dosing. Experience has changed both the injection technique and the dosing so that many treated muscles are just relaxed and not paralyzed. In this way, some muscular activity is conserved, giving the face a more natural appearance.

BTX-A exerts its clinical effect not only by relaxing the treated muscles, but also by allowing the antagonist muscles to act unopposed. For instance, treatment of the superior fibers of the orbicularis oculi (muscles that close the eyelids) will allow the frontalis (forehead muscle) to act unopposed, so resulting in a brow lift.

WHEN NOT TO USE BTX

BTX-A treatment is contraindicated in the presence of neuromuscular diseases that could amplify its effect, such as myasthenia gravis, Lambert-Eaton syndrome, amyotrophic lateral sclerosis, and other myopathies. BTX should not be used during pregnancy and lactation.

BTX FOR THE UPPER FACE

The cosmetic use of BTX began with the treatment of glabellar lines and other areas of the upper face, which remain the most commonly treated areas. The effect of BTX on glabellar lines, horizontal forehead lines, crow's feet, and especially the brow position can ameliorate unwanted facial expressions and signs of aging. More detailed information regarding BTX applications and its uses for the mid and lower face are beyond the scope of this book.

Glabellar Frown Lines

Contraction of the glabellar muscles produces an angry and tense expression. Therefore, the glabella is usually one of the first areas of choice to be treated by BTX-A. Glabellar lines are produced by contraction of the corrugator muscle, the procerus muscle, and the depressor supercilii muscles. The corrugator muscle induces the vertical lines, the procerus muscle the horizontal lines, and the depressor supercilii muscles draw the medial eyebrows down.

In this area, between three and five points are injected. One point for the procerus muscle and one point for each of the corrugator muscles (0.5 to 1 cm above the orbital rim) are the first three. When injecting five points, two additional points for the lateral part of the corrugators and parts of the frontalis muscle (1 cm above the orbital rim) are injected. Often a small injection inferomedial to the medial part of the eyebrow will also be useful.

Usually, the Botox® dose will be 20 to 40 units and the Dysport® dose will be around 15 to 50 units to treat this area.

Crow's Feet

The wrinkles extending laterally from the periorbital area are called "crow's feet". The lateral fibers of the orbicularis oculi muscle that rings the orbit cause these wrinkles. These fibers are arranged in a circular pattern around the eyes and their contraction produces forceful closure of the eyelids. The injections are usually used within this area, each approximately 1 cm lateral to the orbital rim. The patient is asked to smile maximally so that the center of the crow's feet is noted and the first point is injected there after relaxation. Two other injection points are located 1 cm below and 1 cm above that point.

The injections should not be made while the patient is still smiling, as BTX-A may affect the zygomaticus complex and thus cause ptosis (drooping) of the upper lip. Also, the most anterior injection point should not cross the lateral central line (a vertical line drawn through the lateral canthus).

For this area, the Botox® dose is usually 6 to 15 units and the Dysport® dose is 10 to 30 units.

Horizontal Forehead Lines

The horizontal forehead lines are caused by the contraction of a muscle called the occipitofrontalis. This muscle originates from the eyebrow and glabella skin and from the orbicularis oculi fibers and inserts into the galea aponeurotica. When contracted, it not only leads to horizontal forehead lines but also raises the eyebrows and the upper lids and makes the eyes look bigger and more open. Treating the inferior part of the frontalis requires caution, as over-treating may cause brow and even eyelid ptosis. Excessive weakening of the frontalis without a corresponding weakening of brow depressor muscles may result in brow ptosis with a puffy-eyed expression.

It is also important to realize that the ideal female brow is arched, with the lateral aspect more elevated than the medial, whereas the ideal male brow is almost horizontal in shape. Therefore, in females, at least some activity of the lateral frontalis muscle should be conserved.

For this area, usually 4 to 20 injection points are best, with a Botox® dose of 10 to 16 units and a Dysport® dose of 20 to 40 units.

COMPLICATIONS

The safety of BTX-A, when used in cosmetic doses, is excellent. Complications are uncommon and are mostly mild and transient. The majority of the side effects are due to suboptimal injection technique or diffusion of the BTX-A into adjacent muscles.

Drooping of an Eyebrow (Brow Ptosis)

The most troublesome complication, when treating the area between the eyebrows or the forehead, is drooping of the adjacent brow. The medical term for this is *brow ptosis*. As the lower 2.5 to

4 cm of the forehead muscle (frontalis) are responsible for brow elevation, its paralysis will lower the position of the eyebrows and impair brow elevation. At risk are patients with a low forehead and older patients with redundant eyelid skin. To prevent this complication, it is advisable to inject forehead wrinkles as high as possible (at least 1 cm above the orbital rim or higher) and to start with low doses in this area. Another possibility is concomitant injection of the opposing brow depressors, particularly in patients over 50.

Drooping of an Eyelid (Blepharoptosis)
The sinking down of an eyelid (eyelid ptosis) is another complication that may be seen when the injected toxin migrates to the levator palpebrae muscle. This temporary side effect can usually be avoided by careful injection technique.

Mephisto Sign
In some patients, restricting frontalis treatment to the central part of the forehead will mean the central brow falls, but the lateral brow remains elevated, conferring a diabolic expression. The devil in this can easily be put to flight by injecting 1 to 2 units of Botox® or 2 to 6 units of Dysport® in the point of maximum contraction when the patient raises the forehead.

Bruising
One of the most common complications in the area surrounding the eye (periorbital area) is bruising. This area has a rich vascular supply and thin skin. Injections should be placed very superficially, and care must be taken to avoid hitting the superficial vessels that may be seen through the skin.

Formation of Antibodies
The production of antibodies against the toxin may decrease the efficacy of the treatment. This problem is negligible in the cosmetic application of BTX, where very low doses of BTX are used.

SUMMARY

Since the introduction of BTX-A into aesthetic medicine, tremendous progress has been made in all aspects of its use. Over the years, BTX-A has proven to be one of the safest and most exciting drugs in aesthetic medicine. We now understand much better its mechanism of action. Dosing and injection technique have become individualized, which has led to better results with fewer side effects. BTX-A is currently used for many challenging conditions and new applications are constantly being developed.

28 | Mesotherapy

Evangeline B. Handog and Encarnacion R. Legaspi-Vicerra

Contents Overview • History of mesotherapy • Before commencing treatment • Techniques of mesotherapy • Mesolift • Mesolipotherapy • When should mesotherapy not be used • Side effects of mesotherapy • Summary

OVERVIEW

Mesotherapy is used to treat a broad spectrum of medical disorders such as allergies, arthritis, asthma, depression, fibromyalgia, irritable bowel syndrome, immune system deficiencies, and insomnia. It is also used for a variety of conditions associated with chronic pain. The dermatologic uses of mesotherapy include such conditions as acne, hair loss, various types of dermatitis, scars, chronic itching, psoriasis, stretch marks, spider veins, venous insufficiency, and vitiligo.

The cosmetic uses of mesotherapy include aesthetic medicine to treat photoaging and its various manifestations. It is intended for the tightening of loose, saggy skin on the face and neck, reducing the extent of wrinkling. Mesotherapy is also used to treat pigmentary changes. In this chapter, we refer mainly to its cosmetic applications.

Mesotherapy is a nonsurgical aesthetic medical treatment. The term itself was coined in 1958 by Dr Michel Pistor as a treatment employing minute doses of multiple pharmaceutical and homeopathic medications and standardized natural plant extracts, vitamins, amino acids, and other ingredients, which are injected into various levels of the skin depending on the indication of treatment. Mesotherapy may be injected subcutaneously (into the fat layer just beneath the skin) to treat localized adiposity, whereas for skin rejuvenation, the injection is targeted into the dermis.

The technique is called mesotherapy (from the Greek *mesos*, "middle") because the injections are intended for tissues derived from the embryonic mesoderm layer, one of the three primary germ layers in the early embryo, which eventually becomes the supporting and nourishing layers of the skin, containing connective tissue, muscle, subcutaneous fat, and blood vessels.

In mesotherapy, a medicinal "bullet" is delivered directly to a particular target area in the body, as opposed to orally administered medication which must first pass through the gastrointestinal tract and is filtered by the liver before it is released into the bloodstream. For example, when using oral medications intended to treat inflammation in the knee, only a small portion of what is ingested actually reaches the knee itself. In mesotherapy, on the other hand, a much smaller dose of the same medicine can be injected with a tiny needle very close to the target area, with the skin acting as an efficient time release delivery system. In essence, mesotherapy is based on a simple principle: to inject little, seldom, and at the right place.

HISTORY OF MESOTHERAPY

In 1952, a French physician by the name of Dr Michel Pistor developed the technique. In the treatment of an asthmatic patient, he gave intravenous procaine, which was meant to improve the condition. However, due to the limited effect of the medicine on the patient, Pistor employed multiple, local, superficial (3 to 5 mm deep) injections of the medication around the patient's ears. The treatment yielded some improvement and was recognized as the original application of mesotherapy.

The French Academy of Medicine recognized mesotherapy as a specialty of medicine in 1987. Mesotherapy is now a popular procedure throughout European countries and South America, and is practiced by approximately 18,000 physicians worldwide.

BEFORE COMMENCING TREATMENT

Before commencing mesotherapy treatment, several factors should be considered:

1. **Needs of the patient**—Before carrying out mesotherapy, consider whether it would be the most appropriate procedure available for treating the particular problem of the patient.
2. **Type of medications needed**—The specific solution of vitamins, minerals, enzymes, plant extracts, anesthetics, medications, and amino acids to be administered should be carefully considered beforehand.
3. **Frequency of visits**—How many treatment sessions will be required? This depends on the type of medical problem, its extent, and severity. The treatment sessions usually take place every 7 to 15 days.
4. **Number of visits required**—The number of visits will be determined by the patient response to the mesotherapy treatment. The number of visits usually ranges from a minimum of 4 to a maximum of 20.
5. **Technique to be used**—Certain problems require particular mesotherapeutical techniques, of which there are several.

TECHNIQUES OF MESOTHERAPY

The exact technique to be employed in mesotherapy depends on the target area to be treated. The types of techniques include intraepidermal (tremor), superficial intradermic (multipricking), deep intradermic (point per point), and intra-hypodermic.

Intraepidermal (Tremor)

Intraepidermal technique refers to injecting the mesotherapeutic agents into the epidermis. The term "tremor," regarding this technique, refers to the rapid fine movements of the injection. A tuberculin syringe with a 4-mm needle, or a mesogun (depending on what is available), is used to inject the medications into the epidermis (see illustration). Intraepidermal technique is intended for facial rejuvenation. Mesotherapy injections at two-week intervals for a total of 10 treatments is advised. The success of the treatment depends on the accuracy and technical skills of the administering physician in the use of either the mesotherapy gun or the syringe.

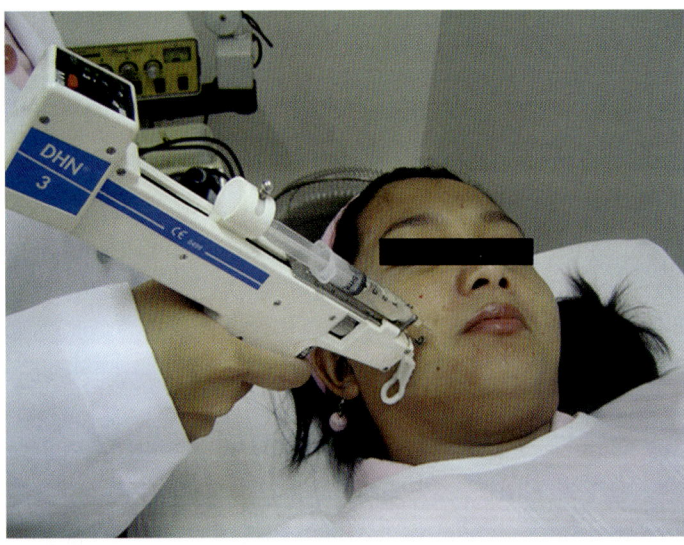

Mesogun.

Superficial Intradermic (Multipricking)

Superficial intradermic or multipricking methods refer to the injection of mesotherapeutic agents into the dermis (see illustration) by multiple rapid injections delivered using a 4- or 6-mm needle.

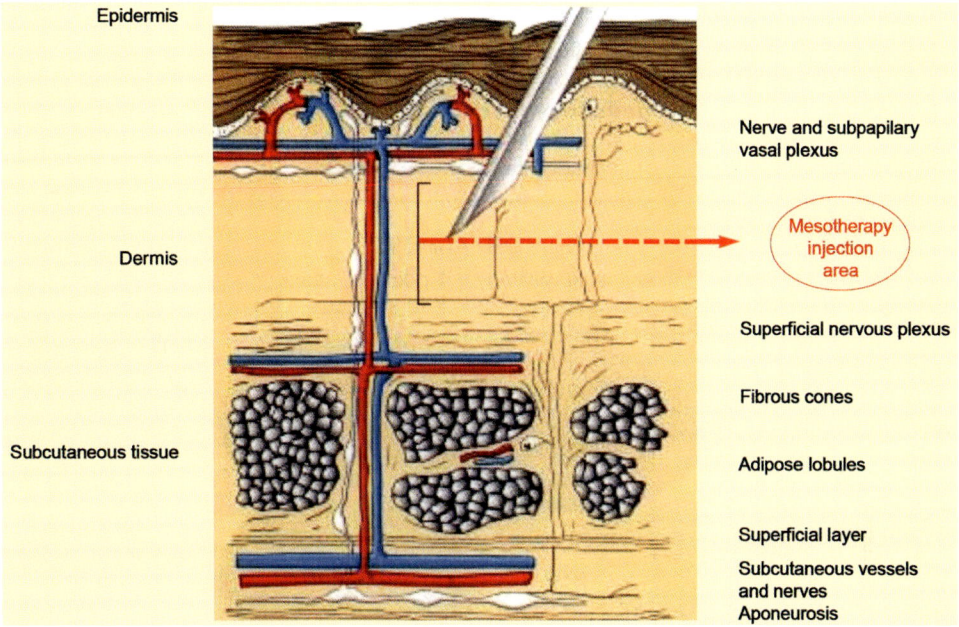

Mesotherapy site of injection.

Injections should produce a wheal—which is a rounded- or flat-topped, pale-red papule or plaque that is characteristically evanescent, disappearing within hours—similar to the purified protein derivative (PPD) wheal, an intradermally administered tuberculin injection used as a test for the diagnosis of tuberculosis. This technique for mesotherapy should be used for injections in the treatment of cellulite. Mesotherapy injections weekly for 10 to 15 visits is advised. The number of treatment sessions depends on the patient response and may be tapered off to once a month for maintenance.

Deep Intradermic (Point Per Point)

Deep intradermic injection or point per point injection technique is employed for arthritis and tendonitis wherein mesotherapeutic medicines are injected into the dermis using a 4-mm needle. Injections are directed to the areas that are inflamed or affected by disease. With this technique, patients may benefit more from immediate relief of pain and inflammation than taking oral medications.

Intra-Hypodermic

Injections into the hypodermis or subcutaneous layer of the skin are used for lower back pain or musculoskeletal pain. Needle length of 13 mm is used to deliver mesotherapeutic cocktails.

MESOLIFT

As one ages, the blood supply to the skin decreases, resulting in a reduction in the flow of oxygen and nutrients to tissues. Similarly, free radicals cannot be eliminated from the bodily tissues as easily as in the young. This, in turn, causes aging and the development of an unaesthetic appearance of the skin.

Mesolift is a mesotherapy procedure that helps minimize wrinkles and improves skin elasticity and tone and texture. It enhances skin contour, lifts sagging skin in the areas of the face and neck, and decreases wrinkles and "crepe" skin in the facial and décolleté areas. Although mesolift is not a substitute for facelift, it can give one a fresher and healthier look, defying the aging process.

The mesolift products may contain hyaluronic acid, highly concentrated vitamins, trace elements, coenzymes, amino acids, and antioxidants that nourish and rejuvenate the skin, promoting the production of collagen and elastin, and stimulation of metabolism. They also improve circulation in the small blood vessels of the skin, strengthening its structure and restoring its firmness. When used as facial creams or face masks, penetration of these compounds into the skin is minimal. Injecting them, via mesotherapy, brings them right into the desired place in the skin and subcutaneous tissues, where they can exert their beneficial effect. The procedure uses a device containing syringe and needle, which acts similar to a manual sewing machine. Multiple small pricks, into a measured depth, that insert into the tissue accurate quantity of the active compound used.

After treatment, the patient's skin looks well rested, radiant, and firmer. Mesotherapy works well in conjunction with other antiaging regimens such as botulinum toxin, laser resurfacing, peels, antioxidants, topical creams, and facelift.

The following tables detail various mesolift cocktail mixtures including hyaluronic acid + vitamin C + vitamin A cocktail, glutathione cocktail, vitamin cocktail, and hyaluronic acid + vitamin C cocktail.

Hyaluronic Acid + Vitamin C + Vitamin A Cocktail

Active components
Phase 1
Hyaluronic acid 3.5 %
Phase 2
Vitamin C
Procaine
Amino methyl silanetriol + DMAE
Vitamin A
Treatment: Remove 2 ml out of 7 ml diluted HA to mix with phase 2 solution

Glutathione Cocktail

Active components
Glutathione
Vitamin C
Glycolic acid or pyruvate
Indications
Photoaging
Melasma
Sun damage
Frequency: Use vitamin C once per week

Vitamin Cocktail

Active components
Vitamin C
Saline solution
Procaine 2%
Indications
Photoaging
Melasma
Sun damage
Frequency: Use vitamin C once per week

Hyaluronic Acid + Vitamin C Cocktail

Active components
Phase 1
Hyaluronic acid 3.5 %
Phase 2
Vitamin C
Procaine
Amino methyl silanetriol + DMAE
Treatment: Remove 2 ml out of 7 ml diluted HA to mix with phase 2 solution

MESOLIPOTHERAPY

Mesolipotherapy can be used to contour different parts of the body. The procedure diminishes the areas of fat by blocking the internal signals of fat uptake that trigger fat release, improving circulation, while vitamins and amino acids are added to tighten the sagging skin and restore a more youthful and athletic appearance. Similarly, mesotherapy may reduce the appearance of cellulite by dissolving excess fat.

Mesolipotherapy is by far the most popular mesotherapy procedure because it offers an alternative to liposuction and is regarded as a safe treatment of localized areas of adiposity. Mesolipotherapy removes fat from adipose tissue without completely destroying it. Thus, if one gains weight after mesotherapy, the fat returns to the treated area, unlike liposuction in which fat can reappear in places that had been thin in the past.

The most thoroughly researched medication used in mesolipotherapy is phosphatidylcholine. Phosphatidylcholine works as a lipolytic substance that initially increases the blood flow in the affected area, causing local breakdown of fat. This compound and procedure is detailed in chapter 13 on lipolysis.

WHEN SHOULD MESOTHERAPY NOT BE USED

Basically, the ideal candidate for mesotherapy is an adult, 18 to 75 years old, and in good health. Mesotherapy should not be implemented for people in whom any of the following applies:

- pregnant or breast feeding
- insulin-dependent diabetes
- history of recent cancer
- history of blood clots or use of blood-thinning medication
- those on multiple heart medications
- history of severe heart disease or history of heart arrhythmias
- history of stroke

SIDE EFFECTS OF MESOTHERAPY

Mesotherapy is a very low-risk procedure. The treatment is carried out on a fully conscious person and does not require anesthesia. Therefore, there is no need for postoperative recovery times or for the application of heavy compressions. The amount of medications used is extremely minute. However, the side effects of mesotherapy can include:

1. itching, burning, or swelling, which usually subsides within one hour after treatment,
2. pigmentation on the area of injection,
3. allergic reaction to injected drugs, and
4. infections due to poor injection technique.

SUMMARY

Mesotherapy is carried out by injecting various active compounds into subcutaneous tissue and the skin. In every injection, a small quantity of the compound is inserted to target area. Mesotherapy has been used to treat a broad spectrum of medical disorders. When used in the treatment of facial aging, there is evidence that certain compounds, such as hyaluronic acid combined with vitamins, improves the general appearance of the area treated and, to a certain extent, reverses skin aging. More research studies are required to accurately evaluate the extent of beneficial effect of mesotherapy and the optimal compounds to be used in the procedures.

29 | Camouflaging Skin Lesions and Other Disfiguring Conditions

Victoria L. Rayner

Contents Overview • Types of skin lesions that can be hidden using makeup • Techniques of camouflage • Foundation creams • Applying foundation cream • Cover creams • Matching cover creams to the skin • Applying cover cream • Determining the right application method • Recreating skin imperfections

OVERVIEW

This chapter deals with camouflaging skin lesions. The following pages describe a series of aesthetic problems that cannot always be treated effectively. The correct and efficient use of makeup techniques can help the patient considerably, and bring about a marked improvement in his/her appearance.

By studying this chapter, the reader will by no means be qualified to practice as an expert in makeup, which requires skills that take years of experience to acquire. Nevertheless, reading this chapter will provide some idea of the types of techniques in use, and the various possibilities that exist in the field of camouflaging skin lesions. Before trying to hide a skin lesion, it is recommended that a physician be consulted in order to determine the nature of the lesion to make sure it is not something that requires medical treatment. For example, the removal of cancerous lesions is of critical importance, and should be performed not just because of aesthetic considerations. Moreover, sometimes a skin lesion may be the sign of an internal disease. Merely covering up or hiding the lesion, without consulting a doctor, may delay appropriate diagnosis and treatment of the underlying illness.

In addition, one needs to determine whether or not there is some way of removing the lesion permanently (e.g., surgery, laser treatment, bleaching preparation, or some other technique), rather than merely hiding it.

TYPES OF SKIN LESIONS THAT CAN BE HIDDEN USING MAKEUP

Pink-to-Red Lesions

Fine Networks of Blood Vessels
The medical term for a fine network of blood vessels is **telangiectasia** (see chapter 11). It is a relatively common condition, which is usually the result of cumulative damage to the skin from various causes: cumulative exposure to the sun, radiation therapy for various diseases, prolonged use of steroid-containing medications, and others. Sometimes these lesions are a manifestation of certain skin diseases.

Various Growths Derived from Blood Vessels
There is a wide range of growths that are derived from the tissues that form blood vessels. Because these lesions contain a relatively large amount of blood, they usually range from pink to red in color. The term **angioma** is used to describe a group of benign growths that are derived from the tissues that make up the blood vessels. Although these growths are benign, and pose no medical danger to the patient, they may be aesthetically bothersome.

Light-Colored (Hypopigmented) Lesions
Vitiligo is a skin disease that is characterized by light, white/ivory-colored lesions. The reason for the appearance of these areas on the skin is not really known, although we do know

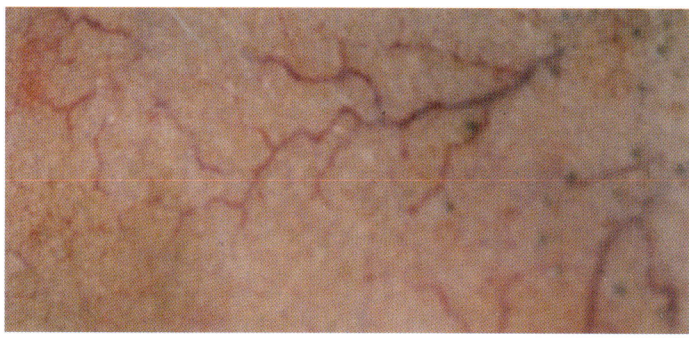

Telangiectasia of the face.

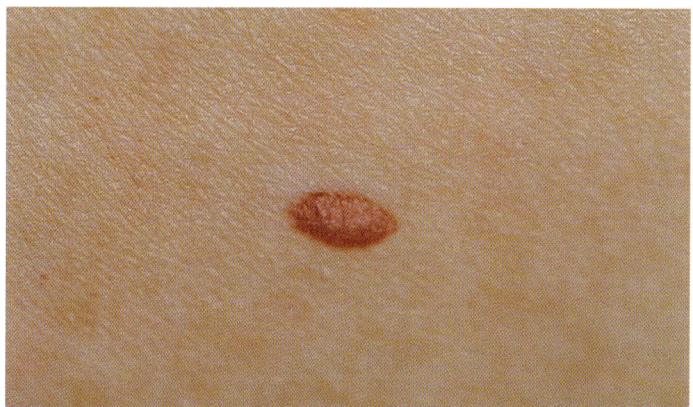

Angioma.

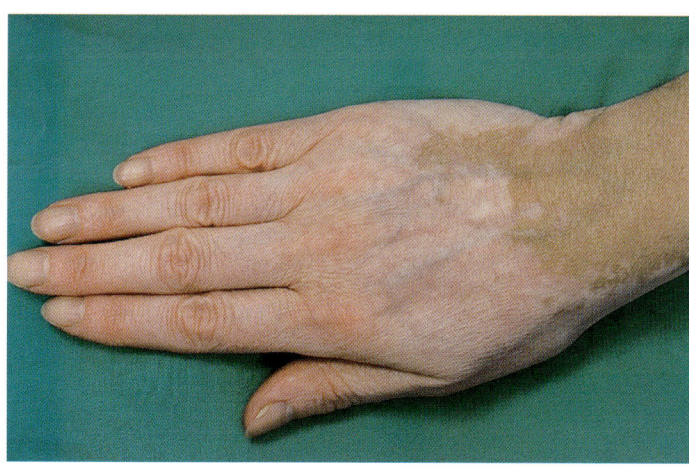

Vitiligo on the skin of the hands.

that in this disease there is some abnormality in the function of the body's immune system. As a result, the patient's immune system attacks his/her own pigment-producing system in the skin.

Another group of light-colored skin lesions includes pale areas of skin that can appear following some inflammatory process or injury. The medical term for these areas is **postinflammatory hypopigmentation**. Following injury or inflammation in a certain region, that area of skin may become paler (hypopigmented), or sometimes even darker (hyperpigmented).

Tan-to-Dark Brown Lesions

A typical example of this type of lesion is the "**pregnancy mask**" (**melasma**, or **chloasma**). Melasma describes a specific distribution of brown pigmentation on the face, which is frequently seen in pregnant women. These are light to dark brown in color. They are usually symmetrical in appearance and occur typically on the upper lip, the forehead, and the chin. For a more detailed discussion of the pregnancy mask, see chapter 20 on bleaching preparations.

Other pigmented lesions of the skin include **freckles**, **sun spots** (liver spots, correctly termed **solar lentigines**), and **nevi** (beauty spots). These lesions are discussed in more detail in chapter 20 on bleaching preparations and chapter 15 on skin tumors.

Scars

Scars may range in color from pale to dark. They may be raised above the skin surface or sunken below the surface, and so that when using makeup to hide scars, these parameters must also be kept in mind.

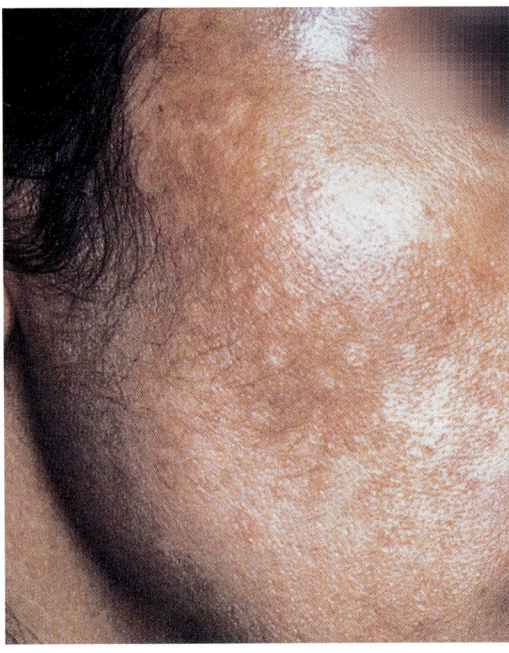

"Pregnancy mask" (melasma).

Transient Problems

All the aesthetic problems mentioned above refer to lesions that are present on the skin for a long time. However, there may be transient injuries or lesions on the skin that are also an aesthetic problem and need to be dealt with by makeup and camouflage. For example, a blow or injury may produce a red, swollen area on the face. Concealing such a lesion would be desirable before some important social event, for instance.

In these cases, it is also important to consult a dermatologist before embarking on cosmetic treatment. In certain skin diseases, one should avoid applying makeup preparations on the affected skin areas.

TECHNIQUES OF CAMOUFLAGE

Attracting attention away from facial or bodily disfigurements by camouflaging can be achieved by using two different techniques. For cosmetic problems that require full concealment, one should use **cover creams**. On the other hand, a variety of skin lesions may require only subtle textural and pigment blending using **foundation creams**.

Selection of the cosmetic solution will depend on the quality of the cosmetic result that can be achieved by each of the above techniques, what the individual can and will apply, the cost of the materials, and how well the procedure fits into his/her daily activities.

When deciding upon the appropriate technique for camouflaging skin lesions, seek the advice of an experienced cosmetician or makeup expert.

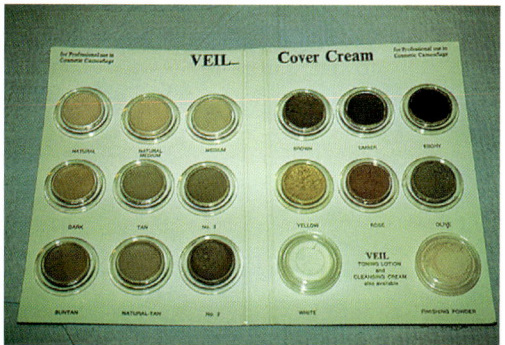 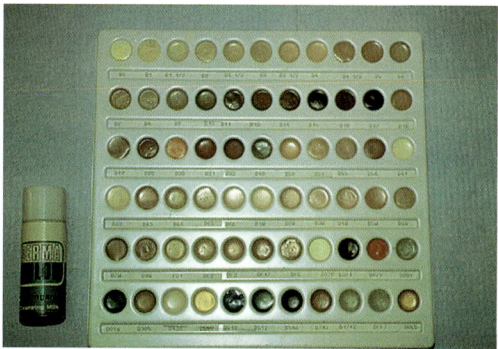

Two examples of cover cream palettes.

FOUNDATION CREAMS

There are two types of foundation creams: clear foundation cream that is applied in order to bind makeup preparations to the skin, and foundation creams that contain various coloring agents, which can be used to cover and disguise unwanted coloration on areas of the face. In this chapter, we shall deal with colored foundation creams.

Colored foundation creams contain less pigment than cover creams. Therefore, when using foundation creams, the best cosmetic result will be achieved by proper selection of the right shade. This can be obtained by using only foundation creams and combining color correctors with the foundation creams.

If a foundation cream alone is to be used, one should keep in mind that it may appear darker in the container than when it is applied to the skin, because the pigment is in its concentrated form. The undertones of the treated skin should be carefully analyzed and identified in order to achieve the optimal color matching.

If the foundation cream does not offer adequate coverage, a **color corrector** can be used. Color correctors are not foundations. They are designed to be applied under a foundation in order to neutralize light-to-moderate skin discoloration. In such cases, only after the application of a color corrector should one use a foundation cream—whose color should more closely match the skin color.

Color correctors are most commonly used to counterbalance ruddiness or sallow undertones of the skin. When using color correctors, one should keep in mind some basic principles of proper color matching:

- Use a green-colored corrector to conceal and neutralize pink or red skin discoloration.
- Use a lavender-colored corrector to normalize a sallow shade.
- Use a gold-colored corrector to tone down gray discoloration.

APPLYING FOUNDATION CREAM

The foundation should be applied to the skin by lightly spreading it on, using a delicate swab or a disposable sponge (wet or dry), or with the fingertips. This spreads it out more evenly over the skin, and helps it penetrate the skin pores, thereby improving its adherence to the skin so that it remains on the skin for longer. Once applied, the foundation should appear well blended.

COVER CREAMS

Cover creams are used to camouflage skin lesions. Basically, they represent a certain subtype of makeup products. They consist of various coloring agents in an oily base.

The coloring agents give the product its covering ability and, in various combinations, provide the required color and appropriate degree of gloss. Substances used for this purpose include various minerals and metal compounds, such as titanium dioxide, iron-based compounds, zinc and magnesium compounds, and other pigments. As opposed to regular makeup products, cover creams are **opaque**, with superior covering capabilities. They are more **stable** on the skin, and remain on the face for longer than ordinary makeup products. This durability is particularly important when hiding scars. The reason is that the ability of a substance to remain on the skin for a long time depends on its ability to get into the skin pores. A scar does not have any pores, so ordinary makeup would normally not remain on scar tissue for a lengthy period.

Matching Cover Creams to the Skin

To successfully match a cover cream to the patient's skin, the camouflage therapist must be able to identify the underlying colors that make up the patient's skin tone. The procedure is performed as follows:

1. The cover cream palette is held by the camouflage therapist alongside the area of skin that is to be camouflaged. The therapist makes a quick scan of each cover cream shade to determine its match to the patient's skin color.
2. If necessary, a second color should be added and blended into the cover cream. No more than two cream shades from the cover cream palette should be selected to match the skin tone. The camouflage therapist has to approximate the percentage that will be needed of each of these shades to produce the correct color match.
3. Once the correct shade or shades have been chosen, the camouflage therapist removes a small amount from the container and places it on the back of his/her hand. The cream is rubbed onto the back of the hand in a circular motion until it is malleable and spreads easily.
4. Three different color combinations of no more than two blended colors are blended and mixed. The formulas are recorded.
5. A small sample of each of the three separate cover cream combinations is applied to the patient's skin.
6. The camouflage therapist examines the patient's face from a distance, trying to choose the best combination of cover cream. The cover cream should meet the edges of the surrounding skin without detection. If the cover cream color combination is the right shade, it will blend so well (not too light or too dark) that it will barely be noticeable. If the cover cream color combination is too dark, a little bit more of lighter color of the two can be added until it matches the patient's skin tone. A pinhead amount of white cover cream can also be used to lighten it up. If it is too light, a little more of a darker shade of the two can be added until the color of the patient's skin tone is matched as closely as possible.

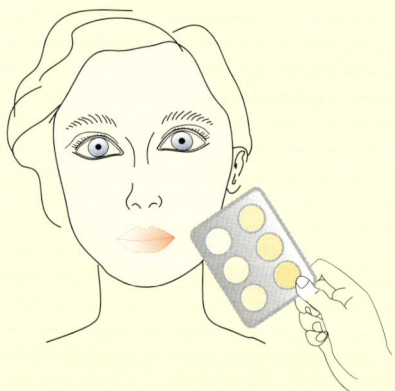

Identifying the underlying colors of the patient's skin.

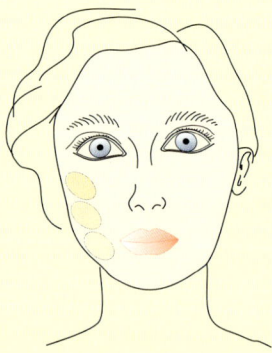

Application of cover cream combinations on the patient's skin.

MATCHING COVER CREAMS TO THE SKIN

It is wise to test several different products to find the product with the optimal shade that is most suitable for the client. To achieve optimal coverage, the makeup should be a little darker than the natural shade of the skin. (It should be remembered that the original shade of the makeup changes somewhat once it is applied to the skin, depending on the degree of moisture and the pH of the skin).

In general, it is virtually impossible to attain a perfect color match. Two products usually have to be used to achieve the best possible color. After the correct formula has been identified and optimal coverage has been achieved by the camouflage therapist, the patient will be able to regularly perform these camouflage procedures himself/herself.

APPLYING COVER CREAM

Application of cover cream involves the technique of dabbing on the cream with the third finger (or with a synthetic sponge) in a patting motion, rather than rubbing. The edges of the cover cream should blend with the surrounding skin to avoid areas of demarcation. The cover cream layer needs to be stabilized and waterproofed by the application of a colorless powder on its surface to prevent the cover cream from sliding on the skin. After the problem area has been covered, makeup should also be applied to the other side of the face in order to achieve a more natural and symmetrical look. Attempts should not be made to cover a lesion or area with the "perfect" coverage, which may give the face a strange and unnatural look. Remember that every normal, healthy face has a certain degree of natural imperfection. Some examples of the use of cover cream are shown below.

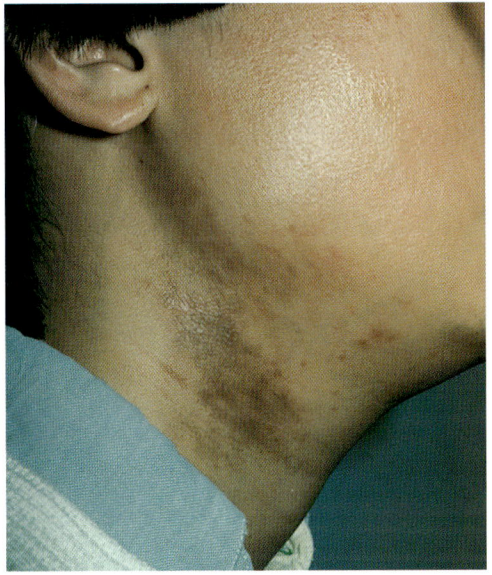
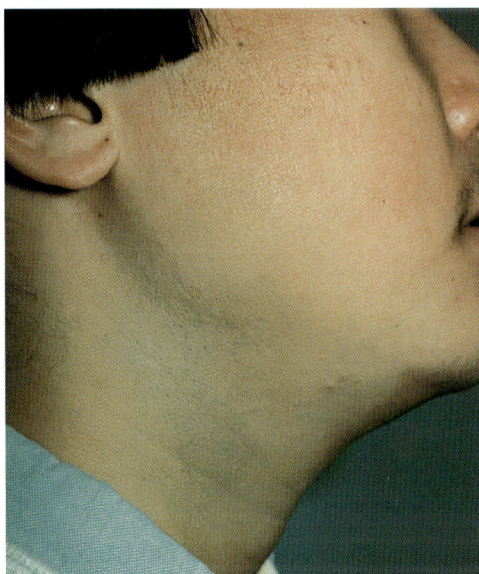

Camouflage of a hyperpigmented scar; before and after.

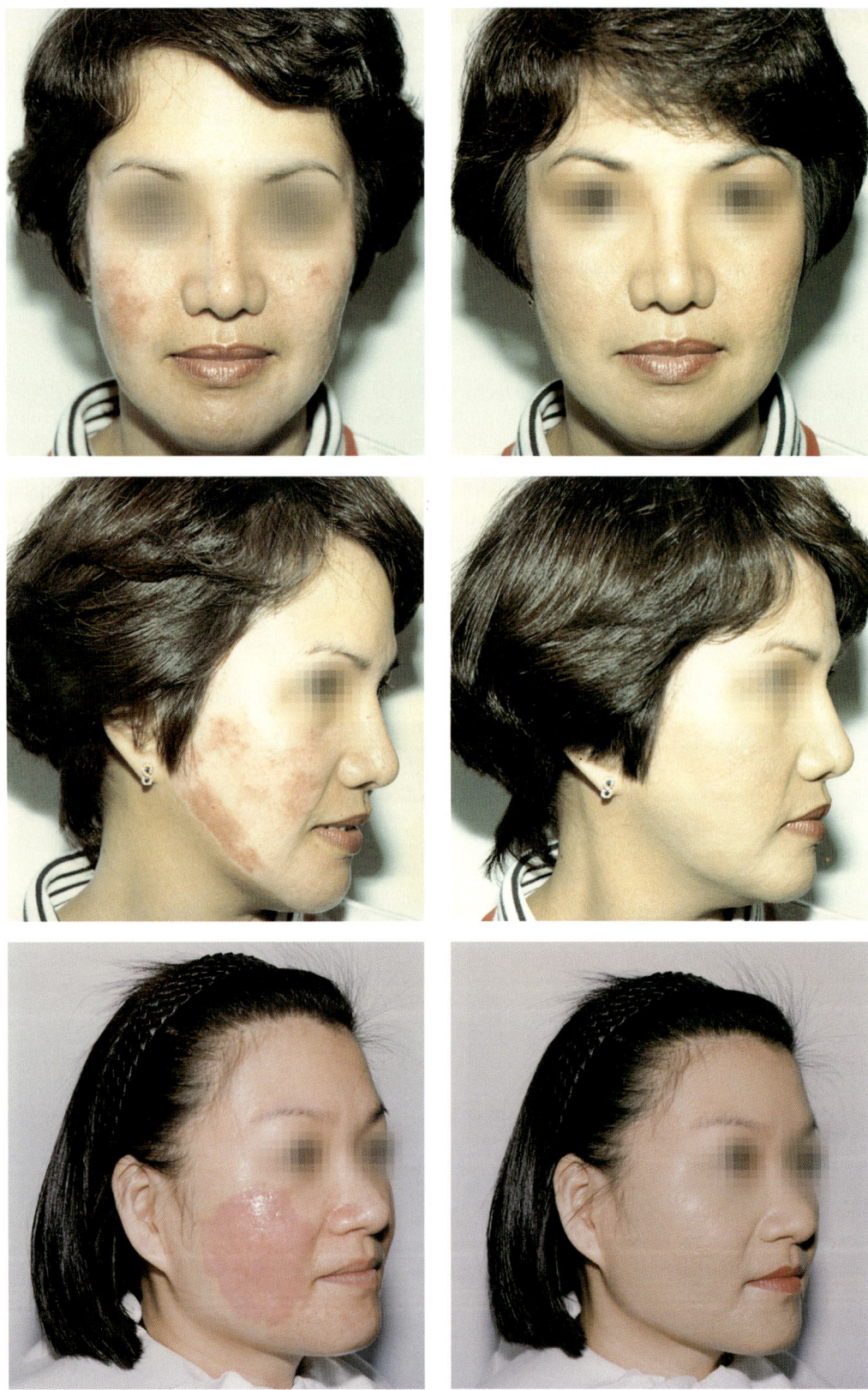

Camouflage of burn wounds.

DETERMINING THE RIGHT APPLICATION METHOD

There are three distinct types of skin with regard to the level of moisture: dry, oily, and normal. Each requires a different cover cream application method to ensure the best result.

Dry Skin
If the skin is dehydrated and dry in texture, the cover cream should be applied and left to remain on the skin for up to 10 minutes before being set with powder. The powder should be colorless and quickly brushed off after application to prevent the area from looking scaly.

Oily Skin
The cover cream should be applied and powdered, and the talc should be left sitting on top of the cover cream mixture for up to 10 minutes to absorb the oils in the product before the powder is brushed off.

Normal Skin
The cover cream should be applied and powdered, and the powder should be brushed off immediately to produce the most natural effect.

RECREATING SKIN IMPERFECTIONS

In certain instances, to provide the most natural cosmetic result, one must recreate the appearance of imperfections on the skin. Freckles, beard stubble, and broken veins can all be reproduced with the use of cosmetic sponges. To stipple-in freckles, broken veins, or beard stubble over a cosmetic camouflaged area, one would simply press a wedge-type cosmetic sponge into a cover cream mixture. To determine the amount of pressure required to imitate the skin irregularity, the sponge should be pressed down on the back of one's hand before applying it to the skin area. Using the stipple sponge as an applicator, powder is afterward applied to set and waterproof the application. To reproduce broken capillaries, a rose cover cream can be used; to imitate freckles, a golden-brown mixture can be used; while for beard stubble one should select (depending on the beard color) a brown, dark brown, gray, or black cover cream.

30 | Hair Structure and Its Care
Emilia Hodak

Contents Overview • Definition: hair follicle • Types of hair • How many hair follicles are there? • Hair structure • Transverse section of the hair shaft • Life cycle of the hair • Hair growth rate • Hair care: factors which affect hair growth • Hair loss and baldness

OVERVIEW

The social, psychological, and sexual significance of the scalp and body hair is immense. Any change in the pattern of the hair—too much hair, too little hair, change of color—may have far-reaching emotional consequences for the person involved. This chapter presents facts about the scalp and body hair and general suggestions regarding hair care.

DEFINITION: HAIR FOLLICLE

The hair follicle is an elongated tube-like structure in the skin. It is lined by cells, and the hair grows out of the base of the follicle.

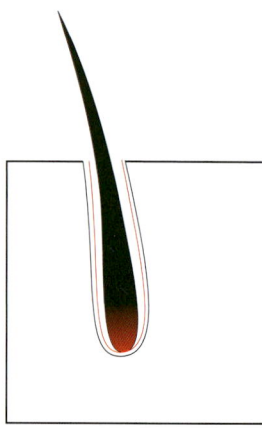

Schematic representation of a hair follicle.

TYPES OF HAIR

Vellus Hair
This is fine, short, light-colored hair. Its length rarely exceeds 2 cm.

Terminal Hair
Terminal hair is longer, thicker, more pigmented, and coarser than vellus hair. Before adolescence, terminal hair is found only on the scalp, the eyebrows, and the eyelashes. During sexual maturation, in response to hormonal changes, some hair follicles from which vellus hair previously grew start to produce terminal hair.

Intermediate Type
Apart from the two types of hair noted above, there are some hairs that represent an intermediate form. These are somewhere in the wide range between the vellus hair type and the terminal hair type.

HOW MANY HAIR FOLLICLES ARE THERE?

The average number of hair follicles on a person's body surface is approximately 5 million. There is no significant difference in the number of hair follicles between men and women or between different races. The differences in the appearance of hair between men and women are due to the type of hair produced by a follicle. Hair follicles do not develop after birth.

Some regions of the body have no hair follicles: the palms and soles, the red parts of the lips, the umbilicus, the nipples, the skin over the joints of the fingers and toes, and parts of the genitalia. All the other apparently hairless parts of the body are, in fact, covered with fine, almost invisible, vellus hair.

> Number of Hair Follicles on the Scalp
>
> The average number of hair follicles on the scalp is approximately 100,000. This figure is an average and applies to people with dark hair. The number varies, depending on hereditary factors and the shade of hair. Redheads have relatively less, but thicker, scalp hair (the average is 80,000). People with blond hair have thinner hair, but more of it—approximately 120,000 hair follicles on the scalp. With age there is a gradual loss of hair follicles from the scalp, to varying degrees.

HAIR STRUCTURE

The hair consists of an elongated part, which grows from the dermis and protrudes above the surface of the skin, known as the **hair shaft**. Hair grows from a **hair follicle**—an elongated

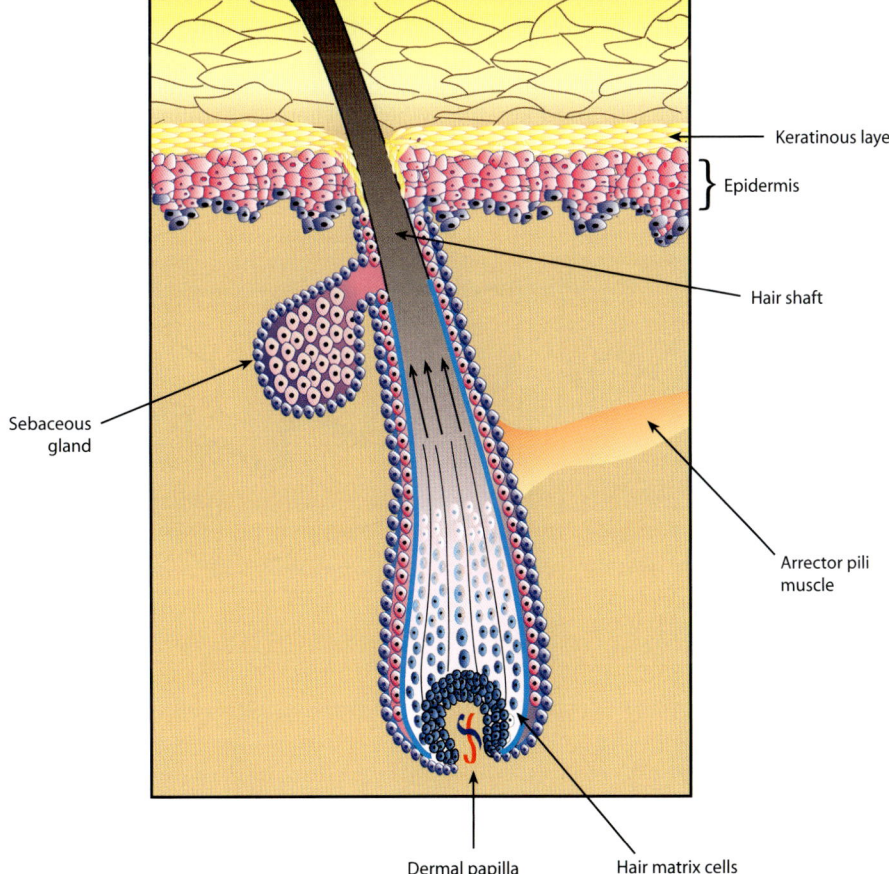

Structure of the hair (longitudinal section).

tubular structure in the skin, which is lined with cells. One or more **sebaceous glands** open into the hair follicle. A fatty substance called **sebum** is produced by the sebaceous glands and passes via a short duct from the gland into the hair follicle. An **arrector pili muscle** is attached to the hair follicle; when this muscle contracts, it causes the hair to stand up. As can be seen from the illustration, the bottom of the follicle is wider and thicker. The region below the lower end of the follicle is called the **papilla**. It is also called the **dermal** or **follicular papilla**; it contains blood vessels that nourish the hair follicle.

At the bottom of the hair follicle are the unique cells that produce the hair itself. These cells have enormous replicating abilities. They divide, and as more and more cells appear, the older ones are "pushed" upward in vertical rows and gradually degenerate. Since the cells degenerate and die as they move up the follicle, the upper part of the hair is made up of dead cells, which remain attached to each other by an intercellular cement-like substance. In other words, the hair that protrudes above the skin is actually made of dead keratinous material. The only living part of the hair are the cells at the bottom of the hair at the base of the hair follicle, which constantly divide and determine the hair quality.

As long as the cells at the bottom of the hair follicle (which form the base of the hair) are healthy and normal, the hair can continue growing. If, for any reason, those cells are destroyed, there will no longer be any hair growing from that follicle.

Hair Formation

The process by which hair is formed resembles the way in which the keratinous (horny) layer of the skin forms. The cells at the base of both the epidermis and the hair follicle divide and then are pushed upward, degenerate, and die. In the course of this process of degeneration, cells accumulate large amounts of a protein called **keratin**. This is, in fact, the major component of the keratinous layer of the skin. Keratin imparts to the outer layer of the skin its horn-like consistency (it is the substance from which horns of mammals are mainly built).

In hair follicles, the cells produce a different keratinous substance—another protein of especially hard consistency, called "hard keratin," which is chemically different from the usual keratin of the skin.

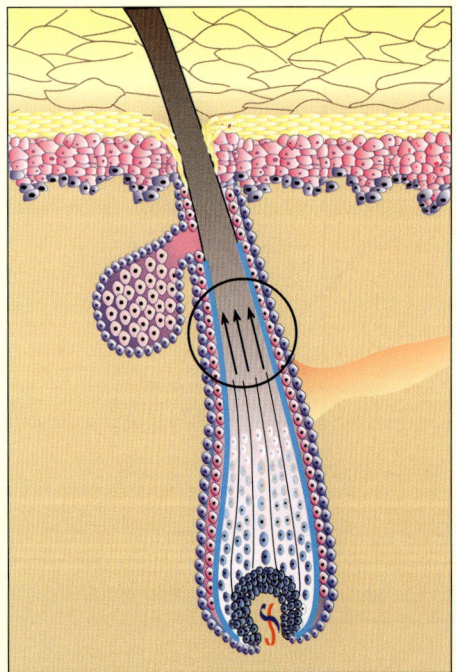

Formation of hair.

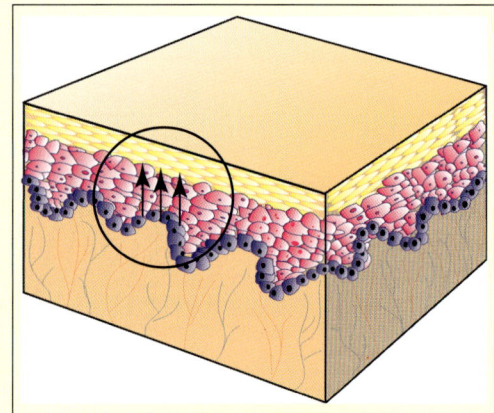

Formation of the keratinous layer of the skin.

HAIR STRUCTURE AND ITS CARE

Hair Color

In the same way that the **melanocytes** (**melanin**-producing cells) in the skin give it its color, the melanocytes in the hair follicle give the hair its specific color. Different types of melanin, which differ from one person to another according to each one's genetic characteristics, determine the hair's final color. Different concentrations and different chemical compositions of melanin produce blond, brown, or black hair.

- A compound called **eumelanin** makes a hair brown to black; when the concentration of eumelanin is relatively low, the hair is blond.
- A compound called **pheomelanin** imparts a red color to the hair.
- When the hair loses its pigment, it becomes grey or white.

Microscopic Structure of the Hair Shaft

The major component of hair is the protein keratin. The hair shaft is made up of many thin fibers of keratin twisted together into thicker bundles, as shown in the illustration.

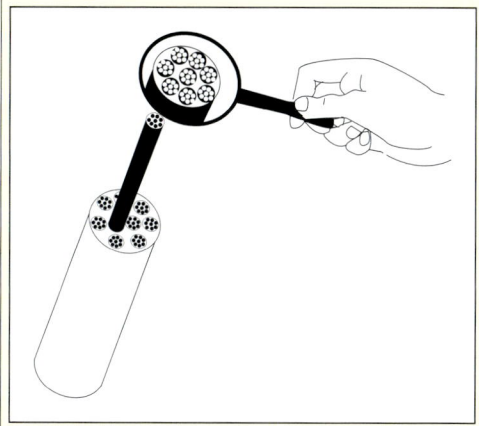

Microscopic structure of the hair shaft: Thin fibers linked into thicker bundles.

TRANSVERSE SECTION OF THE HAIR SHAFT

The hair shaft is made up of three layers:

- the **medulla**,
- the **cortex**, and
- the **cuticle**.

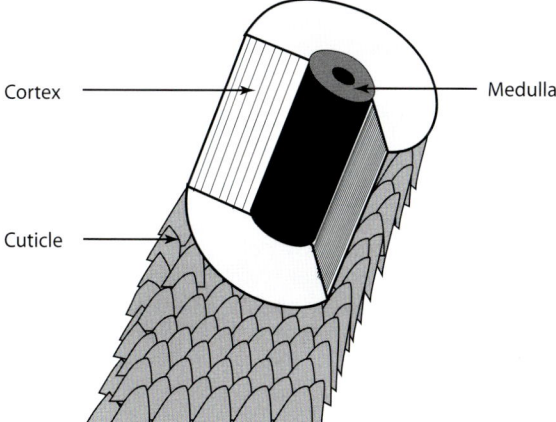

Transverse section of the hair shaft.

Cortex
This is the largest layer of the hair shaft; it is made up of hair cells that are constantly moving upward, and as they do so, they degenerate and die. The cells are connected to each other by a cement-like substance.

Cuticle
This lies outside the cortex, and is a sort of thin outer wrapping. This layer is made up of cells that partially overlap (see the illustration). The cuticle is relatively impermeable, and protects the hair from penetration of foreign materials.

If the cuticular layer is intact, and the cells overlap each other in an orderly fashion (as they are meant to), the hair looks soft and shiny, since light rays are reflected from it evenly. On the other hand, if the cuticle is damaged (for example, by incorrect treatment of hair, such as by excessive brushing, waving, straightening, or dyeing), the cuticular layer loses its uniformity, the hair loses its sheen, and the ends of the hair become frayed and split.

Medulla
This is a thin layer in the center of the hair shaft. Sometimes the medulla is absent or is not continuous along the length of the hair. Its presence or absence may affect the sheen and coloring of the hair.

LIFE CYCLE OF THE HAIR

Every hair follicle has a regular life cycle of growth, rest, and falling out. The cycle of any single hair is not dependent on the others—there is no synchronization. Therefore, it is normal and natural for up to 100 scalp hairs to be shed daily and approximately 100 other hairs will appear in their place.

Some of the complaints of hair loss that are brought to the doctor merely reflect this normal cycle. In such cases, obviously no medical treatment is necessary, other than reassurance and explaining to the patient that this shedding of hair is a well-recognized phenomenon and is quite normal.

STAGES IN THE LIFE CYCLE OF THE HAIR

Anagen: The Active Growing Phase
In the anagen phase, the hair cells at the base of the hair follicle are dividing repeatedly, and the hair grows steadily. This growth phase can last from several months to several years (on the scalp, the average time is approximately three years). The length of this phase determines the maximum length that the hair will reach, and it varies from person to person.

Catagen: The Transition Phase
This relatively brief phase, lasting some two to four weeks, is a transitional phase during which the hair stops growing.

Telogen: The Resting Phase
The telogen phase lasts three to six months. During this period, the mechanism responsible for the replication of the cells at the base of the hair, and the subsequent hair growth, are inactive for several months. By the end of telogen, the hair is only loosely attached to the follicle, and can be easily pulled out simply by brushing or washing the hair, etc. It is hairs in this phase that come away readily from the scalp when pulled.

Resumption of Active Growth

After the resting phase, a new hair appears from the same follicle during the next anagen (growth) phase. As this new hair grows, it pushes the old one, which is shed from the follicle.

Normally, at any given time, approximately 80% to 90% of the hairs on the head are in the anagen (growth) phase, and 10% to 15% are in the telogen (resting) phase. Less than 1% are in the catagen phase. As noted above, the cycles of the different hair follicles are in no way related to each other. Hence, in a normal scalp, the normal shedding of the hairs in the telogen phase is not noticeable.

The duration of the various phases of the cycle differs in different parts of the body. For example, scalp hair has different cycle periods to those of body hair.

Life Cycle of a Hair

1. Active growth phase (anagen): Cells at the base of the hair follicle divide repeatedly, and the hair grows steadily.
2. Transition phase (catagen): The hair follicle becomes shorter.
3. Resting phase (telogen): Cells at the base of the hair follicle are not dividing; the hair is shorter, located more superficially—nearer to the skin surface.
4. Resumption of the growth phase (new anagen phase): From the same follicle, from a growth center lower down (compared with the "old" hair), a new hair starts to grow.

Life cycle of a hair

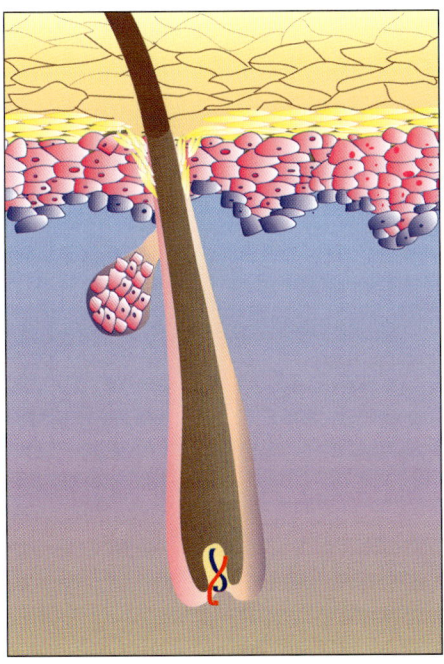

(A) Active growth phase (anagen).

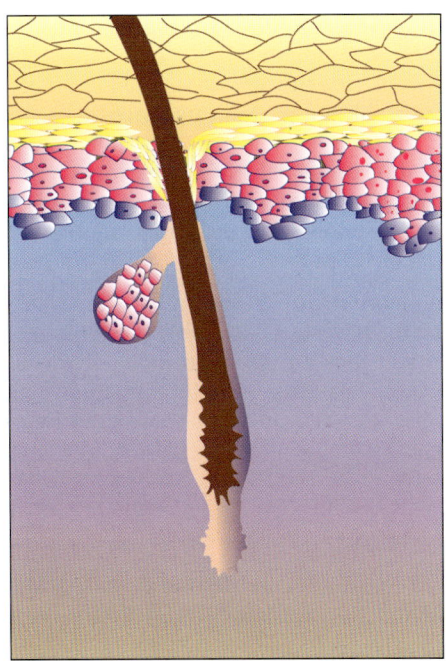

(B) Transition phase (catagen).

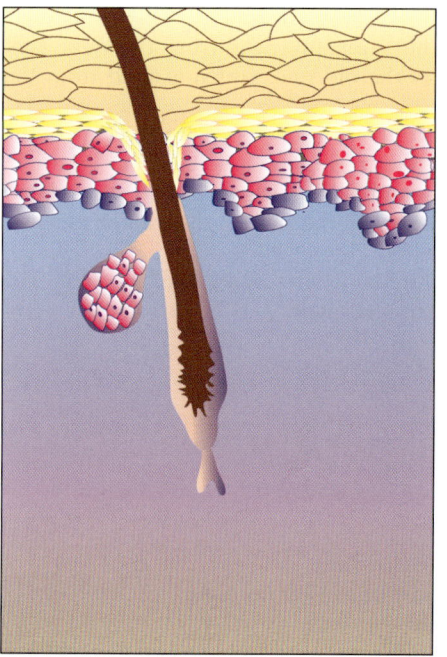

(C) Resting phase (telogen).

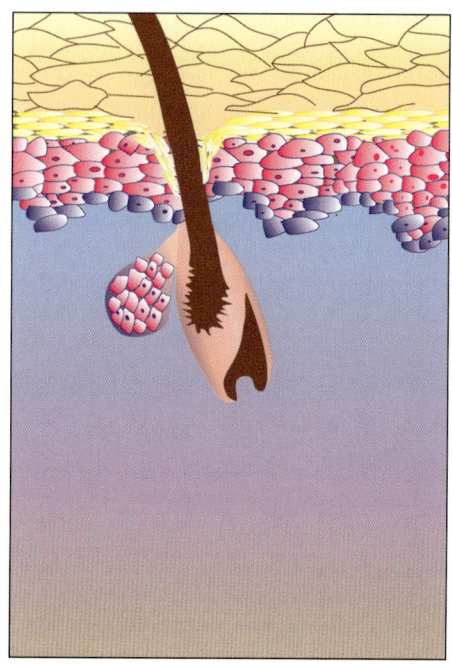

(D) Resumption of the growth phase (new anagen phase).

Normal and Abnormal Hair Loss

The hairs that normally fall out are in the **telogen** phase. A telogen hair is club shaped—i.e., a thin shaft, with a wider "blob" at the base. As opposed to anagen hair, its base is devoid of pigment. This can be seen clearly with a magnifying glass or microscope.

Because telogen hairs have this shape, people tend to mistakenly think that the hair has come out "with the root," and that a new hair will not grow in its place. In fact, just the opposite is true—a club-shaped hair that has fallen out is normal, and is a manifestation of the natural and reasonable shedding of up to 100 telogen hairs each day. How can a doctor tell for certain when hair loss is normal and when it is abnormal? The signs of abnormal hair loss are as follows:

- when more than 100 telogen hairs are shed in a day,
- when the hair starts to visibly thin out, or
- the hairs that are shed are not telogen hairs. Certain medical problems may lead to this abnormal status. A dermatologist can identify this abnormality by examining the shed hairs.

A telogen hair.

HAIR GROWTH RATE

Scalp hair grows at a rate of up to 0.4 mm a day during a growth period of three to five years; its average length is 70 cm, but it can grow up to 100 cm. Body hair grows at a slower rate than scalp hair, at 0.2 mm/day, and the growth period is two to six months. These hairs ultimately reach a length of 1 to 3 cm.

Both the period of active growth and the rate of growth vary from person to person. Largely, hereditary factors determine the length of the growth period and rate of growth. The length of the growth period and the rate of growth also vary with age. They differ between males and females—body hair of women grows more slowly than that of men, whereas scalp hair grows faster in women than in men. Nutritional, hormonal, and other constitutional factors also affect hair growth.

A fast growth rate and relatively long growth period are determined genetically, which explains why some women's hair is particularly long, while other women's hair never grows beyond shoulder length, even if they do not cut it.

HAIR CARE: FACTORS WHICH AFFECT HAIR GROWTH

Factors that may affect hair growth include:

- pulling or stretching the hair,
- local pressure on the scalp,
- certain externally applied substances, and
- local heat.

Pulling or Stretching the Hair

Cutting the hair has no effect on growth, which takes place at the bottom of the hair follicle. On the other hand, pulling the hair and exerting some tension on the root could cause damage to the root, weakening it and making the hair shed more readily.

Tension on the hair can occur as a result of combing the hair back and fastening it tightly with a clip or pin. Loss of hair in this way is usually apparent at the temples or the forehead, because that is where the hair is under the maximal tension. A similar phenomenon can occur following the use of hair rollers.

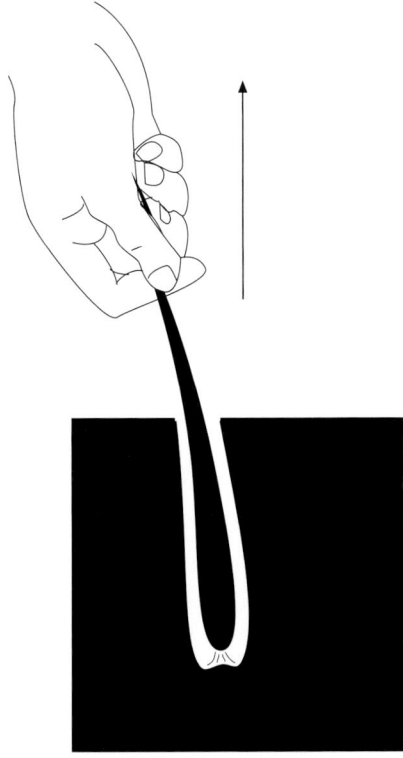

Pulling on the hair applies tension to the root and may damage it.

Similarly, curly hair can be pulled and possibly damaged by being combed in the opposite direction to its natural growth. In addition, hair loss can occur due to:

- overvigorous brushing,
- overvigorous massaging and rubbing of the scalp and hair when washing it, or
- drying the hair by rubbing it too vigorously (the correct way to dry hair is to absorb the water by gently patting the head with the towel).

With time, any of the above can cause damage to the hair and increase hair loss. If someone already has a tendency to hair loss, he/she should take particular care to wash the hair gently and dry it by gentle patting, to minimize the already existing damage.

Local Pressure on the Scalp
This is a relatively uncommon problem, which is probably caused by interference with the local blood supply to the scalp. In infants who sleep on their backs, a bald area often appears at the back of the head. A similar phenomenon may be seen following some major surgical operations, in which patients lie on their backs without moving for long periods.

Externally Applied Substances
Many externally applied products on the cosmetic market claim to revive hair roots by supplying basic "building" materials, and in that way encourage and accelerate hair growth and prevent hair loss. Most of those substances do not even reach the hair root, nor are they absorbed into the root, which is located deep in the dermis. There is no proof that these products have any effect on hair growth. A medication that *has* been shown to affect and accelerate—to a certain extent—hair growth following its local application is a substance called **minoxidil**.

On the other hand, certain toxic substances, whether absorbed into the body or applied locally, may damage the hair follicles. Therefore, care should be taken when selecting a product for dyeing, straightening or curling the hair, and to ensure that it is produced by a reputable, recognized cosmetics manufacturer.

Among the numerous depilatory products available on the market for removing excess hair, there are substances that can dissolve the keratinous substance of which the hair is made. These products have no effect on the living part of the hair (see chapter 33).

Local Heat
Heating of the scalp usually occurs as a result of using equipment to dry, curl, or straighten hair (electric rollers or hair "irons"). A shower that is too hot and vigorous also does not benefit the hair. The resultant high temperatures near the hair root can cause damage.

HAIR LOSS AND BALDNESS

Apart from the common male baldness, there are many possible causes of hair loss and baldness in men and women, such as hormonal factors, dietary deficiencies (of various vitamins or iron), exposure to toxic substances, infections, and other diseases.

This is not a problem that cosmeticians should attempt to manage. The best thing that a cosmetician can do when asked about a hair loss problem is to refer the client to a dermatologist. **The investigation of hair loss and baldness should be performed only by a physician.**

31 | Shampoo

Avi Shai, Robert Baran, and Howard I. Maibach

Contents Washing hair: overview • Surfactants • The best shampoo • Components of shampoo • Dandruff and antidandruff preparations • "Gentle" shampoos • Washing the hair • Appendix: details of shampoo ingredients

Note: It is recommended that this chapter be read after reading chapter 5 on skin cleansing.

WASHING HAIR: OVERVIEW

The scalp and hair are normally lubricated by sebum, which is secreted from the sebaceous glands. This oily secretion protects the hair and skin against water loss and gives the hair its sheen. On the other hand, there is some disadvantage to the oily layer on the scalp—dust, soot, and other environmental pollutants tend to stick to it, as do particles of keratin from the skin.

The same principle that applies to cleansing the skin also applies to shampooing hair; in order to remove the dust, soot, and other grime, as well as the cells of the keratin layer that have peeled off, the oily layer on the scalp and hair must be removed, since these particles are embedded in it. In addition, the same principle that applies to the action of soaps and surfactants for cleansing the skin also applies to shampoos for cleaning the scalp and hair. The surfactants, the active ingredients in shampoos, surround and trap tiny droplets of fat (that contain the grime), and these are removed from the scalp and hair by rinsing with water.

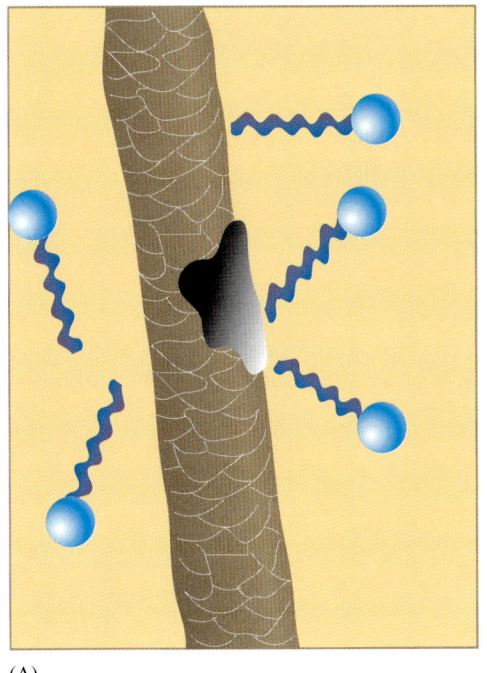
(A)

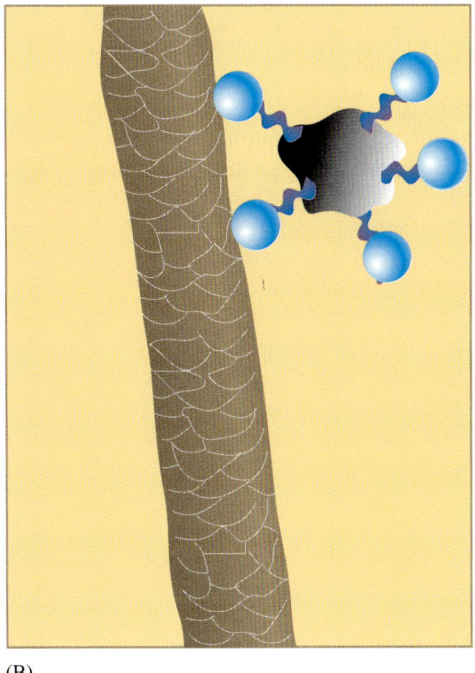
(B)

*The principle of action of shampoo is identical to that of soap: (**A**) A particle of fat and grime adherent to a hair shaft. (**B**) Surfactants trap the fat particle and remove it from the hair.*

Shampoos are designed to replace ordinary soap. The basic compounds within shampoos are surfactants.

> **Why Should One Not Use Normal Soap?**
>
> Normal soap has two major drawbacks and so it is not recommended for washing the hair:
>
> - Normal soap has a high pH, which may damage skin and hair.
> - The use of normal soap with tap water produces calcium salts that adhere to the hair. This causes the hair to look and feel dull, brittle, and disheveled, making it hard to comb.

SURFACTANTS

Surfactants (surface-active agents), which are water-soluble compounds, constitute the major component of soaps and shampoos. Surfactants clean by virtue of their chemical structure. They "surround" the fat, with its embedded grime, by forming chemical structures called micelles, so that on rinsing with water, the fat and dirt can be removed from the hair or skin. There are four main groups of surfactants, distinguished from each other by their chemical structure and electric charge:

- anionic surfactants
- cationic surfactants
- nonionic surfactants
- amphoteric surfactants

Different surfactants have different properties, and vary in their abilities to clean, create lather, and impart luster or softness to hair. Shampoos usually do not contain just one surfactant, but a combination of several, designed for use on different types of hair. For example, anionic surfactants have good cleaning properties. Therefore, anionic surfactants are commonly found in most shampoos. On the labels of most shampoos will be found the names **sodium lauryl sulfate** and **sodium laureth sulfate**, which are anionic surfactants.

> **Natural Surfactants**
>
> Natural surfactants are made up of saponins, which are derived from various plants. Saponins are good at creating foam, but less effective at cleaning. They are, therefore, usually used in combination with synthetic surfactants to achieve effective cleaning and good cosmetic results.

THE BEST SHAMPOO

As noted above, a shampoo is not only meant to clean, but to fulfill several other functions, in accordance with the demands of the customer. A shampoo should be adapted to the individual in terms of the following aspects:

Hair type

- Is the hair dry or oily?
- Is the hair thin?
- Has the hair been bleached, dyed, or permed?

Specific scalp problems

- Does the user have dandruff?

Safety requirements

- Does the preparation irritate the eyes?
- Does the preparation irritate the scalp?

Personal preferences of the user: These may include:

- the shampoo's consistency and texture (a shampoo may be in the form of a liquid or a cream),

- the presence of a particular fragrance,
- the ease and convenience of application of the shampoo,
- the ease with which it spreads through the hair,
- the amount of foam it produces and its quality and texture,
- how easy is it to rinse off,
- the degree to which it makes the hair soft, supple, and shiny, and
- how easy is it to comb and manage the hair after using the shampoo.

Similarly, the shampoo should be appropriate for the season of the year, for the frequency of use, and for other specific demands of the consumer.

COMPONENTS OF SHAMPOO

Up to this point, we have confined our discussion to the role of surfactants in washing hair. However, if a shampoo were to contain only cleansing agents whose task it was to remove the fatty layer from the hair and scalp, the hair would end up becoming dull, coarse, and hard to comb and manage. What other constituents are there in shampoo?

- a mixture of several surfactants. (A single surfactant usually cannot guarantee that a shampoo will achieve what is required. Note that some surfactants have properties other than simply cleaning. Some have good foaming capabilities, and some are effective in conditioning and softening the hair.)
- moisturizers, as needed, when the hair tends to be dry,
- conditioners,
- foaming agents,
- water softeners (chelating agents),
- thickeners,
- pearlescents,
- coloring agents,
- fragrances,
- preservatives, and
- "special" ingredients.

Surfactants
The role of surfactants has been discussed above. Different surfactants have different properties, and vary in their abilities to clean, create lather, and impart luster or softness to hair.

Moisturizers
In many cases, moisturizing agents have to be added to the shampoo because cleansing with a surfactant results in the removal of the natural oil. Without oil, the hair becomes dull and loses its softness, which makes it hard to comb and manage. The hair becomes more fragile and tends to split at the ends. This phenomenon of dry hair is usually the result of several factors: dry weather, exposure to wind, air pollution, swimming pools containing chlorine, and the use of "hard" shampoos that dry the hair. These characteristics are even more pronounced in hair that has been bleached or dyed. Shampoo removes the unwanted oil and grime from the hair and scalp, but it also removes the oil that the hair needs, which gives it luster and softness.

Therefore, shampoo should be tailored to the particular type of hair—someone with oily hair requires a shampoo that is more effective in removing oil, while someone with dry hair requires a shampoo with a less vigorous, gentler cleaning effect, and an added moisturizer.

In general, tailoring the shampoo to the user, in terms of the amount of moisturizer it contains, should be related to the type of skin on the scalp—if the scalp is dry, the hair tends to be dry; with an oily scalp, the hair also tends to be oily.

Conditioners
The purpose of conditioners is to make the hair soft, shiny, and easier to comb and manage. Conditioners are a particularly important component of shampoos used for dry or damaged hair (following coloring, waving, etc.).

In general, many dermatologists advise using a conditioner after washing the hair with shampoo, rather than using a shampoo that contains a conditioner. This is because two different functions are involved here: cleansing and conditioning. A shampoo that contains conditioner has to fulfill several functions, the chief being cleansing the hair. Such a shampoo cannot achieve the efficiency of a pure conditioner used independently after washing and cleaning the hair. Furthermore, remnants of shampoo that remain on the hair after using a conditioner-containing shampoo must obviously contain cleansing agents, and should be avoided. Hair conditioners are discussed in more detail in chapter 32.

Other Components
These include foaming agents, chelating agents, thickeners, pearlescents, dyes, fragrances, and preservatives.

Foaming Agents
Foaming agents act by producing bubbles in the water, creating lather. Note that there are many shampoos that clean effectively without producing lather. However, the inclusion of foaming agents in shampoos may be seen as an advantage from the marketing point of view, since the current public opinion seems to associate lather with efficient cleaning. In fact, there is no need for an extensive lather to clean effectively: the effectiveness of a shampoo is mainly determined by how the hair looks and how the user feels after washing the hair, and not by how much lather it produces.

Water Softeners (Chelating or Sequestering Agents)
Water softeners bind ("chelate") calcium and magnesium ions present in water, and thereby prevent their attachment to fatty acids, which would create salts that are not easily soluble. Without the addition of water softeners, the salts that form would affect the cleansing ability by coating the hair. This coating stays on the hair as a thin layer and makes the hair lose its luster.

Thickeners
These make the shampoo thicker. Thickeners have nothing to do with the cleansing properties of the shampoo. However, they make the shampoo look more attractive. Apart from that, people tend to think that the thicker a shampoo, the more effective it is, and the richer in active ingredients. The consistency of a shampoo is not necessarily related to its effectiveness. Nevertheless, there is some advantage to a shampoo that is thicker in consistency, in that a thicker shampoo is less likely to dribble down and get into the user's eyes.

Pearlescents
These are added to shampoos to change their appearance and give them a "pearly" sheen.

Dyes and Fragrances
The reason for using dyes or fragrances is to make the product look and smell good. However, it is preferable not to use shampoos that incorporate synthetic dyes or perfumes that are particularly strong. These may irritate the scalp, cause allergic reactions, or even damage the outer layers of the hair.

Preservatives
These are substances incorporated to preserve the shampoo, and include various preservatives, antioxidants, and emulsifiers, whose task is to stabilize the mixture of ingredients that make up the shampoo (some surfactants also act as emulsifiers).

Special Ingredients in Shampoo
Special substances in shampoo may include various vitamins (e.g., vitamins B and E), plant extracts, egg, honey, jojoba, aloe vera, and others. The shampoo industry has to cater to the ever-changing whims of the public, and the use of these ingredients may have significant effects on sales, especially if some particular ingredient happens to be in vogue at the time.

At present, most interest is centered around substances from the vitamin B group (particularly vitamin B_5 and B_6). Cosmetics and pharmaceutical companies report that the regular use of substances containing these vitamins strengthens the hair, moisturizes it, and gives the hair a healthy sheen. They claim that the hair becomes more supple and less fragile. However, there are no reports in the scientific literature or studies that support these contentions, and these claims have not yet been tested by accepted scientific criteria.

With regard to the use of these substances, it should be remembered that **the hair shaft is made of dead keratin. The external hair can neither be "nourished," nor its growth influenced by something applied to it.**

However, applying them to the external hair can affect its appearance (but not its growth!). The hair will look shinier and "silkier," and will be easier to comb and manage. If, then, shampoos that contain these special ingredients may have some advantage over standard shampoos, in terms of the appearance and manageability of the hair, their use is basically up to the user's personal preference. It is reasonable to assume that, in many cases, users will prefer these preparations.

Whether these "exotic" ingredients penetrate the living tissue, i.e., the hair root, and affect hair growth has never been proven. In any case, if a substance is to have some effect on the hair root, it is better applied to the hair in the form of a solution, which will remain there for several hours, rather than as a component of a shampoo. In the case of a shampoo, any component will be in contact with the scalp for a very short time only, and most of it ends up going down the drain, together with the shampoo and water.

DANDRUFF AND ANTIDANDRUFF PREPARATIONS

Although dandruff is not a disease or a serious problem, it is disturbing to the sufferer and poses an aesthetic nuisance. Dandruff is common—approximately 80% of the population has dandruff at some stage in their lives, mainly between the ages of 20 and 40 years. Because it is so common, one can think of it to some extent as being a normal phenomenon, so long as it is not excessive or becomes a nuisance.

What Is Dandruff?

Dandruff is, in effect, particles of keratin that are shed from the skin. There is a constant turnover of epidermal cells in the skin. At the base of the epidermis, new cells are constantly being formed and migrate to the surface, where they are eventually shed. As long as the rate of this turnover is reasonable and normal, it is hard to actually see the shed cells. If, however, the rate of turnover increases, more and more dead keratinous cells are produced, which adhere to particles of keratin, and become visible to the naked eye as they are shed from the skin.

Dandruff can appear in normal (neither dry nor oily) hair. Sometimes, if the scalp is particularly dry, and the dry skin peels, this can look like dandruff. Nevertheless, dandruff is more common in oily hair. Most dandruff scales are gray to white in color, but if the scalp is very oily, then larger scales are formed, which are oily and have a yellowish color.

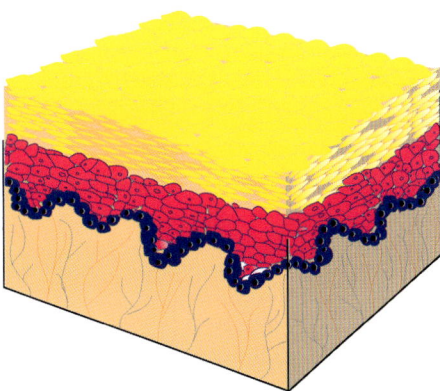

Microscopic appearance of the skin covered by a layer of dandruff scales.

> Seborrhea and Seborrheic Dermatitis
>
> - In **seborrhea,** the sebaceous glands are overactive, producing an excess of sebum. The hair looks oily. This is usually associated with dandruff.
> - **Seborrheic dermatitis** is a chronic skin inflammation that occurs in areas with extensive sebaceous glands. In adults, it tends to appear in the scalp, face, and upper trunk. In seborrheic dermatitis, the affected areas of skin are red and covered by oily scales.
> - **Cradle cap** is a severe form of seborrheic dermatitis in infants that looks like a greasy, scaly layer on the baby's scalp.

What Causes Dandruff?

This subject remains somewhat controversial, but most researchers see dandruff as a mild form of seborrheic dermatitis. The exact reason for the appearance of dandruff is, however, not clear. Hereditary and hormonal factors also seem to be involved. There is also a seasonal effect, with the problem tending to be worse in the winter months. Dandruff is exacerbated by emotional stress or physical ailments (such as a febrile illness).

It has been suggested that dandruff (and seborrheic dermatitis) is associated with the presence of a microscopic yeast called *Pityrosporum ovale* in the hair follicles. Some shampoos designed for treating dandruff contain substances aimed at eradicating this yeast from the scalp.

In the same way that different shampoos are based on variations of the same basic constituents (surfactants), with each manufacturer producing its particular combinations of constituents, so are shampoos for the treatment of dandruff.

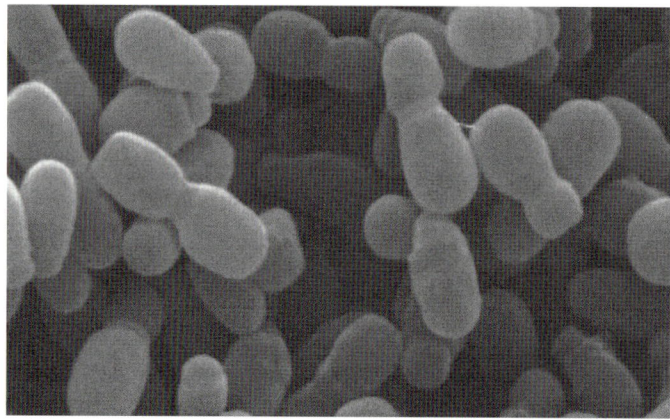

Pityrosporum ovale visualized by scanning electron microscopy.

The guiding principle in the treatment of dandruff, as far as the consumer is concerned, is that if a shampoo of a given type has not helped, one can switch to a shampoo of a different type. In most cases, one will eventually find a shampoo that does achieve a definite improvement.

As already mentioned, if the scalp is particularly dry, and the dry skin peels, this can look like dandruff. In that case, most antidandruff shampoo will not be of much help. It would be advisable just to use shampoo intended for dry hair.

Antidandruff Ingredients in Various Shampoos

Zinc Pyrithione and Pyridine Derivatives

These substances slow down cell turnover—meaning that fewer scales are produced. Furthermore, these substances are effective against *P. ovale*, which is now considered, if not the cause, at least an additional factor in the development of dandruff. They are present in many nonprescription shampoos.

Quaternary Ammonium Surfactants
These compounds belong to the cationic surfactant group. They have antibacterial and antifungal effects. In addition, they decrease the production of free fatty acids which cause of the irritant effect of sebum, so they have a soothing effect.

Sulfur Derivatives, Including Selenium Disulfide
The main effect of sulfur derivatives is **keratolytic**, i.e., they dissolve the keratin of the keratinous layer of the skin, thereby preventing the formation of visible flakes. In addition, they slow down the rate of turnover of the epidermal cells. Sulfur derivatives are best used for short periods of treatment, since they may result in the breaking of hair shafts.

Tar
It is not clear how tar works in the treatment of dandruff, but it is probably related mainly to the slowing down of epidermal cell turnover. Hence, products based on tar are also useful in other inflammatory skin conditions, such as *psoriasis*, in which there is excessive cell turnover. Tar also has a degree of antiseptic activity and is also antipruritic (prevents itching). The medical ramifications of using tar in shampoo for long periods are controversial. Usually, these products are well tolerated. However, the European Community decided recently that cosmetic products containing tar should be removed from the market.

Piroctone Olamine
Piroctone Olamine substance decreases dandruff by slowing down epidermal cell turnover. It is also claimed to be effective against *P. ovale*.

Antifungal Medications
Antifungal medications act directly on the microscopic yeast *P. ovale*. Because they contain antifungal medications, some are available only on a doctor's prescription. Shampoo preparations containing antifungals may eliminate production of dandruff in cases where nonprescription shampoo preparations do not show any beneficial effect. Since they contain an active medication, some should only be used for a limited period. The usual recommendation is to wash the hair twice a week for up to a month, and no more. Such a course of treatment should be sufficient to eliminate the yeast and prevent dandruff.

Use of Antidandruff Shampoos
To obtain the best results from any antidandruff shampoo, the shampoo should be left on the scalp for approximately three to five minutes, or according to the manufacturer's instructions, and then rinsed off. If the preparation is in contact with the scalp for a shorter period, its effect will be reduced.

In more severe cases, when there is no improvement with the above shampoos, a dermatologist should be consulted. The dermatologist may advise applying an oily preparation containing **salicylic acid** to the scalp for a number of hours before rinsing. Salicylic acid dissolves the scales attached to the scalp. In cases of seborrheic dermatitis, a dermatologist must be consulted.

"GENTLE" SHAMPOOS

So-called "gentle" shampoos are shampoos for people with delicate skin or, more particularly, for babies. They also are designed not to cause stinging of the eyes, which results from certain ingredients in shampoos getting into the eyes. The special nature of these preparations is based on the following:

- They are not supposed to contain ingredients that may cause irritation, particularly perfumes and certain preservatives.
- Many contain a relatively higher concentration of **betaines**, which are surfactants from the amphoteric group. These surfactants are relatively gentle, and do not tend to cause skin or eye irritation.

WASHING THE HAIR

Method of Washing

Hair is composed largely of dead keratinous material. Thus, for example, cutting a hair, which is dead keratin, has no effect on the active cells at the base of the hair follicle, and can have no effect on the growth or vitality of the hair. However, pulling the hair can affect the root. Hence, when applying shampoo, this should be done gently and not roughly, and there is no need to massage the hair or scalp vigorously when washing it. By the same token, the hair should be dried gently and not roughly.

People with sparse or thin hair should be even more gentle when drying their hair, and it should be patted dry rather than rubbed. When washing hair, very hot water should not be used, since repeated use of water that is too hot can damage the hair. Shampoo should be kept away from the eyes, even the gentle shampoos that usually do not cause eye irritation. Every last bit of shampoo should be washed out of the hair to avoid irritation of the scalp. Therefore, it is advisable to rinse the hair for three to four minutes after washing it.

Recommended Frequency of Washing

There is no specific recommended frequency for washing hair. Each person has his/her optimal time scale, depending on whether the hair is dry or oily, how much physical exercise the person engages in, their occupation, and their degree of exposure to dust, soot, and other environmental pollutants. People with oily hair, particularly if they are exposed to dirt, soot, etc., during the day, may need to wash their hair daily. If the hair is gently washed, there is no reason for avoiding a daily shampoo.

APPENDIX: DETAILS OF SHAMPOO INGREDIENTS

Moisturizers are discussed in chapter 4.
Conditioners are discussed in chapter 32.
Foaming agents: The main substances used for this purpose are **fatty acid alkanoamides**, which produce a soft lather, and various surfactants that are able to produce a strong lather.
Water softeners: The most widely used are EDTA and citric acid.
Thickeners: The most widely used substances are "natural" gums (such as tragacanth and karaya), hydrocolloid substances, acrylic polymers (such as carbomer), and salts such as sodium and ammonium chloride.
Pearlescents: The most commonly used substances are **alcohol sulfates** and **fatty acid esters.**
Dyes, fragrances, and preservatives are discussed in chapter 3.
Emulsifiers stabilize the mixture of ingredients that make up the shampoo (some surfactants also act as emulsifiers).

32 | Hair Conditioners
Itzchak Shelkovitz-Shilo

Contents Overview • What happens if the outer surface of a hair is damaged? • What activities damage hair? • Principles behind the action of a hair conditioner • Types of hair conditioner • How to use a hair conditioner • Frequency of use of a hair conditioner • Hair styling: mousses and gels

OVERVIEW

The **cuticle** is the outer layer of the hair shaft (see chapter 30, "Hair Structure and Its Care," for further information). Its integrity and health determine the appearance of scalp hair. The properties of hair, such as its softness, luster, and pliability, are determined mainly by what happens on its surface. Hair conditioners treat the external surface of the hair.

WHAT HAPPENS IF THE OUTER SURFACE OF A HAIR IS DAMAGED?

The luster of hair is the result of the light reflecting off each individual hair. If there is damage to the surface of the hair, there is less reflection of light and the hair loses its shine and luster. If the external surface of the hair is damaged, the hair shaft develops negative electrostatic charges along its length. As a result of the electrical charge, the hairs repel each other, which makes it very difficult to comb or manage the hair.

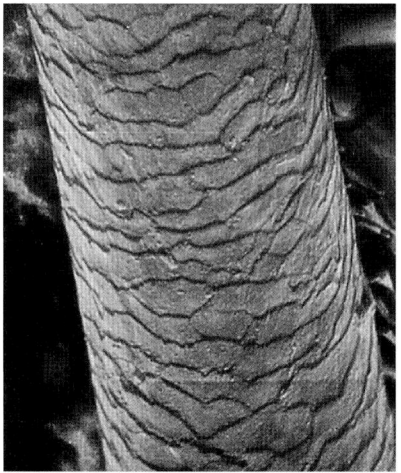 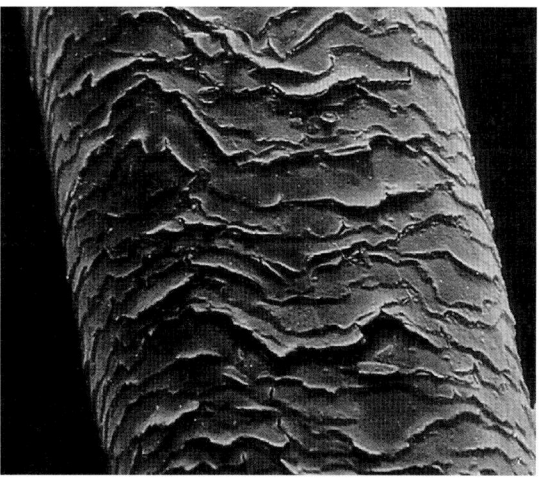

Hair shaft: Normal (left) and with early signs of damage (right), as seen under a scanning electron microscope.

The smoothness and softness of a hair are thought to be related to the orderly and uniform arrangement of the cuticle. A normal, healthy cuticle looks like the arrangement of roof tiles. Should the cuticle be damaged, the surface of the hair shaft becomes irregular and disorganized, and the hair becomes rougher and coarser. The hair becomes more brittle, and the ends tend to fray and split.

WHAT ACTIVITIES DAMAGE HAIR?

Hair can be damaged by:

- washing the hair too frequently (however, if the hair is short and the shampoo mild, there is only minimal damage),
- too frequent combing and brushing,
- overuse of a hair dryer,
- perming,
- dyeing with permanent dyes,
- bleaching and,
- exposure to certain environmental conditions, such as the sun's radiation, wind, and swimming pool water.

All of the above activities damage the cuticle of the hair shaft. As a result, the hair becomes rough, loses its luster, becomes stiff and fragile, and is harder to comb and arrange.

Note: The above list refers to agents or activities that affect the external hair, which is above the surface of the skin. This means that all of these agents damage the dead keratinous layer of the hair shaft, but usually have no effect on the hair cells deep inside the hair follicle. Hence they *usually* have no effect on the growth of the hair, so that after exposure to the above damaging agents, as the hair grows out, it will gradually regain its original, healthy appearance.

Nevertheless, if the above activities are exaggerated and excessive, some damage may occur to the living cells inside the follicle, which will affect hair growth. For example, excessive use of a hair dryer can result in the heating up of the area, which can damage the living cells in the hair follicle. Activities that tend to pull on the hair, or put it under tension, can also cause damage to the deeper cells in the hair follicle, and affect growth.

PRINCIPLES BEHIND THE ACTION OF A HAIR CONDITIONER

Hair conditioners are designed to prevent damage to the outer covering of the hair. The principles behind the actions of all types of hair conditioner are identical. The main functions of a hair conditioner are:

- to create a coating that covers the outer, rough layer of the hair—this coating gives the hair its smooth, uniform look;
- to neutralize the electric charges on the surface of the hair. By doing this, the hair does not look so unruly, and becomes much easier to comb and style; it also makes the hair look thicker and less wispy, and prevents knots.

Note: The active ingredients in conditioners affect only the surface of the hair. They do not penetrate the interior of the hair, and certainly do not affect the hair follicle. Their effect is only temporary and is lost within a few days (depending on environmental conditions). When the hair is washed, the conditioner is removed from the surface of the hairs. The effect of a conditioner is purely cosmetic, and it does not have any medical benefits.

As with shampoos, apart from the active ingredient (which is the conditioner itself), conditioners also contain a variety of ingredients with various functions. They may contain fragrances, preservatives, moisturizers for dry hair, dyes, etc.

TYPES OF HAIR CONDITIONER

Hair conditioners can be of the following types:

- cationic surfactants
- cationic polymers
- protein conditioners

CATIONIC SURFACTANTS

In general, the surface of the damaged hair carries negative electric charges. Since cationic surfactants carry a positive electric charge, they are attracted to these negative charges and become attached to the surface of the hair. Thus, the outer surface of the hair acquires a uniform coating. At the same time, the electric charges are neutralized.

Since cationic surfactants contain long fatty chains, they produce a fatty layer on the surface of the hair that gives it a soft, smooth feeling, and a shiny appearance. Cationic surfactants are useful for hair that has been damaged as a result of dyeing, bleaching, or perming. The more the outer surface of the hair is damaged, the more negative electric charges its surface carries, and the stronger the bond with the conditioner. The cationic surfactant is therefore attached most strongly to those areas of hair that are the most severely damaged, so the end result is that the surface of the hair develops a smooth, uniform look.

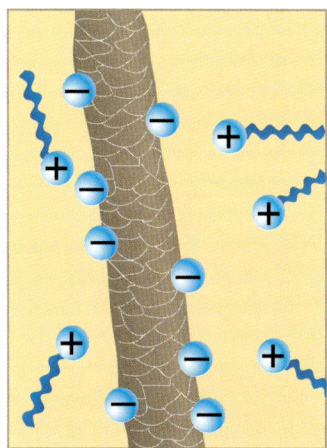

Mode of action of cationic surfactants.

CATIONIC POLYMERS

In general, polymers are chemical compounds built up of long chains of many small, identical building units. The cationic polymers that are used in hair conditioners contain substances such as:

- silicones,
- polyamides,
- polyamines, and
- substances based on cellulose.

They become attached to the surface of the hair as long units of polymer chains. Cationic polymers fill in the defects in the hair shaft, thus allowing light to be reflected more completely from the hair, since the hair surface is now smooth.

These products are also cations (i.e., they carry a positive electric charge), so they also reduce the negative static electric charge on the surface of the hair. Shampoos containing cationic polymers are recommended for normal hair. Dermatologists do not recommend their use on delicate hair.

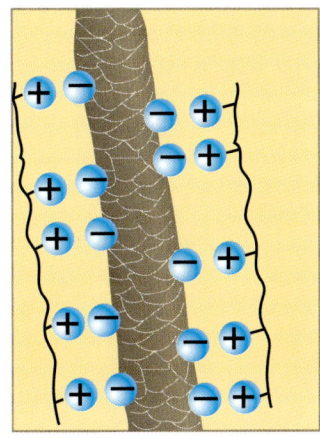

Mode of action of cationic polymers.

PROTEIN CONDITIONERS

The protein in these conditioners is extracted from animal tissues (proteins such as keratin, collagen, casein, and others) or from other sources, such as silk or certain plant proteins. In their raw form, these proteins are made up of large molecules. In preparing conditioners for the hair, the proteins are chemically broken down into smaller components. In that form (peptides or amino acids), they can attach themselves to the hair and fill in the cracks and gaps. This strengthens the hair shaft and repairs the split ends. It must be remembered that the hair shaft is not living tissue, so that it cannot bind the protein conditioners permanently. When the hair is washed, these substances are washed out of the hair shaft.

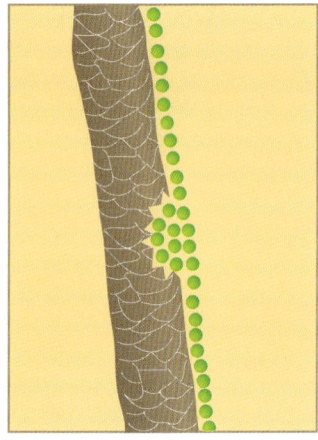

Protein conditioners penetrate into the cracks of the hair shaft.

HOW TO USE A HAIR CONDITIONER

Hair conditioners are meant to be used after washing the hair with a shampoo. They should be applied **only to the hair**, and not the skin of the scalp. Most conditioners should be left on the hair for two to three minutes, and then rinsed off. For people with severely damaged hair, there are "deep conditioners," which are left on the hair for several minutes (in accordance with the manufacturer's instructions) until being rinsed off.

FREQUENCY OF USE OF A HAIR CONDITIONER

The frequency with which a hair conditioner is used varies in accordance with the user's personal preference. People with healthy hair do not necessarily need a conditioner. If the hair has been damaged as a result of bleaching, perming, or exposure to dry weather, then a conditioner is helpful. If the hair tends to be unruly, difficult to manage and dull, then a conditioner should be used. Conditioners should not be used too much, since if an excessive amount settles on the hair, the hair tends to lose its shine.

HAIR STYLING: MOUSSES AND GELS

Mousses and gels have a different task to that of a conditioner. **Mousses** are meant to help style the hair and help the hair keep its shape. They cover the hair with a thin, uniform coating that can protect the hair from unwanted external influences such as strong wind or strong sunlight. To create a specific hairstyle, **gels** are used. They make the hair firm, so that it can be styled into complex shapes, depending on the desired appearance.

33 | Methods for Temporary Hair Removal
Zehava Laver

Contents Overview • Epilation and depilation • Methods of hair removal • Shaving • Mechanical scraping • Plucking • Chemical depilatories • Eflornithine cream • Bleaching

OVERVIEW

People are becoming increasingly concerned with the aesthetic aspects of their appearance. Men and women may be bothered by the presence of unwanted hair in certain areas. Most of the many methods currently available for hair removal provide only a temporary solution; other methods intended for the permanent removal of hair are discussed in chapter 34. The present chapter reviews accepted methods for the temporary removal of hair.

Note that all people have hair follicles on most of the surface of their skin. The number of hair follicles in men and women is similar. The differences in the appearance of hair between men and women lie in the hair type: a hair follicle can produce a fine, thin, light (lacking pigment) hair that is almost invisible. This is called **vellus hair**. In contrast, other hair follicles may produce a long, thick, dark hair that is readily visible to the eye. That type of hair is called **terminal hair**. In children, the only terminal hair is on the scalp, the eyebrows, and the eyelashes. Facial hair in women and children is of the vellus hair type, which is not visible to the eye. The facial hair in men is of the terminal hair type, visible to the eye. Excess hair in women refers to the fact that the thin, fine, almost invisible hair in various parts of the body becomes coarse, dark, and visible.

Causes of Excess Hair

- **High levels of male hormones (e.g., testosterone) in the blood and body tissues:** Women normally have low basal levels of testosterone, but certain hormonal disturbances can occur, resulting in a rise in testosterone. In these cases, excessive hair will appear in places where hair is typically seen in males (such as facial hair). The appearance of excessive hair may be accompanied by other characteristics suggesting a hormonal basis for the problem, such as a deepening of the voice, irregularity of the menstrual cycle, persistent acne, an increase in muscle mass, and changes in the distribution of body fat.
- **Increased sensitivity of the hair follicles to normal hormone levels:** In this case, excess hair appears, although the woman's basal level of testosterone will be within the normal limits. This phenomenon is attributed to increased sensitivity of the hair follicles to normal testosterone levels. The exact nature of this increased sensitivity is still unclear. The phenomenon is partly hereditary and occurs more commonly in certain ethnic groups.

In every case of excess hair in a woman, it is not sufficient to merely remove the hair cosmetically; the woman should also be referred for a medical endocrinological (hormonal) evaluation, which will include examination by a gynecologist and/or an endocrinologist.

There are many women who need or desire to remove hair from various parts of the body even without having any medical problem. This chapter discusses the accepted methods for the removal of hair.

EPILATION AND DEPILATION

Epilation
Epilation is a technique whereby the hair is removed by its root. However, not all epilation techniques will also destroy the active cells at the hair root. Depending on the particular type of epilation method, the hair may be eliminated temporarily or permanently. Electrolysis, for example, is a method of epilation that aims to eliminate hair permanently (see chapter 34). On the other hand, plucking the hair (using wax or a thread) is a method of epilation where the hair is only removed temporarily.

Depilation
Depilation is a method of hair removal that does not involve the root of the hair, but a region higher up the hair shaft, at or near the surface of the skin. Examples of depilation are shaving and the use of depilatory creams. All depilation methods remove hair only temporarily.

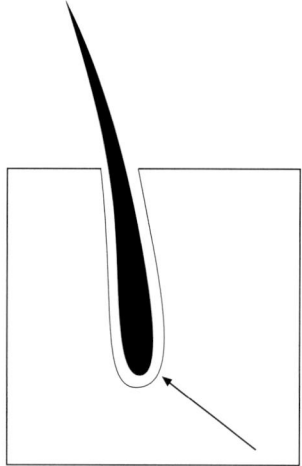

In epilation, the hair is removed by the root.

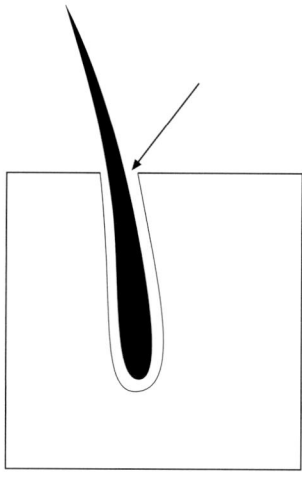

In depilation, the hair is removed at or near the skin surface.

METHODS OF HAIR REMOVAL

Methods of hair removal include:

- shaving,
- mechanical scraping,
- various methods of plucking (tweezers, thread, warm wax, melted sugar, cold wax, or special instruments), and
- chemical depilatories.

SHAVING

Shaving is fast, simple, convenient, and painless. Many women use this method for shaving their legs and armpits. It can be used on the face, but women, in general, prefer not to shave the face because of the masculine connotation of that procedure.

Note: The myth that shaving the hair increases the rate of growth and produces thicker hair is without foundation. The upper part of the hair that is found above the surface of the skin does not contain any living material. This upper part is composed of lifeless keratinous tissue, and therefore cutting or shaving it cannot result in the growth of coarse, thick, dark hair, and does not encourage hair growth. When a hair (which, as stated, is merely dead keratinous material) is cut, there is no effect on the hair root where the active cells that cause the hair to grow are found. The mistaken impression arose, perhaps, because the short hairs (stubble) that are seen on the skin after hair is shaved are straight, prickly, and relatively thick compared with their length. As the hair grows longer, it loses its "prickliness."

Advantages of Shaving

Shaving, being not painful, quick and safe, can be used over wide areas of skin and on any type of skin and any hair—fair or dark.

Disadvantages of Shaving

- The main disadvantage of shaving is that the hair grows back relatively soon after and has to be reshaved.
- Skin may be nicked.
- There may be skin irritation.
- Bacterial infection in the shaved area may occur. These infections (medically termed as **folliculitis**) tend to occur more frequently in the groin.

To prevent cuts, skin irritation, and infections, it is advisable to use a new, sharp blade; to soften the skin by wetting the area to be shaved and covering it with a liberal layer of lather; and to shave as gently as possible, with minimal pressure of the blade on the skin.

In cases where the skin tends to be injured, each stroke of the blade should be directed toward a new area of hair, and a stroke of only a few millimeters should be used each time—this is preferable to trying to cover wide areas of skin in one movement. In this situation, once the hair has been "soaked" in water and lather, the excess lather should be removed so that the precise location of the short hairs, and their direction of growth, can be seen in order that they can be shaved correctly.

MECHANICAL SCRAPING

Another method, equivalent to shaving, is mechanical scraping. In its classic form this is done using a **pumice stone**. As with shaving, this procedure needs to be repeated every few days. Vigorous scraping, which may result in redness and irritation of the skin, should be avoided. A similar technique is to rub the skin gently in a circular motion with a **depilatoric glove**, whose surface is composed of fine sandpaper. An antiseptic alcohol solution should be applied before scraping the skin. Following the scraping, moisturizers containing "soothing" preparations (such as aloe vera or witch hazel) should be applied.

PLUCKING

In shaving, the hair is cut off at the skin surface, at the level of the dead keratinous component of the hair; therefore, there is no effect on processes that occur in the live region of the hair root. On the other hand, by plucking, the hair root is **actively pulled out**, and the consequences are unpredictable and change from person to person.

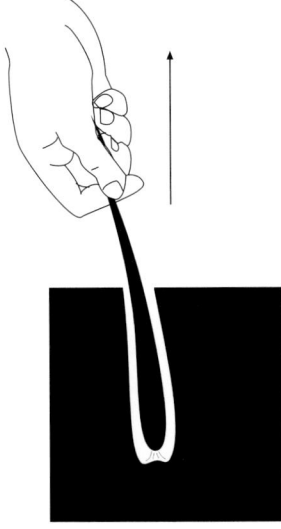

Pulling a hair out by the roots by plucking.

Repeated plucking can cause some damage to the hair root. In most cases, plucking has no effect on the shape or structure of the hair (for example, many women pluck their eyebrows without this causing coarse, dark, thick hair to grow back). However, the reaction of the eyebrow hair to plucking is unpredictable, differing from one person to another. Sometimes plucked hair follicles of the eyebrows tend to grow hairs that turn in different directions, deviating from the natural direction of the eyebrow hair. On the other hand, and relatively more commonly, following repeated plucking, the hair tends to become finer and thinner. Note that in the area of the eyebrows, after plucking (or repeated plucking), the hair may not grow back. Often the recovery period following the plucking of eyebrow hair is relatively long, and may last for more than one year. Therefore, unnecessary plucking in this area should be avoided. Many women who succumbed to fashion trends of the past are now forced to draw-in their eyebrows because the eyebrow hair has thinned out owing to repeated plucking.

> Does the Hair Become Thicker and Coarser After Plucking?
>
> Sometimes there is the impression that, following plucking, the hair becomes thicker and coarser. In most cases, that appearance is not a result of the plucking, but rather a reflection of the normal life cycle of the hair: a hair follicle that is plucked while it is in the resting (telogen) phase, will later be in the active (anagen) phase, with new hair growing from it. The new hair grows, and because it is in the active anagen phase, it can look thick, dark, and coarse. However, this is merely a reflection of the particular phase of the hair's life cycle at that time, and is not related to the plucking.

Plucking can be done using:

- tweezers,
- thread,
- warm or cold wax or warm melted sugar, and
- special instruments.

Possible Disadvantages of Plucking
- There may be pain, which some people cannot tolerate.
- Folliculitis (inflammation of the hair follicles) may occur. This is caused by microscopic injuries during plucking and subsequent infection by bacteria.
- Scars may develop in the areas of plucked hair.

Main Advantage of Plucking
As opposed to shaving, the smooth, hairless skin left behind after plucking remains that way for a longer time. The hair tends not to grow back for a few weeks in areas that have been plucked.

Using Tweezers or a Thread
Plucking with tweezers or a thread is used where there is a small number of hairs to be removed (such as the eyebrows, chin, etc.), or where there are isolated hairs in some part of the body (for example, around the nipples). The thread is coiled around the hair and allows it to be plucked out easily and efficiently.

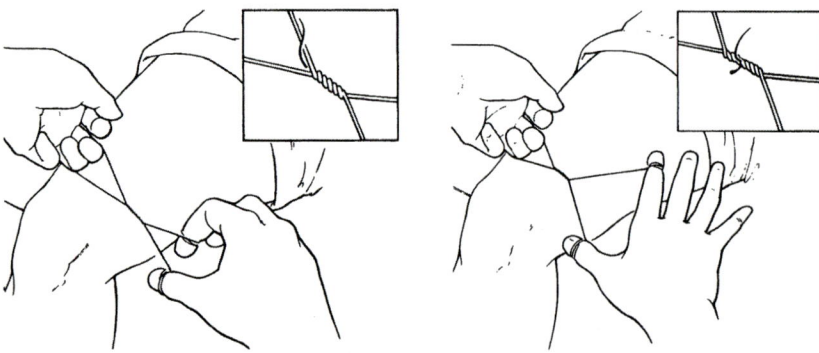

Plucking a hair using a thread.

Warm Wax

Using wax to remove hair is, in fact, a form of plucking that can be done over relatively large areas of skin. The wax that is used is obtained from beehives. The treatment is performed as follows: The wax is heated until it melts, and smeared over the area where the hairs are about to be removed. The wax solidifies within a minute, and the hairs become stuck to the wax and "trapped" in it. The layer of solid wax can then be peeled away rapidly from the skin, pulling away the hair trapped within it. Using wax detaches hairs from the skin near the root—deeper than the effect of shaving, which removes the hair at the skin surface—so the effect lasts longer than with shaving. It takes a few weeks for plucked hairs to reappear above the surface of the skin. A few days after using wax, new hairs may appear. This is not regrowth of the plucked hairs, but growth of new hair that happened to be in the active growth phase of its life cycle. These hairs were due to appear in that area regardless of the wax treatment.

Disadvantages of Warm Wax
- Wax is only partly effective, since it cannot trap and hence cannot remove short hairs that have just reached the surface of the skin; hairs of less than 2 mm in length are usually not caught up in the wax.
- Irritation or allergic reactions may occur, ranging from mild irritation (manifested by transient redness and slight stinging) to moderate and severe reactions. If there is merely a mild skin irritation, it is sufficient to apply soothing preparations (such as 1% hydrocortisone cream or aloe vera preparations) on the affected skin. In the case of more severe reactions, the patient should be referred to a dermatologist.
- Folliculitis (inflammation of the hair follicles) may appear following waxing. It is manifested by the appearance of many small, red lesions, or by the presence of many small lesions containing pus, where the hairs grow. In this case, the patient must be referred to a dermatologist.
- The technique may be painful; different people feel the pain to different degrees.
- Careless use of hot wax may burn the skin.
- Waxing may cause the appearance of superficial small blood vessels on the skin.

In most women who have used wax for years, specific or significant problems do not occur. There have been reports that, after prolonged use of wax, there is less regrowth of hair, and the hair that does regrow tends to be finer and thinner. Theoretically, that is possible, because repeatedly plucking out of a hair by the root does damage the root. Nevertheless, most women who use wax find that they have to continue treatment time after time, for years.

Instructions for Using Warm Wax

- Thoroughly clean and dry the skin.
- Some people recommend sprinkling a light layer of talc on the skin to absorb any residual moisture or oil, so the wax will stick better to the skin.
- When using warm wax, make sure that it is not too hot by testing a drop on the back of the hand.
- Never use wax on injured or diseased skin.
- There is no point in advising wax treatment for someone who has recently shaved the area or used a chemical depilatory agent, since the hair in the area will be too short and will not become stuck in the wax. In such a case, wait two or three weeks until the hair has grown longer.
- Smear the wax on the skin in the direction of the hair growth.
- Wait a few minutes for it to cool and harden, and remove it by peeling if off against the direction of the hair growth.
- Following the treatment, it is advisable to disinfect the skin with alcohol.

Warm Melted Sugar

This is not popular, because it is painful. The technique is based on applying warm, melted sugar, which is sticky, then pulling it off together with the hairs that have stuck to it. A strip of material is used to help pull out those hairs that have stuck to the sugar. The method is similar to warm wax treatment.

Cold Wax
Cold wax works the same way as does warm wax. The hair is trapped in the cold wax, which is then quickly peeled off, thus plucking out the trapped hair. To be precise, the correct chemical term for "cold wax" is, in fact, not wax at all, but a mixture of various sugars. Usually these preparations also contain citric acid. This combination of compounds produces a thick and sticky substance, which is generally quite effective in pulling out hairs. In general, the stickier the substance, the easier it is to remove the hair, and the less painful it is.

Special Instruments for Plucking
Instruments on the market for plucking hair are based on the action of a spiral spring. The hair is caught up in the spring and pulled out. The pros and cons of this technique are the same as those for plucking hair in general, but the design of these instruments allows hair to be removed quickly from larger areas, such as on the limbs.

CHEMICAL DEPILATORIES

These preparations are usually marketed as creams or ointments, but some are also available as gels or foams or in a roll-on form. Chemical depilatories contain chemical substances that dissolve the keratin fibers from which the external part of the hair is made. The hair comes off at or just below skin level. The hairs tend to break in those places where the keratin is slightly deficient or unevenly distributed.

Chemical depilatories affect only the external part of the hair and not the living root. Therefore, within a few days, the hairs growing back can be noticed.

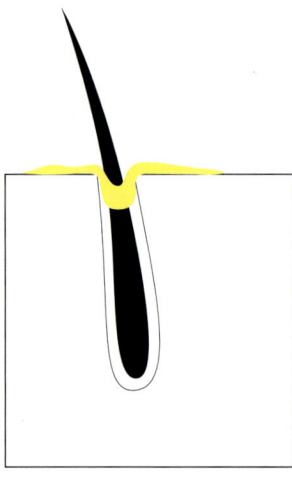

Hair comes away at the skin surface when treated with depilatory cream.

Main Types of Preparations

Sulfides
Barium sulfide and strontium sulfide have been used since 1800; they act rapidly and effectively. However, when using these substances, a compound called hydrogen sulfide (H_2S) is formed, which has a repulsive "rotten egg" smell and irritates the skin.

Thioglycolates
Thioglycolates form the main component of the preparations that are currently used. The basic ingredient of depilatory agents is a salt of thioglycolic acid. These compounds act on the fibers of the hair, dissolving and disrupting the keratin.

Thioglycolate salts tend to cause less skin irritation than do the sulfides, and their odor is also less offensive compared with sulfides; however, it takes longer for the hair to come away from the skin. Because thioglycolates rarely cause skin irritation, they are designed for use on areas of sensitive skin, such as the face. The length of application time is determined by the manufacturer, and is usually between 5 and 20 minutes, depending on the nature of the preparation and the strength of the hair. These preparations work well on fine hair.

Enzymatic Depilatory Agents

There is no problem of odor or skin irritation with enzymatic depilatory substances. The basic component is an enzyme called **keratinase**, which dissolves the protein of the keratin that makes up the hair. The enzyme is produced by certain bacteria. These compounds are less effective than sulfides and thioglycolates.

Instructions for Using Depilatory Agents

- Follow the manufacturer's directions carefully; the instructions may vary depending on the type and concentration of the preparation.
- Do not leave the preparation on the skin for longer than is specified in the instructions.
- Do not apply to the face a cream meant for the legs.
- Do not use these creams on damaged skin; in any case of skin disease, a dermatologist should be consulted.
- The first time a preparation is used, it should be tried on a small area of skin (usually the arm) first to confirm that there is no abnormal sensitivity to the substance. Evaluation of the test area should be done after 24 to 48 hours. If, after that trial application, there is no skin irritation (redness, swelling, itching, or burning sensation), the substance can be used over wider areas of skin.
- Clean and dry the skin thoroughly before using the depilatory agent.
- The skin adjacent to the area to be treated can be protected by covering it with a fatty preparation, such as petroleum jelly.
- After leaving the depilatory agent on for the required time, wash it off with lukewarm water.

Advantage of Depilatory Agents

The main advantage of using depilatory agents is that they, as opposed to other methods, are painless.

Disadvantages of Depilatory Agents

- There may be skin irritation—chemical depilatories may affect not only the hairs but also the superficial layers of the skin. This irritation is due to the fact that both the hair and the skin are composed of keratin. The degree and extent of irritation depend on the type of preparation (more common with the sulfides) and its concentration. Mild irritation may be treated by application of 1% hydrocortisone cream or aloe vera preparations. In more severe cases, the person should be referred to a physician.
- They can give rise to an unpleasant odor.
- Regrowth of the hair can occur following the use of a depilatory agent. Although the hair is removed at a deeper level than with shaving, within a few days, the hairs growing back can be noticed.

EFLORNITHINE CREAM

Eflornithine cream (Vaniqa®), launched in 2004, is a product intended to minimize facial hair growth in women. It is available only on prescription. Eflornithine affects the active cells within the hair follicles by inhibiting an enzyme called ornithine decarboxylase, which plays a role in controlling hair growth. The efficacy of eflornithine has been demonstrated in several research studies. The cream is not said to permanently remove hair, but to slow down hair growth so that women who apply it regularly will be able to decrease the frequency of using other methods intended for hair removal. There is some evidence that it can lighten dark facial hairs. It should be noted that while using eflornithine, they still will have to use hair removal measures, but less frequently. When treatment is discontinued, hair is expected to grow again to pretreatment levels within two to three months.

The product is intended for facial skin only. A thin film should be applied on the affected areas twice a day. It is not advisable to clean the treated area for four hours thereafter. Should no beneficial effect be seen within four months of treatment, it should be discontinued.

Adverse Effects and Precautions

The main adverse effect that has been reported thus far (the product is relatively new) is local irritation. In this case, it is recommended to discontinue the treatment. It may also induce the development of acne on the treated skin areas. There is insufficient data as to the safety of eflornithine in pregnancy and breast-feeding, so it should not be used under these circumstances. It should not be used in children younger than 12 years.

BLEACHING

This is another method of dealing with the problem of excess hair. It is intended for women with a fair complexion who wish to "camouflage" hair on the face and arms. The hair is still there, but is less obvious and almost invisible.

A bleaching preparation can be made by mixing hydrogen peroxide with ammonia in a low concentration. The effect of the solution starts immediately after the two substances are mixed. There are many preparations on the market for bleaching hair. The preparation should be applied, and left on the area to be treated for 5 to 15 minutes, according to the manufacturer's instructions.

As is usual with cosmetic agents, the first time a bleaching preparation is used, it is advisable to try it out on a small, unexposed area of skin. Only when it has been confirmed that the substance is safe should it be used over a wider area. If there is a burning sensation, the bleach should be washed off with water. The application can be tried again a few days later with a weaker solution once the burning sensation has disappeared completely. If the treatment was not adequate to achieve the desired result, it can be repeated a day or two later, with the bleach being left on the skin a little longer.

34 | Permanent Hair Removal: Electrolysis
Zehava Laver

Contents Permanent removal of hair • Electrolysis: overview • Equipment needed for electrolysis • Instructions for electrolysis • When should electrolysis not be performed • Complications of electrolysis • Effectiveness of electrolysis

Note: To better understand the boxed sections in this chapter, the reader should review chapter 30 on the structure of hair, particularly the section dealing with the growth cycle of hair.

PERMANENT REMOVAL OF HAIR

Electrolysis has been proven to be effective in permanently removing hair. Another technique for dealing with excess hair is by the use of a laser. Laser treatment stops the active growth period of the hair for long periods. The use of lasers for removing hair is discussed in chapter 25. Apart from these two methods, there are other techniques on the market that claim to remove hair permanently. Some are based on a series of treatments with gel preparations that contain various substances (some contain aromatic oils) combined with equipment for heating the gel, and the hair is then removed with wax.

Note: Apart from laser treatment and electrolysis, the results of no other techniques for the permanent removal of hair have been published or proven in the accepted scientific literature. Hence, we have no objective way of assessing whether those methods are effective.

The term "permanent removal of hair" applies only to the treated hair follicles, and even then the results are not absolute. In the area of skin treated by electrolysis, there may be hair follicles that were not treated by the electric needle (i.e., follicles that were not in the stage of active growth) or hair follicles that were ineffectively treated. However, when speaking about a single hair follicle that has been effectively treated, irreversible damage is expected to have occurred, and this follicle will not grow a new hair.

ELECTROLYSIS: OVERVIEW

Electrolysis is an effective method for the permanent removal of hair, based on inserting a fine metal needle into the hair follicle, with the aim of destroying the active cells in the hair root. At this point, let us recall that a **hair follicle** is an elongated, tube-like depression, in which a hair grows. At the base of the follicle are the active cells of the hair root, responsible for its growth. Hence, to destroy these active cells, a fine metal needle is inserted through the opening of the follicle and advanced until the tip reaches the base of the follicle. At this stage, an electric current is passed down the needle to destroy the active cells at the hair root. The hair breaks off at the root and can then be easily pulled with fine tweezers.

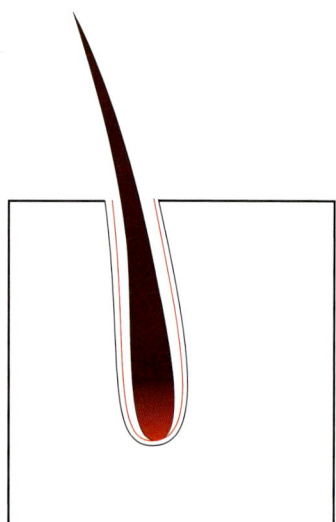
Hair follicle (shown in red).

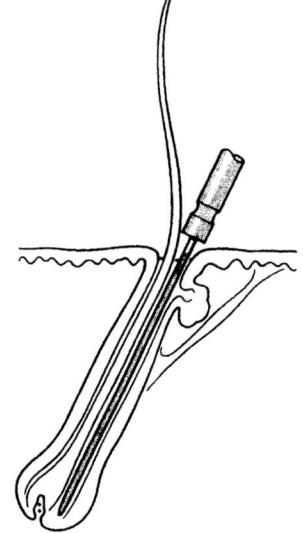
Insertion of a needle to the base of the hair root.

The great advantage of this technique derives from the fact that a follicle that has been effectively treated by the electric needle cannot grow a hair again, provided that the active cells in the root have indeed been destroyed.

Note: The illustrations on pages 250, 252 and 253 are presented by courtesy of Dr RN Richards, from the book *Cosmetic and Medical Electrolysis and Temporary Hair Removal*, 2nd edition, by RN Richards and GE Meharg (Medric Ltd, 1997). This book is recommended for those who are interested in additional information on electrolysis.

EQUIPMENT NEEDED FOR ELECTROLYSIS

Several types of electrolysis equipment are in use in cosmetic clinics. We shall discuss the general features of each one:

- direct electrolysis,
- electrocoagulation,
- blend, and
- instruments for home use.

Direct Electrolysis

This method, less commonly used nowadays, is based on the use of a direct electric current (galvanic current) that destroys the cells in the hair follicle. It is done using a prolonged electric current, of a minute or more, for each hair, rendering it a rather painful procedure. Despite this, the method is much more effective than other electrolysis techniques.

Direct Electrolysis

The remarkable effectiveness of this technique stems from the mode of action on the hair cells. The electric current results in the production of a chemical substance—**sodium hydroxide (NaOH)**—that destroys the cells of the hair root. The sodium hydroxide trickles down the length of the follicle, reaches the cells at the root, and destroys them.

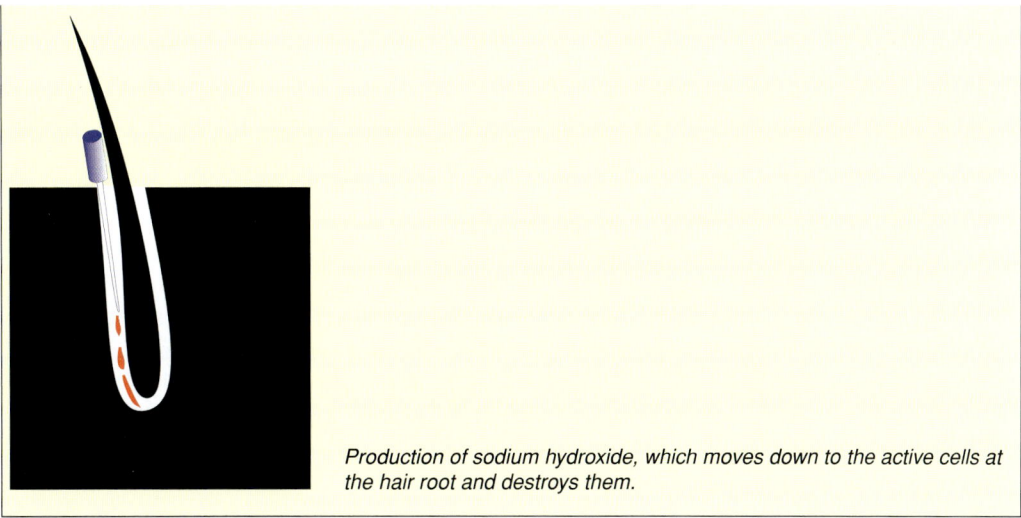
Production of sodium hydroxide, which moves down to the active cells at the hair root and destroys them.

Electrocoagulation
This is a newer technique, which is now commonly used in cosmetic clinics. It uses a high-frequency electric current to destroy the hair root by creating heat in the follicle. Other names for this method include:

- diathermy,
- thermolysis,
- high-frequency alternating method, and
- short wave

Electrocoagulation involves the use of a high-frequency alternating current. The current passes along the needle and heats up the tissues of the hair follicle, destroying them. With this instrument, the current is applied for only a few seconds.

Another technique, known as **high-speed flash thermolysis**, involves applying the current for less than a second. The significant advantage of this technique compared with ordinary electrocoagulation is its speed. Using this procedure, it is possible to remove up to 200 hairs in an hour. However, it causes less destruction to the tissues at the base of the hair and is less effective in removing coarse hairs.

Blend
The so-called 'blend' method combines direct electrolysis and electrocoagulation and is more effective for the removal of coarse hairs.

Instruments for Home Use
The principle of use of these instruments is similar to the techniques described above, but the electric current is provided by batteries. The needle is inserted into the hair follicle until the end of the needle reaches the hair root, the electric current is then applied to destroy the root.

The main disadvantages of home use are that, since the user is not a professional, it is difficult to treat certain areas, such as the face; the user must get accustomed to working with a mirror; and treating oneself tends to be slow. In general, this method is not recommended for areas with extensive hair.

Needles
Use only disposable needles. The length and diameter of the needle should be appropriate for the type of hair being removed. If the needle is too thick, it cannot be inserted into the hair follicle. On the other hand, if the needle is too small, the treatment will be less painful, but also less effective. The upper part of the needle should be covered by insulating material, to prevent damage and scarring to the upper layers of the skin. A relatively flexible needle, made of two

parts, is preferable to a rigid needle. This enables it to be inserted into the hair follicle more precisely.

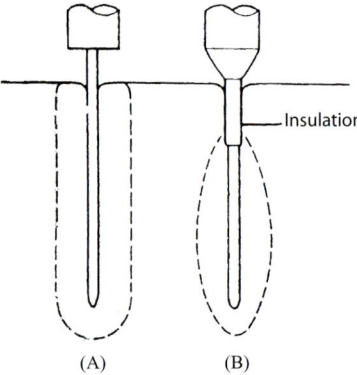

(**A**) An epilation needle. (**B**) A needle with insulating material at its upper end: This insulation prevents unnecessary damage to the upper part of the hair follicle (there is no point in destroying this part, anyhow), and to the skin surface. The cells one wants to destroy are in the hair root, at the base of the follicle.

Why Shave the Region To Be Treated?

The reason for shaving the area to be treated is that one can identify those hairs that are in the **anagen** phase. Those are the hairs that grow back after shaving. As opposed to the scalp, where 60% of the hairs are in anagen, only 30% to 50% of body hairs are in the anagen phase. Identifying those hairs that are in the anagen phase allows the treatment to be carried out only on those hairs. Electrolysis carried out on anagen hairs is very effective, whereas if carried out on hairs in the telogen phase, it is much less effective.

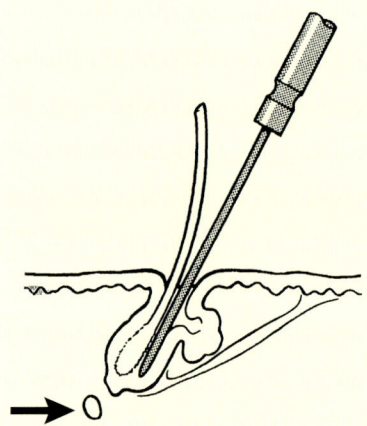

Ineffectual insertion of the needle into a follicle that is in the telogen phase. The new hair will grow from the part of the follicle indicated by the arrow: The needle cannot get to that place while the hair is in the telogen phase.

The reason why electrolysis on hairs in the telogen phase is less effective is that, in that situation, the base of the follicle where the needle tip reaches is actually the root of the old hair. When a hair is in the telogen phase, it is almost impossible to reach the place from which the new hair will start growing.

INSTRUCTIONS FOR ELECTROLYSIS

- In order to enable the operator to achieve the high level of concentration needed, the client should be lying down, with the operator seated nearby, as comfortably as possible.
- Bright light and a magnifying glass are essential for effective treatment.
- The region to be treated should be shaved three to five days before the treatment.
- Apply antiseptic solution (e.g., chlorhexidine, alcoholic solutions) should be applied before and after the treatment. Following electrolysis, some cosmeticians apply a substance with a cooling and soothing effect, such as witch hazel. Some recommend the application of 0.5% to 1% hydrocortisone cream, which has anti-inflammatory properties.

- Insert the needle into the opening of the follicle and advance it gently and precisely as much as possible within the follicle. A sensation of touching a "barrier" is felt when the needle has reached the base of the follicle.
- Use the correct current strength, in accordance with the manufacturer's instructions. In the newer instruments, in common use these days, the duration of the current is controlled automatically.

> **Minimizing the Pain Associated with Electrolysis**
>
> The degree of pain experienced during electrolysis varies, depending on the pain threshold of the individual patient, and on the region of the body being treated.
>
> Consider using **EMLA cream** for patients who have a low pain threshold or for treatment of particularly sensitive areas, such as the upper lip, the groins, and around the nipples. EMLA cream (Eutectic Mixture of Lidocaine and Prilocaine) contains local anesthetic agents—a mixture of lidocaine and prilocaine. The cream is applied to the skin approximately 60 minutes before the treatment, and an occlusive dressing applied over it. EMLA may reduce the pain considerably. While using EMLA, one should be cautious: minimizing the pain means also losing an important parameter of the degree of possible damage to the skin.

During electrolysis, try to avoid the following pitfalls:

- **Avoid activating the electric current while the needle is located superficially in the follicle.** If the needle is too superficial (not deep enough) and does not reach the hair root, the electric current will not destroy the active cells that form the hair. Furthermore, there is a risk of damage to the skin, resulting in scarring.

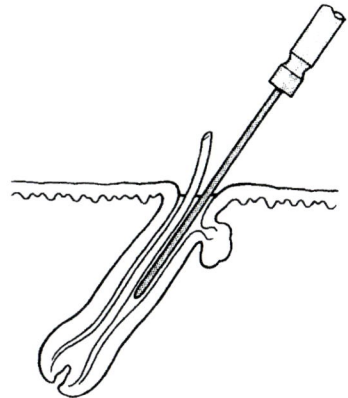

Too superficial a placement of the needle.

- **Avoid puncturing the follicle wall.** If the needle passes through the wall of the follicle, into the surrounding tissue, there will be damage to the skin tissue, and hair growth will not be affected. This tends to occur in a "crooked" hair follicle, in which case the operator will find it hard to insert the needle correctly. A deviation of 1 or 2 mm from the correct direction of the electrolysis needle may result in damage to the follicle wall or to the skin near the follicle.

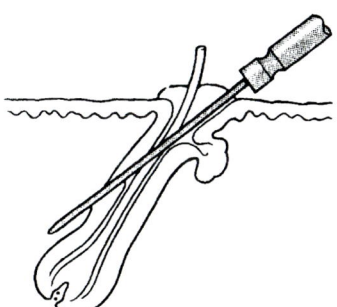

Needle passing through the wall of the follicle and "missing" the active cells in the hair root.

- **When electrolysis is performed in the armpits and groin, take extreme care.** In these areas, certain anatomical structures (e.g., nerves and lymph nodes) are located near to the surface of the skin. It is advisable to fold the skin between two fingers in order to elevate the area being treated from the skin surface to prevent possible damage to these structures.

WHEN SHOULD ELECTROLYSIS NOT BE PERFORMED?

Electrolysis should not be performed on injured skin or skin affected by any disease. If the client suffers from any disease (e.g., heart disease, especially those with a cardiac pacemaker), obtain a doctor's written permission before using electrolysis. Clients suffering from an infectious disease (e.g., AIDS or viral hepatitis) can undergo electrolysis, but extra care must be taken not to get jabbed by the needle and disposable needles be used. (Disposable needles should be used for every patient.)

Electrolysis should not be used to remove hairs growing from nevi (moles). The cells that make up a nevus are **melanocytes**, which are the cells that produce the pigment melanin. Some of the destructive skin tumors, such as melanomas, arise from melanocytes. One cannot predict the possible influence of an electric current on these cells, and hence it should be avoided. In such cases, the patient should be referred to a dermatologist or a plastic surgeon, who will remove the nevus in its entirety.

Do not carry out electrolysis on hair that is next to cartilage (e.g., the ear or nose). Check with the patient whether he/she has a tendency to form raised scars, or dark hyperpigmented scars (ask about previous operations or injuries, and what the scars look like). If there is a possibility of these problems, treat a few hairs in an area that is not readily visible, wait a few months, and then evaluate the outcome. In someone who tends to produce raised scars after the slightest injury, a dermatologist's opinion should be sought before embarking on electrolysis.

Women with excess hair (**hirsutism**), may have a hormonal problem, which could have significant medical implications. In such cases, a medical opinion must be obtained to determine whether, in fact, such a problem exists. Should that be the case, the physician may consider hormonal treatment together with, or prior to, the electrolysis treatment.

COMPLICATIONS OF ELECTROLYSIS

In general, most of the complications from electrolysis arise from damage to the skin while carrying out the procedure. That is not surprising, since the damage results from the very mechanism that is used to destroy the hair root. **The aim of treatment is that the deliberate damage caused by the electrolysis should be confined to the hair root alone.** However, it is obvious that incorrect placement of the needle, or using a current that is higher than necessary, will cause damage to the tissues around the follicle. This damage will be manifested as an **inflammatory reaction**, such as reddening and mild swelling in the area of the follicle.

Used correctly, it is rare for electrolysis to result in scarring. If there is mild, superficial damage to the opening of the hair follicle, small scabs may appear over the openings of the treated hair follicles. These scabs usually disappear within a few days. However, should there be a more severe reaction, permanent scars may result. Scars may result from inserting the needle too superficially, whereby the electric current then passes next to the surface of the skin; using too strong an electric current; not applying the current at all, or not applying it to the base of the hair, the scar appears following the hair being pulled out or infection.

In certain people, usually those with dark skin, there may be a tendency to produce excessive scarring following injuries, operations, etc. These scars are dark in color and raised. Particular care must be taken when treating these people. If it is suspected that the patient does have that problem (either from the patient's history or by examining his/her skin), then electrolysis should be avoided. A test can be performed by treating a few hair follicles in an area that is not readily visible, and then waiting to see the outcome. In any case, it is advisable to consult a dermatologist before deciding upon electrolysis treatment in such patients.

Other Possible Complications
Other complications can include the following:

- Infection may develop in the treated area, due to inadequate sterility measures or because of tissue damage. In the case of infection, a physician will need to prescribe antibiotics, which may involve the external application of an antibiotic cream or ointment, or in more serious or widespread cases, antibiotic capsules or tablets.
- Infection may be spread from one patient to another, hence the importance of using disposable needles.
- A rare occurrence is for a needle to break inside the skin. This uncommon event does not usually pose a serious problem, and the broken-off needle can usually be removed from the skin without too much difficulty. If the point of the needle is in the skin and cannot be removed, a doctor will have to deal with it.

EFFECTIVENESS OF ELECTROLYSIS

Since electrolysis is mainly performed by cosmeticians, rather than doctors, the results of treatment are not subject to statistical analysis. There is relatively little information on this subject in the medical literature. Furthermore, the outcome will vary from operator to operator, since it depends very much on his/her skill and experience.

In general, the process is slow, exhausting, and expensive, since the needle has to be inserted separately into each hair follicle. The advantage of electrolysis, however, is that if performed correctly and effectively, it will destroy the hair follicle permanently.

Most clients can have between 50 and 100 follicles dealt with at one treatment session. Accordingly, several months of treatment are needed to remove all the hair from a relatively small area of skin, such as the upper lip or the chin. In cases of marked hirsutism, it may take two or three years of weekly treatments to achieve the desired result.

Various estimates suggest that approximately 30% to 40% of the hair will reappear following electrolysis. Direct electrolysis, using a direct (galvanic) current, is much more effective. However, some dermatologists do not agree with these results, and maintain that the outcome of electrolysis treatment is not nearly as good as that.

Has the Hair Root Been Permanently Destroyed?

Since the hair is pulled out and removed during the treatment in any case (whether the electric current was on or not), a certain period must elapse before one can ascertain whether the hair root was destroyed for good.

- If the hair was in the telogen phase, it will grow back a few weeks later.
- If the hair was in the anagen phase, several months will have to elapse before one can be certain whether the hair root was destroyed permanently or not.

Reappearance of Hair

Hair that reappears in an area that was treated by electrolysis can be the result of the following:

- hair follicles that were not treated correctly,
- hairs that were in the early growth phase (early anagen), and were not visible above the surface at the time of the electrolysis, so those follicles were, in fact not treated at all,
- hairs that were in the telogen phase at the time of treatment, and were not treated, or that the treatment was not effective and they are now in the anagen phase, or

- in cases where vellus hair is slowly changing to coarser hair. This occurs more frequently in women with a hormonal problem, and in such cases, the underlying medical problem should be diagnosed. The only way to prevent endless cosmetic treatments is to treat the basic hormonal problem, since there is no point in treating hair with an electric needle if, all the while, there is a constant stimulus acting that keeps making the hair darker, coarser, and more obvious.

35 | Nails

Marina Landau and Robert Baran

Contents Overview • Composition of the nails • Structure of the nails • General care of the nails • Common nail problems • Cosmetic treatment of nails • Artificial nails

OVERVIEW

Human nails are the equivalent to the claws in other mammals. In human nails, however, the functions of the nails as tools or weapons have, with evolution, become less important. The function of the nails in humans is basically to protect the fingers and to assist in delicate manual activities.

The presence of aesthetically pleasing healthy nails is very significant. Nails that are well cared for complement a pleasant overall appearance, and also reflect one's general health status. To some extent, the condition of the nails may also reflect a person's social status.

COMPOSITION OF THE NAILS

The nails are made up largely of **keratin**—the same protein that makes up the hair and the skin surface—although here we are talking of a special variant of keratin. Nails are composed of "**hard keratin**," which is similar in its chemical composition to the substance that animals' horns are made of. This form of keratin contains much more sulfur than the normal skin keratin. In addition, nails contain small amounts of elements such as calcium, iron, and zinc.

The relative flexibility of nails is due to the presence of compounds called **phospholipids**. These are fatty compounds that also contain polysaccharides and proteins. Phospholipids represent the major component of cell membranes in the body.

Water can pass through the nails readily—more so than through the skin—so that repeated contact with water and cleansing agents causes nails to become relatively dry and more brittle.

The strength of the nails is not only related to their composition but also to their shape. The convex shape of normal nails makes them stronger than they would be if they were flat.

STRUCTURE OF THE NAILS

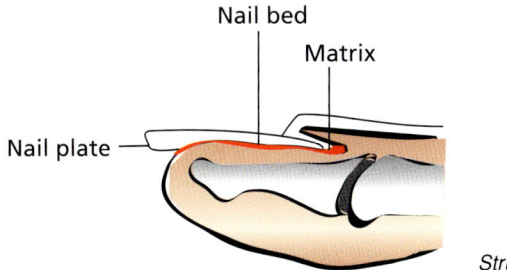

Structure of the nail.

Nail Plate
The nail plate is the external, visible part of the nail.

Nail Matrix
The definition of the term "matrix," in its broad sense, is "an environment or tissue that gives origin or form to something." The term "nail matrix" refers, therefore, to the root of the nail. This is the living, active part of the nail. The cells of the nail matrix are in the area of the **lunula**

(see below) and under the skin fold at the nail base. Matrix cells are continuously dividing, and thus the nail grows.

Any injury or damage to the nail matrix may distort the nail. Severe, permanent damage to the nail matrix will result in permanent deformity of the nail, even to the extent of its total loss.

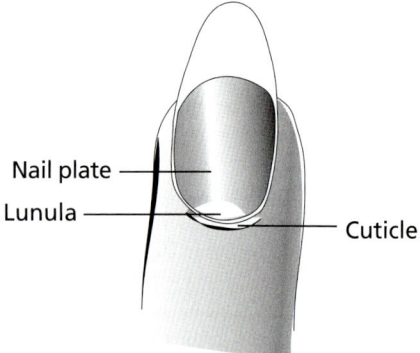

The lunula and cuticle of the nail.

Lunula

The lunula is the pale, crescent-like structure found at the base of the nail. It represents the visible front part of the nail matrix from which the nail grows.

Similarities Between Hair Growth and Nail Growth

The cells at the base of hairs and nails divide continuously, resulting in the growth of the hair or nail. Both the visible part of the hairs and the visible part of the nails are made up of dead keratinous material.

Differences Between Hair Growth and Nail Growth

In the nail, as stated earlier, the keratin that is formed is of a different type to that of the hair but, in contrast to hair, which has growth cycles, nails grow continuously and steadily throughout our lives.

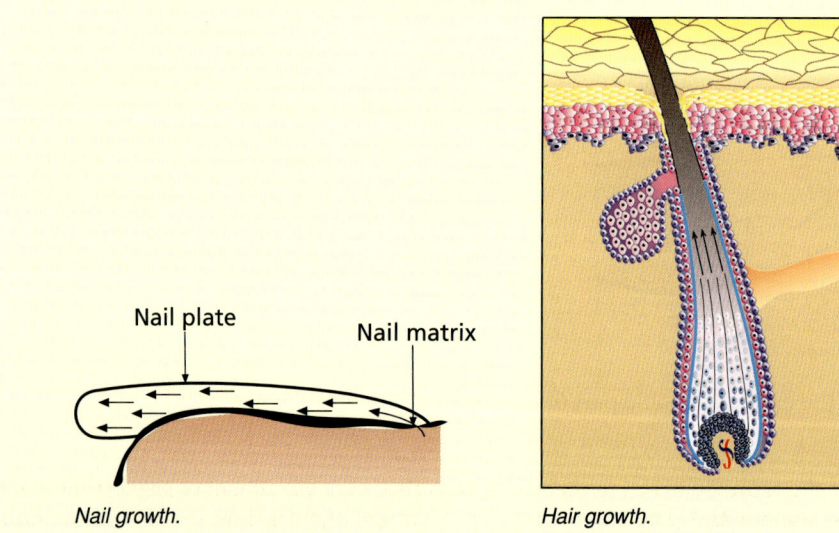

Nail growth.   *Hair growth.*

> **Some Data Regarding Nail Growth**
>
> Fingernails grow approximately 3 to 4 mm per month. Toenails grow more slowly, at approximately 40% to that of fingernails. Nail growth is influenced by the weather: it is accelerated in warm weather and becomes slower in cold temperatures.
>
> Rate of nail growth is influenced by age: nails grow faster in younger people. Advanced age is accompanied by a gradual slowing down of the rate of nail growth. Using the fingers (e.g., typing) stimulates nail growth, so in right-handed people, the fingernails on the right hand grow a little faster than those of the left hand. Some medications may alter the rate of nail growth. Nails grow faster during pregnancy.

Nail Bed
The nail bed is the soft tissue underneath the nail plate. It contains many tiny blood vessels, giving the nail its pink color. The actual nail plate itself (as can be seen at the edge of the nail that protrudes beyond the edge of the finger) is white.

Cuticle
The cuticle is the skin fold at the base of the nail.

GENERAL CARE OF THE NAILS

Nail Care
- Nails should not be regarded as instruments (e.g., for opening lids, tabs of drink cans, etc.). Long nails that protrude beyond the edges of the fingers tend to break more readily, so it may not be such a good idea to grow long nails.
- Nail biting should be avoided.
- Repeated exposure to water eventually leads to drying out and damage to the nails. The nails become more brittle and tend to split at their ends. Also, continuous exposure to soap and cleansing agents leads to dryness and damage.

  Therefore, when washing dishes or performing some activity involving exposure to various chemicals, it is advisable to wear protective gloves (as explained in detail in chapter 14, "Inflammation, Dermatitis, and Cosmetics"), particularly if there is frequent exposure to water or chemicals.

Cutting Nails
Hands should be rinsed in warm water prior to cutting nails in order to soften the nails. While cutting, the nail should be rounded at its front edge; however, its sides should be left straight.

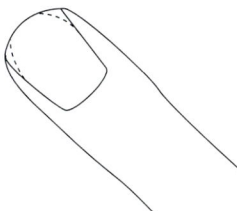

Improper cutting of the nail (indicated by the dashes), with an attempt at rounding off the nail's natural, straight line.

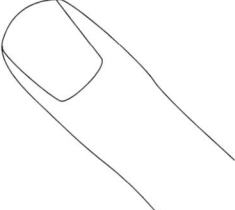

The proper way of cutting the nail.

Unnecessary rounding off of the corners of the nail should be avoided. The nail should not be cut beyond its natural line of growth. If care is taken to cut the nails this way, they will be stronger. Furthermore, this prevents the occurrence of an **ingrown nail**, which is the painful penetration of the nail into the surrounding tissues.

COMMON NAIL PROBLEMS

Nail Deformities

Deformation, or a change in nail shape, may indicate a medical problem which, in some cases, may be diagnosed merely from the shape of the nail. Covering or hiding the misshapen nail(s) with artificial nails may interfere with the correct diagnosis of the problem by a physician—thus further damage may occur, leading to permanent nail deformity. Therefore, seek medical advice from a dermatologist if there is nail deformity. Only after the medical evaluation has been completed may artificial nails be used.

In many cases, nail deformity is the result of fungal infection. In recent years, many effective medications against fungal infections of the nails have been developed. In most cases, these infections can now be cured.

Note: The earlier the patient sees the doctor, the better the chances are of full recovery. The longer a nail deformity has been present, especially if it involves the nail matrix, the less the chances are of complete recovery.

Brittle Nails

As mentioned above, changes in the shape of the nail may reflect some medical problem (skin disease or internal disease). Nevertheless, not every change in the nail necessarily means that there is an underlying medical problem.

Brittleness and splitting of the nails are common, and occur more often in women than in men. Although it is true that excessive brittleness of the nails may be due to a general illness (including malnutrition and anorexia), the most common cause is dryness of the nails as a result of repeated exposure to water and cleansing agents. Even simple washing of the hands, if carried out too frequently, can cause brittleness of the nails. Excessive exposure to cleansing agents (such as dishwashing liquid) or over-frequent use of nail polish removers damage the keratin, the water content of the nails decreases, and they become more brittle. The main principles of treatment of brittle nails include:

- prevention of exposure of the nails to repeated wetting, cleansing agents, and other chemicals—if necessary, protective gloves should be used (it is important to use gloves that have an inner lining made of cotton and
- the use of moisturizers and nail hardeners (see below).

In addition, there are those who recommend taking various vitamins or other basic elements (mainly metals) as treatment for brittle nails (biotin and zinc are commonly recommended). A physician may consider the use of substances such as these in certain cases of brittle nails. More data regarding nail fragility is presented in Appendix III of the book.

COSMETIC TREATMENT OF NAILS

General: Manicure

The term **manicure** describes the variety of treatments related to the care of fingernails. The word is derived from the Latin *manus* = hand, *cura* = care (similar to the term **pedicure**—care of the foot and the toenails: *pes/pedis* = foot). Manicure includes the following:

Cutting the Nails Correctly

As discussed above, the nail should be rounded at its front edge; the corners should not be rounded off, but left squared. Cutting the nails correctly helps to strengthen them and prevents the development of ingrown nails.

Smoothing the Free Edge of the Nail

Smoothing the free edge of the nail is done by using a nail file or an emery board, in order to prevent splitting and breakage.

Care of the Cuticle
The cuticle is the skin fold at the base of the nail. The management of the cuticle basically consists of cutting away excess skin in such a way as to make this part of the nail look neater (if necessary). This is done after gently freeing the cuticle from the nail plate. Soaking the fingers in warm water for several minutes to soften the skin is recommended before trimming the cuticles. It is also advisable to use special cuticle-softening oils.

Freeing the cuticle from the nail plate and its trimming is done by specially designed fine instruments and cuticle retractors (the majority of these are stick retractors made of orangewood; however, some are made of metal). These instruments must be used with extreme delicacy and with great care. Incorrect use may cause mechanical damage to the nail structure and produce permanent deformation. If the instruments are not adequately sterilized before use, there is a risk of introducing bacterial or fungal infection into the nail. In any case, such manipulations should only be done by experienced personnel. Many dermatologists, in fact, are against any unnecessary manipulations in the area of the cuticle, and advise against cuticle retractors—even those made of orangewood. If the manicure requires attention to the cuticles, this should be done after softening the skin by soaking and by pushing back the cuticle using a moistened cloth.

A manicure also includes the correct and proper use of cosmetic preparations, such as nail polish, nail moisturizers, and others, which are used on the nails.

Nail Polish

Nail polish is used for color—both for beautification and to cover up blemishes—and for strengthening weak nails. The main constituent of nail polishes is **nitrocellulose**, a stable substance that mechanically strengthens the nail. It is derived from plant cellulose and is dissolved in organic solvents. Once applied to the nail, the solvents evaporate, leaving a thin film of nitrocellulose that is hard and waterproof.

Other substances used in nail polishes, apart from nitrocellulose, include compounds based on **vinyl**, **methylacrylate**, and **cellulose acetate**. However, these compounds are not as tough and do not produce the same surface hardness as nitrocellulose.

Other Compounds in Nail Polishes

Nitrocellulose has several disadvantages. The thin film produced by nitrocellulose has low gloss, is brittle, and adheres poorly to the nail plate. To overcome these drawbacks, other compounds are added to nail polish preparations:

- **Solvents** whose function is to keep the product in liquid form for long periods and prevent it from drying out in the bottle. The most commonly used solvents are alkyl esters, glycol ethers, and alcohols.
- **Resins** that improve the adhesion of the product to the nail. They also give the polish its characteristic glossy appearance.
- **Plasticizers** that are chemical flexibilizers. They provide flexibility and softness to the nail and the nail becomes less brittle. Plasticizers may also improve adhesion and gloss. The most common plasticizers used in the cosmetic industry are dibutyl phthalate, camphor, and castor oil.
- **Coloring agents** that give the nail plate the desired color. Guanine, derived from the scales of Atlantic herring, produces a pearlescent shade. Bismuth oxychloride and mica coated with titanium dioxide impart an iridescent appearance to the nail.
- Some nail polishes contain **nylon fibers** to thicken and strengthen the nail.
- Some nail polishes contain **proteins, gelatin**, and various **vitamins**.
- Some nail polish preparations contain tiny **pellets**, often made of nickel (and sometimes of **copper**) to help in mixing the polish before use. Most of them are now coated to prevent possible reactions in those who are allergic to copper or nickel.

Application of Nail Polish

Nail polish should be applied evenly over the nail surface. Care should be taken to prevent it from getting on the skin folds and the areas around the nails. Ideally, it should be applied from the base of the nail towards the edge. If too much nail polish has been applied and it has got onto the areas around the nail, the excess should be carefully wiped off with a cotton applicator soaked in nail polish remover.

Undesirable Side Effects of Nail Polish

Prolonged use of dark-colored nail polishes can eventually lead to **staining** of the nails. As the coloring agents in the nail polish permeate the nail plate, their color changes from the original shade of the nail polish, for example, a nail polish that was originally red usually stains the nail yellow. With time, of course, the problem resolves as the nail grows out. To some extent, this problem can be avoided by applying a colorless base coating to the nail before the nail polish itself.

Allergic reactions can take the form of redness, burning, itching, sensitivity, or swelling. The reaction may not be limited to the area immediately around the nail. In fact, **local** reactions to nail polish are relatively rare. On the other hand, since the fingers come into contact with other areas of the body (e.g., while scratching the nose or rubbing the eyes), the allergic reaction may appear in those areas also. Hence, skin inflammation may appear on the eyelids, on various parts of the face, or on the genitalia as a result of using nail polish. If this sort of reaction occurs, a dermatologist should be consulted. There are tests that can be done to identify the specific component of the nail polish that caused the reaction.

Nail Hardeners

The purpose of nail hardeners, as its name suggests, is to harden brittle nails. In fact, nail hardeners are a variant of nail polish, except that they are clear, with no colored additives. They also have a slightly different composition. Substances likely to be present in nail hardeners include acrylate polymers, and a mixture of proteins and salts of various metals. Gelatin has the reputation of being useful as a nail hardener, but its true effectiveness is controversial.

- Some nail hardeners contain **formaldehyde**. In high concentrations, formaldehyde can cause serious side effects and damage to the nail structure. In the United States and most European countries, nail hardeners that contain more than 5% formaldehyde are prohibited. In addition, while using nail hardeners, one should use nail shields that protect the skin around the nail plate. In recent years, formaldehyde has been replaced by other substances, such as polyesters, polyamides, and acrylate polymers.
- Some nail hardeners contain **nylon fibers**, which harden the nail plate even further.

In general, nail hardeners should be applied only to the outer edges of the nails; it is that part of the nail which is most likely to split or break, and there is no sense in covering the entire nail plate with hardener. Also, as with nail polish, care should be taken to avoid getting the nail hardener on the areas around the nail or on the nail fold.

> ### Modern Nail Hardeners
>
> In recent years, a new nail hardening ingredient has been developed which may have certain advantages as compared to formaldehyde. The ingredient, dimethylurea (DMU), is considered to have much fewer adverse effects than formaldehyde in a concentration of 2%. Other alternatives to formaldehyde hardeners are aluminum chloride (5% in water) and nail creams with a high lipid content intended to reduce the probability of nail fragility.

Nail Moisturizers

The purpose of these products is to add moisture to the nail plate. They usually contain proteins, fatty acids, lanolin, and amino acids. Newer products contain vitamins and various plant extracts. Moisturizers are applied to the nail with a brush or by massaging them into the nail.

Nail Polish Removers

The most commonly used solvent for removal of nail products is **acetone**. Other solvents are based on alcohols. Some also contain fatty compounds such as lanolin, which are said to produce an impermeable layer on the nail in order to increase the moisture content of the nail. Nail polish should be taken off by using paper tissue or cotton wool dipped in the remover.

Side Effects of Nail Polish Remover

Nail polish removers can cause the nail plate to dry out, and can cause irritation of the surrounding tissues. Drying out of the nail can lead to nail brittleness. To avoid these problems:

- nail polish remover should not be used too frequently—no more than once a week,
- removers containing fats, which lessen the drying effect, should be used, and
- the hands should be washed thoroughly after using polish remover.

Note: Nail polish removers are basically poisonous and inhaling its fumes could be dangerous.

ARTIFICIAL NAILS

It is not uncommon for artificial nails to cause undesirable side effects. The possibility of these side effects should be considered before using artificial nails. If artificial nails are used to hide defects in the natural nails, it is advisable to obtain a dermatologist's opinion first. Often there is an effective medical treatment for a deformity of the nails. Furthermore, in these cases, not only may the artificial nails be ineffective, they may even aggravate the situation.

Nail Tips

Nail tips are popular because they are easy to use. They are produced in a variety of shapes, sizes, and colors. The nail tips are glued by using **acrylic glue**. They are usually made of nylon or plastic. These compounds do not cause allergic reactions. However, the acrylic glue can cause skin irritation and allergic reactions. Furthermore, using nail tips can lead to excessive brittleness of the natural nails, to splitting, and to changes in their color. A stronger glue containing **ethyl 2-cyanoacrylate** provides better adhesion but can cause damage and disfigurement to the natural nail.

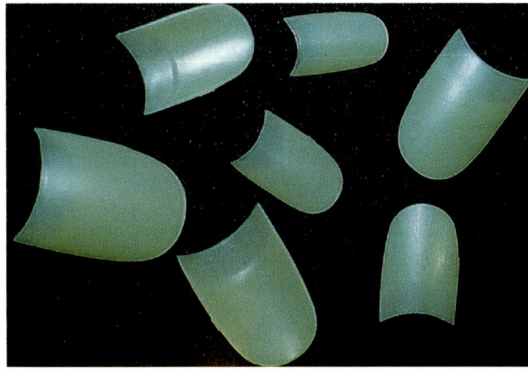

Preformed plastic nail tips.

Nail tips should not be left on for more than a few hours at a time (up to a maximum of 18 hours a day). They must be removed before retiring to bed. Covering up and "sealing off" the natural nail for prolonged periods with nail tips may cause degenerative changes or fungal infections in the natural nail.

Removing the glued-on nail tips without taking due care may result in pulling off some layers of the natural nail. The nail tips must be removed carefully, using a fatty nail polish remover.

Nail tips are often used as extensions of sculptured nails. Professional nail technicians usually coat these tips with artificial nail products to create longer-lasting nail extensions. Most nail technicians feel it is too time-consuming to sculpt nails, and these tips speed the process.

Nail Sculpturing

This method is intended to achieve a stronger, longer, more attractive nail, which can be built up to any desired length. The sculpturing is achieved by using **acrylic polymers** that are built on to a metal form attached to the existing nail plate, as will be described below. Nail sculpturing is usually carried out in cosmetic offices, but there are kits for home use. The result is quite appealing and aesthetically pleasing, especially if the underlying nail was deformed or disfigured. The sculptured nail is an almost perfect continuation of the natural nail and is almost impossible to distinguish from it.

Method of Nail Sculpturing
(1) The nail is cleaned.
(2) The nail is abraded with a nail file or a pumice stone to clean the plate more thoroughly and remove leftover cosmetics (e.g., nail polish) that have adhered to it. In addition, this roughens the nail's surface, which improves adhesion of the sculptured nail.
(3) Some dermatologists suggest the application of antibacterial and antifungal solutions to the surface to prevent bacterial or fungal infection.

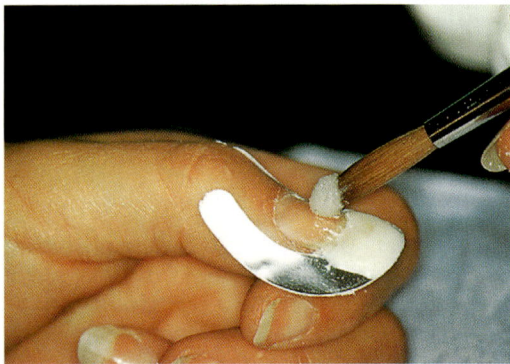

Metallized paper board template for nail sculpturing.

(4) A flexible template is inserted under the natural nail plate, on top of which the nail will be built.
(5) The sculptured nail is made by applying layers of acrylic polymers onto the surface of the natural nail with a brush. The polymers can then be shaped into the desired length and width.

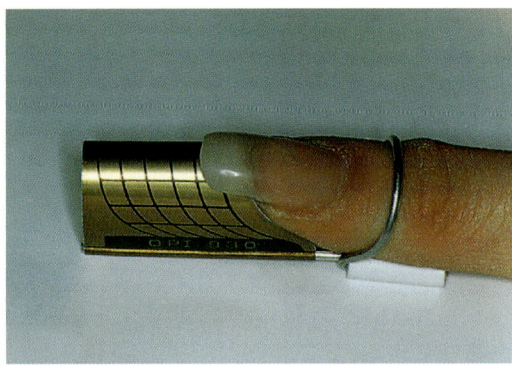

Teflon template for nail sculpturing.

The acrylic material on top of the nail plate is clear, but over the free edges of the nail it looks opaque. This appearance mimics the natural appearance of a nail closely.

Sculptured nails can be removed with nail polish remover. Light-cured gels are resistant to solvents, and where these have been used, the nail should be removed slowly with a medium-grit file (not a drill).

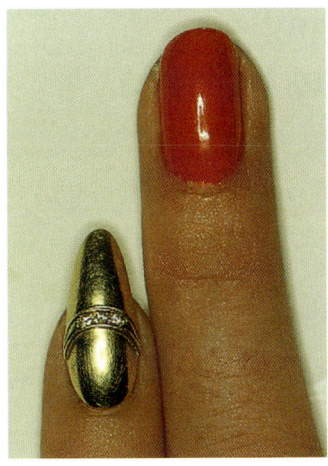
Preformed nail in gold plate.

Undesirable Side Effects of Artificial Nails

Prolonged use of any type of artificial nail can damage the natural nails. Artificial nails cover the natural nail and do not allow the various substances that accumulate under them to evaporate. This may result in softening of the natural nail, with the appearance of **onychodystrophy**—deformation of the nail.

With sculptured nails, since the adhesion between the artificial nail and the natural nail is stronger than that between the natural nail and the nail bed, a condition known as **onycholysis** can occur, in which the nail plate lifts off from the nail bed. The white appearance of the nail plate in onycholysis is due to this separation of the nail from its bed.

There may be allergic reactions to one of the components of the substances used to build up the artificial nail. These reactions usually appear about two or four months after nail sculpturing. Sometimes the reaction occurs later—even after a year. The first sign of an allergic reaction is usually itching of the nail bed.

The use of artificial nails can also lead to a condition known as **paronychia**—a bacterial infection of the tissues around the nail.

It can happen, albeit rarely, that the whole of the natural nail is lost as a result of using artificial nails.

Concluding Comments

Here are some concluding comments regarding artificial nails:

- It is best not to use them, if possible.
- If a patient wants artificial nails because of an unsightly appearance of the natural nails, a dermatologist's opinion should be sought beforehand. It is possible that the problem can be solved medically.
- Whatever type of artificial nails is used, they should be removed as soon as possible.
- If side effects occur, the artificial nails should be removed immediately by using nail polish remover, or with a medium-grit file, if light-cured gels have been used.

Appendix 1: Applying Cosmetic Preparations to the Face and Neck

Avi Shai, Howard I. Maibach, and Robert Baran

How should one apply topical preparations? This question is often asked by cosmeticians regarding the application of moisturizing preparations, sunscreens, creams, and cleansing emulsions for the facial skin. In various books on cosmetics, one finds illustrations and pictures showing how to correctly apply preparations to the face and neck area.

Many dermatologists feel that there is no significance to the direction or the way in which the preparations are applied (in straight or circular motions). However, most dermatologists agree that it is important that the application be done gently in order to avoid repeated, unnecessary stretching of the skin. Other dermatologists may tend to be more rigid about the methods they recommend for applying cosmetic preparations to the facial skin:

- Applying the preparation from the center of the face and outwards is easier.
- It is preferable that the preparation be applied parallel to the natural skin lines of the face and neck, and not perpendicular to them. In this way, one avoids repeated stretching of the skin in a way that later encourages the appearance of wrinkles.

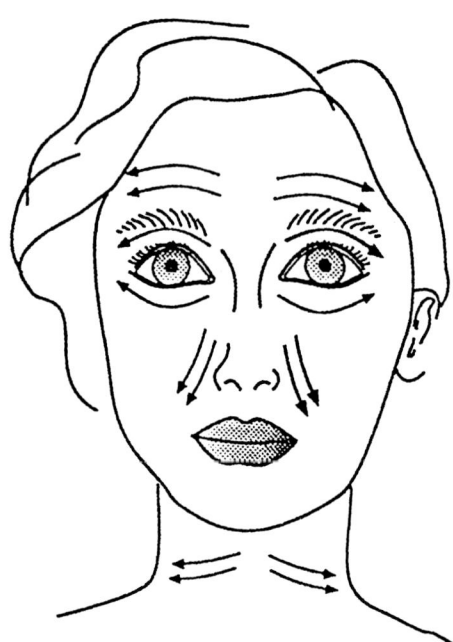

Preferable directions of application.

According to the above-stated principles, the preferable directions for applying preparations to the skin are as illustrated in the diagram above.

WHAT ARE NATURAL SKIN LINES?

Natural skin lines are created according to how the collagen fibers are arranged. The directions in which facial muscles are used determine the direction of the natural skin lines (see diagram). Later in life, these skin lines appear as skin wrinkles.

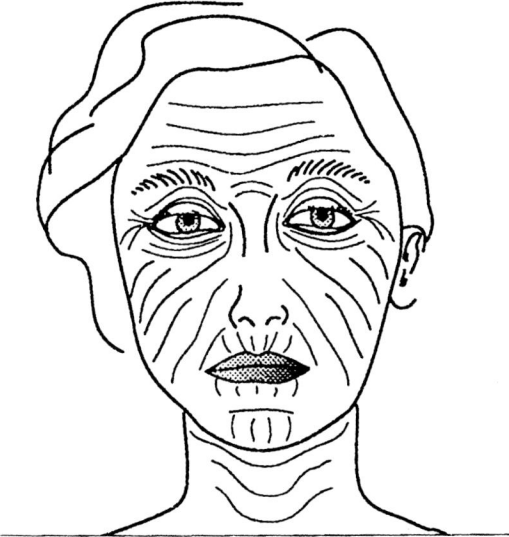

Later in life, natural skin lines appear as skin wrinkles.

As mentioned above, cosmetic preparations should be applied as gently as possible, parallel to the natural skin lines and in the direction of the face and neck wrinkles.

Appendix 2 | Camouflaging Disfiguring Conditions

Victoria L. Rayner

There is no denying that appearance is one of the most powerful factors influencing social interactions. Patients with congenital or acquired physical deformities that alter their body image often experience a diminished feeling of social worth, which erodes their self-esteem. Many of these patients are ashamed to admit to their physicians the depth of anxiety they feel. In many instances, when patients do summon the courage to talk about their embarrassment to their doctors, they are told that there are no medical or surgical solutions available to improve their outward appearance (at least to the extent that will restore their self-esteem). For such patients, cosmetic intervention can be an invaluable resource.

THE ART OF CAMOUFLAGE THERAPY

Camouflage therapy, although still considered comparatively new as a medical specialty, has its roots buried deep in history. By tradition, makeup has long signified camouflage. Throughout the centuries, it has often been used as war paint. Since early times, decorative cosmetics were used by warriors as a form of protection to disguise their original appearance by making themselves appear more fierce and threatening. Even today, makeup is still used as a form of camouflage by soldiers.

Camouflage therapy involves the masking of physical irregularities, with specially formulated cosmetics called cover creams to produce a normalized appearance. This may be achieved by total concealment or subtle textural and pigment blending.

Stage makeup is considered the mother of camouflage makeup because it encompasses a series of methodical procedures that involve lighting and shadowing which are very similar to corrective makeup techniques. By using a modified version of basic theatrical makeup techniques, facial features can be made to appear altered and imperfections diminished. A well-trained camouflage therapist will have carefully studied facial anatomy, highlighting and shading, pigment mixing, and prosthetic makeup. The results a patient can expect will only be as good as the level of expertise of the camouflage therapist.

PATIENTS MOST LIKELY TO BENEFIT FROM CAMOUFLAGE PROCEDURES

Patients who benefit the most are those with scarring from burn injuries, hyper or hypopigmentation, vitiligo, telangiectases, portwine stains, and scarring from lacerations. Camouflage solutions can also be devised for patients recuperating from postoperative trauma—dermabrasion, chemo-abrasion, laser treatments, rhytidectomy, rhinoplasty, and blepharoplasty.

The most difficult abnormalities to correct are stretch marks and protruding scars. Cover creams cannot provide satisfactory coverage for hands and feet because, although waterproof, they can still be rubbed off. Patients with active acne should be discouraged from using oil-based cover creams, because of the high oil content.

Pancake makeup can be substituted to obliterate scarring. Although not waterproof, it will still provide a more opaque coverage than traditional over-the-counter makeup brands.

CAMOUFLAGE MATERIALS

Cosmetic preparations for camouflage procedures have a thick paste-like consistency. They are more opaque than over-the-counter brands of enhancement makeup. To ensure complete coverage, they must be waterproof. Not all cover creams are alike, and they vary in covering capabilities. For this reason, camouflage therapists should work with various brands. At least three palettes from different cosmetic manufacturers are required to offer patients a full range of shades to choose from.

Cover creams can be applied in various ways by using different types of applicators (sponges, brushes, or by using a light touch with the middle finger of the hand). Special theatrical sponges can be used to stipple on cover cream solutions to imitate freckles or beard stubble.

Color correctors are sometimes used as camouflage makeup solutions to counteract ruddiness or offset sallow undertones in the skin. Cream rouges and pigmented powders are needed to restore a natural color tone to the complexion after the application of cover creams to give the skin a healthy appearance.

Because camouflage makeup must be oil-based to be waterproof, soap and water will not remove it. A water-in-oil-based cleansing solution is required.

HOW CAMOUFLAGE THERAPISTS WORK

The goal of cosmetic rehabilitation is to promote self-assurance to patients by providing a cosmetic form of concealment for both permanent and temporary disfigurements.

Camouflage therapy begins with a patient assessment that includes demographic data, medically related information as it pertains to the disfigurement, prescribed medical therapies (topical and systemic), any follow-up surgeries that may be indicated, history of allergies and sensitivities, and the patient's reason for his or her visit. Additional documentation includes a medical description of the proposed treatment site and any other pertinent physical observations, treatment goals, and a record of the cosmetic method used to resolve the patient's aesthetic problem.

Other clinical considerations would include data on the patient's individual goals for treatment, social and leisure activities (the camouflage solution must compliment the patient's lifestyle), his or her peer group, place of employment (to assess the appropriate light source), and any hobbies or sports the patient may be involved in. This information helps the camouflage therapist to determine the special cosmetic needs required according to the patients lifestyle. Patients are also questioned about any prior experience they may have had in applying medical makeup.

The next step of the camouflage process is photographic documentation. Pictures and line drawings are utilized as a record of the cosmetic application process and the camouflage makeup results. The photographs that document the patient's appearance before and after the procedure are included in the patient's file and are also forwarded to the referring physician with the camouflage therapist's written report.

TRAINING AND CERTIFICATION

Only individuals with broad clinical backgrounds and who possess the appropriate credentials should perform cosmetic rehabilitation services. The reason for this is simple: Although the practical aspects of the therapy are elementary, the understanding of patient management is essential to prevent further psychological trauma to patients who may be suffering from the public's reaction to the appearance of their disfigurements.

The best training programmes are those offered through accredited institutions.

For more information about the use of cosmetics to normalize the appearance of disfigurements, the following reading materials are recommended:

SUGGESTIONS FOR FURTHER READING

1. Frost P, Horwitz S. Principles of Cosmetics for the Dermatologist. St. Louis, MO: CV Mosby, 1982.
2. Sieldel L, Copeland I. The Art of Corrective Cosmetics. New York, NY: Doubleday, 1984.
3. Allsworth J. Skin Camouflage: A Guide to Remedial Techniques. Cheltenham, U.K.: Stanley Thornes, 1985.

4. Trust D. Overcoming Disfigurement: Part Three. The Cosmetic Component. Wellingborough, U.K.: Thorsons, 1986.
5. Noyes D, Mellody P. Beauty & Cancer. Los Angeles, CA: AC Press, 1988.
6. Rayner LV. Clinical Cosmetology: A Medical Approach to Esthetics Procedures. Buffalo, NY: Milady, 1993.
7. Edut O. Body Outlaws: Young Women Write About Body Image and Identity. Seattle, WA: Seal Press, 2000.
8. Lucas G. Why I Wore Lipstick to My Mastectomy. New York, NY: St. Martin's Griffin, 2004.
9. Wilhelm S. Feeling Good About the Way You Look. New York, NY: Guilford Press, 2006.
10. Ciaramicoli AP, Ketham K. The Power of Empathy. New York, NY: Dutton, 2000.
11. Rumsey N, Harcourt D. The Psychology of Appearance. Berkshire, UK: Open University Press McGraw Hill, 2005.

Appendix 3 | Fragile Nails

Robert Baran and Avi Shai

The nail plate represents a natural perfection of strength and flexibility. Changes in nail consistency and structure may result in nail fragility.

EXTERNAL CAUSES OF NAIL FRAGILITY

Fragility and splitting of the nails are common, and occur more often in women than in men. The most common cause is dryness of the nails as a result of repeated exposure to water and cleansing agents. Even simple washing of the hands, if carried out too frequently, can cause fragility and brittleness of the nails. Excessive exposure to cleansing agents, such as dishwashing liquid, damages the keratin, and dries out the nails. Hence, they become fragile.

Nails may also be damaged following exposure to other chemical agents such alkalis, sugar solutions, and various solvents. Not infrequently, repeated trauma or exposure to hot water may cause a certain level of damage to the nails.

Drying, with subsequent fragility, may be aggravated by the over-frequent use of some nail polish removers and, less frequently, by some nail polishes. Certain nail treatments (not always desirable) performed by manicurists include soaking the fingers in warm soapy water, which leads to similar outcomes.

The nail plate is also subject to daily assaults, and requires five to six months to regenerate. Factors that slow down the rate of nail growth, such as aging, affect the general health of the nails, increasing chances of fragility. As a result, nail fragility is more common amongst the elderly. As the level of nail cholesterol sulfate tends to decrease in women (as compared to men) with age, they are more prone to fragile/brittle nails.

SYSTEMIC DISEASES

Nail disorders, in many cases, may indicate a certain systemic disease. For example, liver or kidney diseases may affect the appearance of nails in unique patterns.

Nail fragility may be induced by anaemia, arsenic intoxication, certain infectious diseases, hormonal disorders, diseases of the nervous system, arthritis, and conditions such as osteoporosis. Malnutrition and anorexia may induce excessive fragility as well. In addition, there are also certain inherited defects associated with thinning and excessive brittleness of the nail plate.

Iron deficiency can also result in the softening of the nail with subsequent deformity. In addition, deficiencies in vitamin A, C, B_6, and zinc have been documented as causing nail fragility.

Contrary to general opinion, the calcium content in the nail has little influence on nail hardness.

SKIN DISEASES AND NAILS

Certain skin diseases may also affect the nails and significantly reduce the rate of their growth, with subsequent thinning of the nail plate and increased fragility. This may happen in conditions such as *psoriasis*, *lichen planus*, and certain types of dermatitis.

Impairment of circulation with decreased blood supply to the fingers may induce fragility as well. An interesting observation is the presence of nail abnormality in a disease called *alopecia areata*, which mainly affects the hair. This confirms the well-known association between disorders of the nails and hair.

LOCAL TREATMENT FOR NAIL FRAGILITY

Exposure of the nails to repeated wetting must be avoided as much as possible.

Housework can be particularly damaging, because it usually involves exposure to cleansing agents and other chemicals. Protective gloves should be used. It is important to use gloves that have an inner lining made of cotton.

After exposure to water, a light, highly penetrable oil such as olive oil or jojoba oil should be applied to the nails to seal and moisturize. Mineral oils and lubricating creams, although effective in sealing and holding in moisture, wear off more rapidly than lighter, thinner oils.

The use of nail hardeners may be considered as well.

SYSTEMIC TREATMENT FOR NAIL FRAGILITY

In case of an identified specific problem, treatment should be directed accordingly. For example, if low levels of iron are found, supplementary iron should be provided. However, it has been suggested that taking iron over several months may be of some value to the nails even in the absence of demonstrable iron deficiency. Other researchers suggest taking other compounds such as evening primrose oil, pyridoxine, biotin, and/or vitamin C. The beneficial effect of these suggestions, however, requires further research.

Appendix 4 | Glossary

Acne A disease of the hair follicles and associated sebaceous glands. The onset of acne is frequently related to hormonal changes that occur during adolescence.

Acnegenic An acnegenic substance is one that may cause a skin reaction resulting in acne in the area of its application. In that case, the acne is characterized by pustular lesions (containing pus) that appear one to two weeks after using the substance. Certain cosmetic preparations may contain acnegenic substances.

Acute An acute illness is one that develops rapidly and that is not prolonged; it either resolves or progresses to a chronic phase.

Allantoin A substance widely used in cosmetics. In the past, it was extracted from various plants; nowadays it is mainly synthesized from uric acid. It is said to have soothing properties on the skin, and the ability to heal wounds. It is a common ingredient of moisturizing preparations and products designed to soothe irritated skin.

Allergy A state of excessive sensitivity resulting from an immunological response of the body to some substance. Allergy can occur following inhalation of the offending substance, from swallowing it, or from direct contact of the substance with the skin.

Aloe vera This plant extract is said to have soothing properties. It is present in a wide range of cosmetics, and also in home medications for use in mild burns, wounds, and various skin inflammations.

α-Hydroxy acids Substances derived from vegetable and fruit extracts. Preparations containing α-hydroxy acids may have a beneficial effect on skin aging, particularly those processes owing to excessive sun exposure. α-Hydroxy acids also bleach various pigmented lesions of the skin. In low concentrations, they function as effective moisturizing agents.

Anagen The stage of active hair growth, when the hair cells are dividing and the hair is growing.

Antibacterial A substance that kills or inhibits the growth of bacteria.

Antibiotics Substances that kill or inhibit the growth of bacteria. Antibiotics are produced from certain bacteria or moulds.

Antimicrobial A substance that kills or inhibits the growth of bacteria or other microorganisms.

Antiperspirants Preparations that reduce sweating, which are usually made up of aluminum compounds. These substances penetrate the duct of the sweat gland, block it, and thereby reduce the secretion of sweat.

Antiseptic A substance that kills or inhibits the growth of bacteria or other microorganisms, usually applied to body surfaces or used to disinfect medical equipment.

Apocrine sweat gland Specialized sweat gland present in the axillae (armpits) and groin. The fluid secreted by apocrine glands is relatively thick and contains various organic compounds. These organic substances are broken down by bacteria, giving rise to an unpleasant body odor.

Aromatic oils Oily substances derived from various plants, which are volatile liquids with characteristic fragrances. These oils are reputed to have anti-inflammatory and antibacterial properties, as well as a cooling, soothing effect on the skin. They are found in a wide range of cosmetic preparations, including cleansing preparations (soaps and shampoos).

Arrector pilorum muscle A tiny muscle attached to a hair. When this muscle contracts, the hair stands up straight. The sudden contraction of these muscles creates "goose bumps."

Astringents Preparations that, in essence, impart a feeling of coolness and freshness to the skin. The skin feels "taut," and the skin pores are temporarily constricted. Astringents contain a mixture of alcohol and water, aluminum or zinc salts, and other components such as menthol, camphor, and plant extracts (such as witch hazel).

Atopic dermatitis A skin disease characterized by dryness, redness, and severe itching. This disease is one of the group of conditions known as atopic diseases. Asthma and allergic rhinitis (hay fever) are also included in this group.

Atrophy In general, this term refers to a decrease in size or wasting away of a tissue or organ. Atrophic skin is thin and delicate. Severely atrophic skin wrinkles and becomes transparent, so that the underlying blood vessels become visible through it. Skin becomes atrophic with age. The prolonged use of corticosteroid-containing preparations on the skin can make it atrophic.

Azelaic acid A substance used in the treatment of acne. It is also used for lightening dark skin lesions.

Bacterium A single-celled microorganism, often referred to as a "germ." Bacteria cannot be seen with the naked eye, but can be seen with a light microscope. Of the many types of bacteria in nature, most are not harmful to humans. A small number of bacteria are capable of causing infections in humans (e.g., pneumonia, tonsillitis, cellulitis, etc.)

Benzoyl peroxide An oxidizing substance that attacks bacteria. It is useful in the treatment of acne and is present in many acne preparations, including creams, emulsions, soaps, and others.

Biopsy Removal of a piece of tissue from the body (e.g., a piece of skin) for the purpose of microscopic and laboratory examination.

Calamine A mixture of zinc oxide with a small amount of iron oxide; it has a soothing effect on the skin, and decreases itching.

Cancer A malignant growth or tumor.

Carcinoma This term embraces a wide range of malignant growths of various types. Common skin growths that are carcinomas are basal cell carcinoma and squamous cell carcinoma.

Catagen A stage in the life cycle of hair. It is a brief (about two weeks) transitory phase, when the hair stops growing and the cells at its base start to degenerate.

Cationic surfactants A group of surfactants that are used in shampoos and hair conditioners because of their ability to neutralize the negative electric charges on the surface of the hair (see **Surfactants**).

"Cellulite" A lay term (unrelated to any medical term) describing an unattractive distribution of subcutaneous fat in the body, especially in the thighs and buttocks.

Ceramides These compose approximately 40% of the fatty acids within cells. They play an important role in maintaining the keratin layer of the skin. Recently, ceramides have been increasingly used in the cosmetics industry, both as moisturizing agents and as protective agents for the prevention and repair of damage caused by exposure to various chemicals.

Chloasma See **Melasma**.

Chronic A chronic disease is one that exists for a prolonged period.

Cleansing cream Creams containing cleansing substances (see **Surfactants**) designed to clean the face. They are meant to stay on the face for a short time only, and are then wiped off with a tissue or moist cloth, or rinsed off with water.

Cold cream A cream that gives a feeling of coolness when applied to the skin. It is made up of a simple mixture of oil and water. When applied to the skin, the water separates out from the oil and quickly evaporates from the surface of the skin. This process of evaporation produces a cold feeling on the skin (hence the name of this cream).

Collagen A protein present in the dermis. Collagen is arranged in the form of intertwined fibers which give the skin strength and resilience.

Comedogenic A comedogenic substance is an ingredient of a cosmetic preparation liable to cause acne.

Comedone The basic lesion in acne, resulting from the accumulation of compressed keratin and fat in a hair follicle. An **open comedone** (blackhead) results when the opening of the hair follicle is widened by the material that builds up inside the follicle. A **closed comedone** (whitehead) occurs when the opening of the follicle remains closed.

Conditioners (hair) Substances that produce a layer that coats the hair and gives the hair a smooth and uniform look. Conditioners neutralize the electric charges on the surface of the hair, making it easier to comb and manage.

Contact dermatitis Skin inflammation resulting from direct skin contact with various substances. Contact dermatitis may occur by means of a direct mechanism (when it is called **irritant dermatitis**), or via an allergic mechanism (in **allergic contact dermatitis**).

Cortex (of the hair) The central layer seen in a cross-section of a hair. The cortex is made up of cells that are degenerating and dying as they move up the hair to the skin surface.

Corticosteroids A general name for a group of hormones that are produced naturally in the body. Some corticosteroids have anti-inflammatory properties. Hence, these substances are widely used in dermatology against inflammatory diseases of the skin. Prolonged and excessive use of corticosteroids, whether taken by mouth or by application to the skin, may result in serious side effects. Always consult a physician before using any preparation that contains corticosteroids.

Cosmetician Someone involved in the field of cosmetics, which is directed towards the care, protection, and improvement of the appearance of the skin.

Cosmetics A wide field related to the various aspects of appearance and beauty. It mainly involves the care, protection, and improvement of the appearance of the skin. The origin of the word is from the Greek *kosmos*, meaning "order."

Cosmetologist Someone who is an expert in the research aspects of cosmetics, and who may be a chemist, a biologist, or a physician. This definition varies from one country to another. In some countries, such as in the United States, it is a formal title subjected to the regulations of each state, for which one has to graduate from a school of cosmetics. In other countries, cosmetology is not a formally recognized degree.

Cosmetology A general term covering the research aspects of cosmetics, embracing biological, chemical, and medical aspects.

Couperose An alternative term for **telangiectasis**.

Cream A semisolid **emulsion**. Creams, obtained from a combination of a fatty substance with water, are common bases in cosmetics and dermatology and may contain many different cosmetic and medical substances.

Cuticle (hair) The outermost layer of the hair shaft, which is made up of a layer of individual cells, overlapping each other. The cuticle acts as the protective layer of the hair.

Cuticle (nail) The skin fold at the base of the nail.

Cyst A fluid-filled cavity in the skin. Cysts may occur in acne.

Dandruff (scales) Fragments of keratin that are shed from the skin surface as part of the process of epidermal cell turnover. So long as the rate of cell turnover is normal, one cannot normally see these flakes. If the cell turnover is increased, more and more dead flakes of keratin appear, which may join together into larger, visible pieces, and can be seen as they come away from the scalp.

Deodorants Substances designed to prevent unpleasant body odor. Deodorants contain various combinations of antibacterial substances, substances that adsorb odors, and substances that mask odors.

Depilation   A technique for the removal of hair in which the removal is superficial and takes place at or near the skin surface—in contrast to **epilation**, it does not involve the hair root. Depilation can be carried out, for example, by shaving or by using depilatory creams. Regardless of the method used, depilation is only of temporary value.

Dermatitis   A term used for **inflammation** of the skin.

Dermatologist   A "skin doctor"; a physician who deals with the various aspects of skin diseases.

Dermatology   The field of medicine dealing with the diagnosis and treatment of skin diseases.

Dermis   A layer of the skin containing collagen and elastin fibers. The dermis also contains blood vessels, nerves, sensory organs, sebaceous glands, sweat glands, and hair follicles.

Dihydroxyacetone   A substance present in artificial tanning preparations. Dihydroxyacetone reacts chemically with proteins in the outer (dead keratin) layer of the epidermis. In doing so, it imparts an artificial, brown to yellow suntan-like color to the skin, which lasts for about three to five days.

Eccrine sweat glands   These are scattered all over the body. The sweat secreted by eccrine glands plays an important role in regulating body temperature. This sweat does not cause body odor.

Elastin   A protein present in the dermis. It is arranged in fibers and gives the skin its elastic characteristics so that when it is stretched it falls back into place.

Electrolysis   A method of permanent hair removal, which is carried out by inserting a fine metal needle into the opening of the hair follicle. An electric current is then passed through the needle, intended to destroy the active cells at the hair root.

EMLA (Eutectic Mixture of Lidocaine and Prilocaine)   Contains local anaesthetic agents. It is used before performing painful procedures on the skin (such as removal of hair with an electric needle). EMLA should be applied to the skin some 60 minutes prior to performing the procedure, and an occlusive dressing placed over it. It lessens the pain that may accompany the course of various medical/cosmetic procedures performed on the skin.

Emulsifier   (also called an "**emulsifying agent**")   A substance (natural or synthetic) that separates oil from water. In that way, it stabilizes emulsions (which contain oil and water) so that the oil droplets remain dispersed throughout the water as a homogeneous mixture. In the absence of an emulsifier, an oil-water mixture will separate into two distinct layers.

Emulsion   A mixture of oil and water. An emulsion is a basic preparation that may incorporate many cosmetic substances or medications. If it contains a relatively large proportion of water, it is more liquid (and is then known as a **liquid emulsion**). If the preparation does not contain a lot of water its texture is not liquid, but rather semisolid. In that case the substance is a **cream**.

Epidermis   The outermost layer of the skin. At the base of this layer, new cells are constantly and steadily formed by a process of cell division.

Epilation   A technique for the removal of hair that involves removing the hair together with its root. The removal of hair by epilation may be temporary (e.g. by pulling out the hair) or permanent (e.g. by using an electric needle).

Erythema   Redness of the skin. There may be many reasons for the skin becoming red, for example, in certain diseases or following sun exposure.

Eumelanin   A pigment that is similar in its chemical structure to melanin. It gives the hair a brownish-black color.

Fibroblast   A cell in the dermis of the skin that is responsible for producing the intercellular matrix and collagen fibers.

Folliculitis Inflammation of a hair follicle. The word is made up of *follicle*, and *-itis*, which is a standard suffix in medical terminology meaning "inflammation." Folliculitis can occur, for instance, after shaving, after plucking hair, or after the use of an electric needle as the result of microscopic injuries that occur to the follicle during the shaving or plucking process.

Foundation cream In essence, a foundation cream is a pigmented moisturizing cream. In many cases, it contains a sunscreen. Apart from maintaining the skin's moisture and protecting it from the sun, foundation cream gives the face a smooth, uniform appearance, and conceals skin lesions. It is used for under make up.

γ-Linoleic acid A fatty acid that is said to have anti-inflammatory properties. It also serves as an occlusive substance in the keratin layer of the skin, thereby contributing to the defensive properties of skin.

Gel A common base used in cosmetics and dermatology. Gels may contain a wide range of active ingredients or medications. A gel is similar to a cream in its consistency, but contains less fat; it is therefore used on skin that tends to be oily.

Hair follicle An elongated tube-like depression in the skin from which a hair grows.

Hamamelis See **Witch hazel**.

Horny layer See **Keratin layer**.

Humectants Substances that are effective at absorbing water and commonly used in moisturizing substances. Some humectants (e.g., urea or lactic acid) can penetrate the keratin layer of the skin and increase its moisture content.

Hyaluronic acid A component of the intercellular substance in the dermis. It absorbs water efficiently and is commonly used in moisturizing compounds.

Hydrogen peroxide A strong antiseptic liquid. Hydrogen peroxide is not used as a routine antiseptic for wounds, etc., because it also damages normal body tissues. Its use is limited to especially contaminated, infected wounds, such as bites. Hydrogen peroxide is also used for bleaching hair.

Hydroquinone A substance used for lightening dark skin lesions (such as "pregnancy mask" or "sun spots").

Hypoallergenic A preparation that ostensibly does not contain substances that tend to cause skin irritation or allergic reactions (mainly perfumes and various preservatives). However, even hypoallergenic preparations may cause skin irritation or allergy.

Inflammation A defensive response of the body to certain processes, including various infections and other insults. The signs of inflammation are localized warmth (in the area involved), redness, swelling, and sometimes pain and loss of function of the inflamed organ.

Iodine An active substance that inhibits and kills bacteria and other microorganisms. Iodine can appear in different forms in various preparations, for example, tincture of iodine (a preparation based on iodine dissolved in alcohol) and povidone iodine (a compound containing iodine with a polymer that ensures the slow release of the iodine).

Isotretinoin The commercial name for a medication from the retinoid group of compounds chemically similar to vitamin A. It is used in the treatment of acne. It may only be given on the recommendation of a dermatologist.

Keratin This protein, the major component of the keratin layer of the skin, is also present in hair and nails. Keratin gives the skin its strength and provides protection from external insults.

Keratin (horny) layer The outermost layer of the skin. It is made up of flat, dead cells lying one on top of the other. As new cells are formed in the skin, the outer dead cells are pushed out, directed to the surface of the skin, and are shed from the skin.

Keratinocytes The cells that make up the epidermis. They are also known as squamous cells (Latin *squama* = a scale).

Keratolytic A keratolytic substance is one that can dissolve and remove keratin from the skin. Keratolytic preparations are used for treating areas of thickened skin. Sometimes, in the treatment of acne, keratolytic preparations are used to remove the keratin that occludes the opening of the hair follicle.

Keratosis An abnormal situation characterized by localized or generalized thickening of the keratin layer of the skin. It may appear as part of a cancerous or precancerous process (such as solar keratosis) or various inflammatory processes.

Langerhans Langerhans cells are cells in the skin related to the immune system.

Lanolin A fatty substance that is a complex mixture, derived from sheep's wool. Lanolin is a common ingredient of moisturizing substances.

Liposomes Microscopic spheres made up of **phospholipids**. Recently they have become widely used in dermatology and the cosmetics industry. The aim is to introduce medications and various cosmetic substances into liposomes, so they (the liposomes) act as a carrier to help the active ingredient that is inside them to penetrate the skin.

Liquid emulsion An emulsion that appears in the form of a liquid, derived from a mixture of water and oil (**emulsion**). A liquid emulsion is a base that may contain many cosmetic or medicinal ingredients.

Lotion The simple definition of a lotion is a preparation that contains liquid components. However, the more accurate, scientific definition of lotion is a mixture of oil, powder, and water.

Lunula The pale, crescent-like structure that is found at the base of the nail. The outer part of the nail matrix (the area from which the nail grows) lies under this region.

Malignant melanoma A malignant skin tumor. The mortality rate from malignant melanoma is high. It is therefore extremely important to detect this lesion early and remove it in its entirety. Malignant melanoma arises from **melanocytes** in the skin.

Manicure A term that covers numerous procedures involved in the care of the fingernails. The word is derived from the Latin *manus* = hand, *curo* = to care for.

Medulla (of the hair) The inner layer seen in a cross-section of a hair. Sometimes it is missing and sometimes it is not continuous along the length of a hair. The absence or presence of the medulla can affect the sheen and shade of the hair.

Melanin A pigment produced by melanocytes in the skin. Melanin gives the skin a dark color, and it plays a role in the skin's protection against the sun.

Melanocytes Cells in the epidermis that produce **melanin**.

Melanocytic naevus This is the lesion commonly known as a mole, or as a "beauty spot." It originates from melanocytes—the cells that produce melanin. Melanin is the pigment that gives the skin its dark color.

Melasma (Chloasma) "Pregnancy mask." A specific distribution of pigment on the face, seen in some women. This phenomenon develops more commonly during pregnancy. In melasma, there are light or dark brown areas on the upper lip, forehead, and chin, usually symmetrical. There is presumably a hormonal basis for this phenomenon.

Mesotherapy A nonsurgical aesthetic treatment employing minute doses of medications and/or plant extracts, vitamins, amino acid, and other compounds, injected subcutaneously.

Metastases Groups of malignant cells that break away from the primary cancerous tumor and find their way to other areas of the body. In those areas, the metastatic cells continue to multiply uncontrollably and destroy the surrounding tissues.

Micelle The soap structure that surrounds fat and dirt particles, enabling them to be removed from the skin by rinsing with water.

Moisturizing cream Designed to increase the moisture content of the skin. Moisturizing creams contain occlusive fatty substances or water-absorbent substances.

Nail bed   The soft skin underneath the nail plate.

Nail matrix   The living, growing part of the nail, under the nail base. The cells of the nail matrix are continuously, steadily dividing, and in that way the nail grows.

Nail plate   The external, visible part of the nail.

Neoplasm   (also called **tumor** or **cancer**) A lesion arising from the uncontrolled growth of some tissue in the body. If the growth is benign, it remains confined to the area of the body from where it arose; a malignant tumor, on the other hand, tends to spread aggressively to nearby tissues, and to more distant tissues in the body.

Night cream   Night creams are also called "nourishing creams." They have a very high fat content and are supposed to contain various ingredients that penetrate the skin. For that to occur, the cream has to stay on the skin for several hours. Therefore these creams are applied at night, before going to bed. The "nourishing" components of these creams consist of various active ingredients, which are believed by some to benefit the skin after they penetrate deeply into it.

Nitrocellulose   The main ingredient in nail polish and nail hardeners. It is a very stable substance that provides the nail with mechanical strength. Once the nail polish has been applied, various solvents that it contains evaporate, leaving the nitrocellulose behind as a thin, hard, shiny, waterproof layer on the nail.

NMF (natural moisturizing factor)   A mixture of substances present in the skin that make up approximately 20% to 25% of the keratin layer. This mixture is able to retain the moisture content of the keratin layer.

Nodule   An inflammatory lump in the skin. Compared with a papule, a nodule is deeper in the skin. The distinction between a nodule and a papule is based on how they feel to the touch. Nodules may appear in a wide range of diseases and abnormalities of the skin. Acne may be characterized by the appearance of nodules.

Onychodystrophy   Distortion of the shape of the nail.

Onycholysis   This is when the **nail plate** comes away from the **nail bed**. When that happens, white areas appear on the nail plate.

Organic   In the biological sciences, an organic substance is usually said to be one derived from living matter; in chemistry, an organic compound is one that contains carbon atoms.

Oxygen free radicals   These are byproducts of chemical processes that oxygen molecules undergo. They are normally produced regularly and naturally in many body tissues, but certain factors (e.g., solar radiation, smoking, environmental pollutants, and others) increase their rate of production. Oxygen free radicals can damage various body tissues. It appears that they may be involved in the development of some heart diseases, diseases of the blood vessels, and various malignant diseases. Researchers maintain that free radicals have a cumulative effect that accelerates aging of various body tissues.

Panthenol   Also known as provitamin B_5. It is said to help in wound healing and alleviating skin inflammation. It is a common ingredient in preparations used in the treatment of diaper rash in infants.

Papule   A lesion of about 0.5 cm diameter that is raised above the surface of the skin. The papules seen in acne are typically pink/red in color because of the inflammatory process.

Paraffin   Paraffins are a group of fatty compounds derived from the refining of crude oil. After purification and bleaching, they are common ingredients of moisturizing agents. Paraffins may appear as liquids, semisolids (as petroleum jelly), or solids (paraffin wax).

Paraphenylenediamine   A component of permanent hair dyes.

Paronychia   Infection of the tissues around the nail.

Paste   A mixture of powder and an ointment. Because of its fat content, a paste has good occlusive and skin-protective properties. The powder within the paste effectively absorbs liquids. The main use of pastes is in protecting infants' skin from urine and feces in the diaper region.

Patch test   A skin test to help identify causes of skin inflammation or contact allergy. The test is carried out by using small discs containing various substances, which are attached to the patient's skin. The skin reaction is examined under each disc after 48 to 96 hours.

Pedicure   A term that covers numerous procedures involved in the care of the foot and the toenails. The word is derived from the Latin *pedis* = foot, *curo* = to care for.

Peeling   A technique for removing the outermost layer of the skin by creating a chemical burn. As the burn heals, a new outer layer of skin forms, which is smoother, tauter, more uniform, and pinker than the original surface.

Permanent waving of hair   Setting the hair in the form of curls. Permanent waving is achieved by a series of chemical processes performed on the hair, involving softening the hair, fashioning it into the desired shape, and finally fixing it permanently in that shape. The substances used in a permanent wave are thioglycolates or substances chemically related to thioglycolates.

Petroleum jelly   A semisolid form of **paraffin** (white soft paraffin).

Phenol   A substance used for deep skin peeling. The use of phenol requires giving the patient either intravenous analgesia (pain relief) or a general anesthetic during the procedure. When carrying out skin peeling using phenol, the patient's cardiac (heart) status must be monitored carefully, and he/she must be given intravenous fluids to prevent possible kidney damage.

Pheomelanin   A pigment that is chemically similar to melanin. It gives the hair a reddish shade.

Phospholipids   Fatty compounds containing phosphorus that makes up the two-layered cell walls in the body. In the cosmetics industry, **liposomes**, which are made up of phospholipids, are used to help the active ingredients of various preparations penetrate the skin.

Pigment   A colored substance, such as melanin, the more of which there is, the darker the skin looks. Makeup contains various pigments to give the user a skin shade that is different from his/her natural skin color.

Pityrosporum ovale   A microscopic yeast that is commonly present in the scalp and hair follicles. Dandruff and seborrhoeic dermatitis have been attributed to *Pityrosporum ovale*. Some of the shampoos designed to treat dandruff are formulated to act upon this microscopic yeast on the surface of the scalp.

Polymers   Chemical compounds made up of long chains of many small, identical, individual units.

Psoralens   A group of substances that increase the skin's sensitivity to type A ultraviolet radiation, and hence result in faster tanning. They are used in a number of skin diseases. Not only do psoralens accelerate skin tanning, but at the same time they may also increase all the damaging effects of solar radiation on the skin and are therefore prohibited for use as routine tanning agents.

Purpura   Localized bleeding into the skin. Purpura occurs in various diseases—both skin diseases and general diseases. Among other things, prolonged use of corticosteroid-containing preparations can cause purpura to appear in the treated areas.

Pustules   Small blisters on the skin, which contain pus.

Resorcinol   A **keratolytic** substance that also possesses a degree of antiseptic effect. It is an older treatment for acne.

Retinoic acid   This has a similar chemical structure to vitamin A. Preparations containing retinoic acid are used in the treatment of acne, and for bleaching dark areas of skin. Retinoic acid is also used to repair and halt aging processes in the skin—particularly those processes related to excessive exposure to the sun.

Salicylic acid   This is the active component of aspirin (the chemical name for aspirin is acetylsalicylic acid). When applied to the skin, salicylic acid is **keratolytic** and is used to dissolve and remove excessive keratin from the skin.

Scalpel   A very sharp, special knife used by surgeons.

Sebaceous glands   Glands in the skin that are attached to hair follicles. They secrete their fatty product (sebum) into the hair follicle via a small secretory duct. Sebum provides a fatty layer on the surface of the skin and on the outer surface of the hair, which protects them and prevents them from getting too dry.

Seborrhoea   A state characterized by excessive secretion of the sebaceous glands in the skin, producing an excess of sebum. The skin and hair look greasy. In this situation, there is usually flakiness of the skin.

Seborrhoeic dermatitis   An inflammatory skin condition that occurs in areas with numerous sebaceous glands. Seborrhoeic dermatitis goes on for years, with periods of improvement and flare-ups, and is characterized by redness and the appearance of flaky scales. In adults, seborrhoeic dermatitis tends to appear mainly on the scalp, alongside the nose, and above the eyebrows.

Sebum   A fatty substance secreted by the sebaceous glands, which are connected to the hair follicles. Sebum provides an oily layer that covers the skin and hair, which is protective and prevents drying out.

Skin peeling   See **Peeling**.

Solar keratosis   A lesion that tends to appear in fair-skinned people over the age of 40. The lesions appear on areas exposed to the sun. They are slightly raised, dry, rough and, pink/red, with a fine, scaly surface. Solar keratoses are defined as precancerous lesions that are not considered malignant.

Spermaceti   A fatty substance derived from whales. Its use is banned in the United States.

SPF (sun protection factor)   A measurement of the efficiency of a sunscreen. The SPF is determined by measuring how long the sunscreen delays the appearance of redness in the skin when exposed to the sun.

Subcutis   The fatty layer under the dermis of the skin.

Sunscreens   Preparations designed to protect the skin from the sun's rays. Chemical sunscreens absorb the radiation; physical sunscreens act as a mirror and reflect rays back from the skin.

Surfactants (surface-active agents)   Water-soluble compounds that form the major ingredient of soaps and shampoos. Molecules of surfactant surround the particles of fat and dirt on the skin surface, and thereby allow them to be removed by rinsing with water.

Suspension   A product that is a combination of powder and water. In this case, the powder particles are not dissolved in the water, so the preparation looks turbid rather than clear and homogeneous. Before using a suspension, it must be shaken so as to produce an even distribution of the powder particles in the liquid.

Talc   This is the commercial name for zinc polysilicate. It is an inert substance in the form of a powder, and is used to minimize friction and to absorb moisture. Commercial preparations containing talc also usually contain small amounts of other substances, such as zinc oxide or aluminum silicate.

Tanning   The process by which the skin becomes darker following exposure to the sun. Tanning occurs because the solar radiation causes the **melanocytes** to produce melanin, which is the pigment that gives the skin its dark color.

Telangiectasis (Telangiectasia)   Dilatation (widening) of fine, superficial blood vessels (up to approximately 1 mm in diameter) on the skin surface. This phenomenon appears as the result of cumulative damage to the skin following exposure to the sun, to radiation, etc. Various diseases can also result in the appearance of telangiectases on the skin.

Telogen   The resting phase in the life cycle of a hair, during which the mechanism responsible for the cellular division in the base of the follicle is inactive for several months.

Terminal hair   Coarse, thick, dark hair that is readily visible.

Thioglycolates   These are present in depilatory preparations. They dissolve and break down the keratinous substance of the hair and are used for the removal of excess body hair. Thioglycolates break the sulfur bonds that bind hair fibers. They are also used for perming hair.

Tincture   An alcohol-based solution.

Titanium dioxide   A substance that protects against ultraviolet radiation. It is a basic ingredient in most sunscreen preparations.

Trichloroacetic acid   An acid used for skin peeling.

Triclocarban   An **antibacterial** substance present in various deodorants and soaps.

Triclosan   An **antibacterial** substance present in various deodorants and soaps.

Ultraviolet (UV) radiation   Light rays whose wavelength is beyond the visible violet light. Excessive exposure to type A or type B ultraviolet rays produces cumulative damage to the skin, which may manifest itself as "sun spots," wrinkles, and various skin tumors.

Vanishing cream   A cream with a relatively high water content. Because of its "watery" nature, it washes off readily. As it is easier to apply, to rinse off, and to wipe off the skin, it is generally used as a day cream. The advantage of using a vanishing cream is that, once it is applied to the skin, it is virtually invisible and the thin layer on the face can hardly be seen.

Varicose veins   Dilated veins that appear usually on the lower limbs; varicose veins are the result of faulty functioning of the valves in the veins.

Vellus hair   Fine, thin, light hair that is hardly noticeable.

Venous insufficiency   Abnormal and ineffective function of the venous blood vessels, affecting the blood flow through them.

Vitamin   A compound that belongs to a family of organic substances present in tiny quantities in food, which are essential for the normal physiological function of the body.

Vitamin D   A vitamin that is necessary, among other things, for building up bones and maintaining their strength. Exposure to sunlight promotes production of vitamin D in the body.

Witch hazel (Hamamelis)   This plant extract is said to be able to constrict skin pores. It is a common component of astringent preparations.

Zinc pyrithione   A component of many shampoos designed for treating dandruff.

Index

A

Abrasive cleansers, 42
Absorbent masks, 44
Acetone, 263
Acidity and pH, 35–36
Accutane®, *see* Isotretinoin
Acne
 cosmetics and make-up causes, 66–67
 corticosteroids and, 171
 diet and, 65
 facial cleansing for, 65–66
 facial masks for treatment of, 43, 45
 hair follicle, 60
 inflammatory lesions of, 63–64
 lesions, *see* Acne lesions
 overview, 58
 soaps for, 40, 65–66
 sun exposure and, 66
 treatment
  by cosmetician, 67–69
  by dermatologist, 69–75
  tailoring, 75–76
Acne lesions
 basis for appearance of, 60–64
 closed comedones (whiteheads), 58, 62–63
 inflammatory lesions, 63–64
 open comedones (blackheads), 58, 62
 primary, 60–63
Acnegenic effect of cosmetics, 66
Acrylic glue (for nails), 263
Active ingredients of cosmetic preparations, 14
 animal-derived substances, 131, 132–133
 foodstuffs, 131, 141
 plant extracts, 131
  allantoin, 137
  aloe vera, 133–134
  aromatic oils, 138
  chamomile and calendula, 135
  echinacea, 136
  γ-linoleic acid, 137
  jojoba oil, 137
  lavender, 134
  oil of Australian tea tree, 136
 vitamins, 131, 138–40
  in skin preparations, 139
  vitamin C, 140
Acyclovir, 233
Adapalene for acne, 71
Additional/auxiliary substances in cosmetic preparations, 15

Additives
 in moisturizers, 31
 in soaps, 38–40
Adipose tissue (subcutis), 4, 13
Aftershave preparations, 166
Age spots, *see* Solar lentigenes
Aging, 46–57
 anti-aging effects, 36
  of α-hydroxy acids, 54, 149–152
  of moisturizers, 26, 55
  of retinoic acid, 54, 143–5
 chronological aging, 46–9
 control of, 52–7
 photoaging, 49–50
Alcohol sulfates, 236
Alcohol-based solutions, 17
 as antiseptics, 169
Alkalis and pH, 35–6
Allantoin, 137
Allergic contact dermatitis, 109–110, 112
Allergy
 general, 109
 defined, 273
 to cosmetics, 111–112
Aloe vera, 133–134
α-Hydroxy acids
 in acne, 70
 in bleaching preparations, 164
 in chemical skin peeling, 151–3, 179
 combined with retinoic acid, 153
 guidelines for using, 152–153
 high concentrations of
  chemical peeling of skin using, 151–152
  uses of, 149
 low concentrations of
  as water-absorbing agent, 149
  sun-damaged skin, 150
  uses of, 148
 in moisturizers, 29–30, 149
 moderate concentrations of
  effect on epidermis and dermis, 150
  uses of, 149
 side effects of, 154
 uses
  in preparations, 148
  in United States, 154
  on dark-skinned patients, 154
Alpha-tocopherol (vitamin E), 56
Aluminium salts in astringents, 166
Amino acids in cosmetic preparations, 132
Aminophylline, 100
Amniotic fluid, 132

Anagen phase of hair growth, 224, 225
Angioma, 212, 213
Animal-derived fatty bases in cosmetics, 15–16
    lanolin, 15
    spermaceti, 16
    wool alcohols, 16
Anionic surfactants, 37, 230
Anthemis nobilis (chamomile), 135
Antibacterial substances
    defined, 273
    in soaps, 39
Antibiotics
    defined, 168
    for acne
        external, 70–71
        orally administered, 72
Antidandruff shampoos, 235
Antifungal agents
    classification of, 169
    mode of action of, 168–169
    in shampoo, 235
    uses of, 169
Antihistamines, 113–114
Antioxidants, 56, 138
Antiseptics
    for handwashing and disinfecting skin before medical treatment, 169
    for treating infected areas of skin, 169–170
    hydrogen peroxide and iodine-based solutions, 170
Antiperspirants, 273
Antiviral agents, 185
Apocrine sweat glands, 12
    body odor, 39
Aquamid®, 199
Aqueous solutions in cosmetics preparations, 17
Arborizing telangiectasia, 95
Arbutin, 164
Aromatic oils, 138
Arrectores pilorum muscles, 10, 221–2, 273
Artefill® and Artecoll®, 199
Artificial nails, 266
    nail sculpturing, 264
    nail tips, 263
    side effects of, 265
Artificial tanning, 89
Astringents
    composition of, 166
    uses of, 166–167
Atopic dermatitis, 108, 111
Atrophy
    in aging, 47
    in corticosteroid use, 213
Australian tea tree oil, 136
Azelaic acid
    for acne, 71–72
    for bleaching, 163

B

Bacteria, 274
Bacterial infection
    general, 6
    due to peeling, 184

Barium sulfide for hair removal, 246
Basal cell carcinoma (BCC), 122–123
Base (vehicle) for cosmetic preparations, 14–15
Bases in cosmetics
    aqueous solutions, 17
    combinations, 18
        creams, 19–20
        fatty base with water, 18–19
        lotions, 21
        of powder, water, and oil, 21
        powder with fatty base, 21
        powder with water, 20–21
    fatty bases, 15–17
    powders, 17
Beauty spots, see Nevi
Benign tumor
    definition of, 115
    malignant vs., 116
Benzophenone in sunscreen, 84
Benzoyl peroxide
    for treatment of acne, 70
    in acne soaps, 66
Berloque dermatitis, 161
β-Carotene, 90, 140
β-Hydroxy acids
    adverse effects of, 155–156
    in acne treatment, 155
    keratolytic effect of, 155
    precautions of using, 156
    types of, 155
Betaines, 40, 236
Bio-Aquamid®, 200
Biodegradable fillers, see Fillers
Biopsy, 129–30
Blackheads, see Comedones
Bleaching preparations
    α-hydroxy acids, 164
    azelaic acid, 163
    glabridin, 164
    guidelines for using, 161
    hydroquinone, 162–163
    hydroquinone monobenzyle ether, 163
    Kligman's formula, 163
    kojic acid, 164
    retinoic acid, 163
Blepharoptosis, 206
Blood flow in leg veins, 96
Blood vessels, see also Telangiectasia
    fine networks of, 212
    in dermis, 6
    laser instruments for treating, 188
Body odor, 39–40
Borage oil, 137
Botulinum toxin (BTX)
    complications of, 205–206
    contraindications for, 204
    cosmetic use of, 201
    for forehead, 205
    for glabellar lines and upper face treatment, 205
    indications for, 202–203
    mode of action, 201
    patient selection for, 202
    preparations/products, 203

Bovine collagen, 197
Bronzers, 90
Brow ptosis, 205–206
Bruising in ageing, 48
Burns
   camouflage, 218
   sunburn, 79

C

Caffeine, 100
Calamine
   defined, 274
   lotion, 21
   powder, 17
   in facial cleansing masks, 62
Calendula, 135
Calendula officinalis, 135
Calendula extract, 135
Camouflage therapy
   burns, 218
   cover creams, 215–7
   foundation creams, 215
   recreating imperfections, 219
   skin types, 219
   temporary problems, 214
   types of lesions, 212–4
Camphor
   in aromatic oils, 138
   in astringents, 166
Cancer, see Tumors
Cancerous lesions, management of
      biopsy, 128–130
Carcinoma, 119, 274
Catagen phase of hair growth, 224, 225
Cationic polymers, 239
Cationic surfactants, 239
Cell membranes
   microscopic structure of, 142
   structure of, 175
Cellulite
   cosmetic preparations for, 100
   general, 98–101
   injection lipolysis for, 101
   prevention of, 99–100
   surgical methods for removing excess fat, 101
Ceramides, 132–133
Cetomacrogol, 28
Cetrimide, 169
Chamomilla recutita, 135
Chamomile, 135
Chamomile extract, 135
Chelating agents in shampoo, 232
Chemical depilatories
   disadvantages of, 247
   instructions for using, 247
   types of, 246–247
Chemical skin peeling
   α-hydroxy acids, 151–3, 179
   complications
      bacterial infection, 184
      scarring, 185
   course following, 183–184
   depth of, 180–1

   factors influencing, 181
   pain with, 183
   preparations used in, 179–181
   preparation prior to procedure, 183
   procedure, 228–30
   skin regeneration following, 180–181
Chloasma, see Melasma
Chlorhexidine, 169
Chrome, 109
Chronological aging of skin, 46–49
   changes appear with, 48–49
   degeneration of elastin/collagen fibers, 46
   thinning of skin, 47–48
   vs. photoaging, 48–49
Cleansing creams, 20
   vs. soaps, 41
Closed comedones (whiteheads), 58, 62–63
   release of contents of, treatment by cosmetician, 69
Clostridium botulinum, 201
Cold creams, 20
Cold wax treatment, 246
Collagen fibers, 132
   of dermis, 9
   skin aging and degeneration of, 46
Colored foundation creams, 215
Coloring agents
   in soaps, 38–39
Combination skin, 30
Comedogenic effect of cosmetics, 66
Comedone extractor, 67
Comedones
   closed, 58, 62–63
   defined, 58
   open, 58, 62
   release of contents, 67–69
   softening of, 67
Contact dermatitis
   overview, 109
   allergic, 109
   diagnosis, 112–3
   hand eczema, 110–111
   irritant/allergic, 109
   phytodermatitis and phytophotodermatitis, 110–111
   treatment, 145–146
Contaminated products, identification of, 20
Corticosteroids
   generic and brand names, 172–4
   side effects, 171–2
   in the treatment of dermatitis, 113
   prolonged use
      purpura, 171
      telangiectasia, 171–172
   preparations, types of, 172–174
   uses of, 171
Cosmeceuticals, 2–3
Cosmetic preparations
   definition and classification of, 2
   for cellulite, 100
   organic, 23

Cosmetician
　acne treatment by, 67–69
　defined, 1
Cosmetic products
　active ingredients, 14
　application, 266–267
　aqueous bases, 17
　bases (vehicle), 14
　combinations, 18–21
　definition of cosmetic product, 2
　dermatitis, due to, 111–112
　fatty bases, 15–16
　classification, 2–3
　creams, suspensions and pastes, 19–20
　lotions, 21
　pastes, 21
　powders, 17
　preservatives, 22
　suspensions, 20–21
Cosmetologist, 1
Cosmetology, 1
Couperose, 92
Cover creams
　application of, 217–218
　coloring agents, 215–216
　for different types of skin, 219
　matching to skin, 217
　stability of, 216
Cradle cap, 234
Creams
　general, 19–20
　application, 266–267
　facial cleansing, 41–42
　types of, 19–20
　vs. gels, 22
Crow's feet wrinkles, 51, 205
Cuticle
　of hair, 223–224
　of nail, 258–259
Cysts, 60, 64
　treatment by cosmetician, 69

D

Dandruff
　causes of, 234
　treatment of, 234
Depilation,
　definition, 242
　depilatories, 246–7
　depilatoric glove, 243
Dermal cells, 9
Dermal or follicular papilla, 222
Dermatitis
　atopic, 108
　Berloque, 161
　contact, 109–110
　cosmetic preparations and, 111–112
　defined, 106
　diaper, 138
　seborrhoeic, 108, 234
　stasis, 96

Dermatologist
　acne treatment by, 69–75
　defined, 1
　hyperpigmented blotches treatment, 161
Dermatology, 1
Dermis, 4
　blood vessels in, 6
　long-term effects of sun exposure on, 81–82
　structure of, 8–12
　collagen and elastin fibers, 9
　dermal cells, 9
　eccrine sweat gland, 12
　hair, 10–11
　sebaceous glands, 10
　thickness of, 6
Detergent, 37
Diaper dermatitis, 108
Diaper rash, 21
Diet
　for cellulite, 99
　crash, 99
　healthy lifestyle, 55
Diathermy, 251
Dihydroxyacetone, 89
Diluted chlorine solutions, 170
Doxycycline, 72
Drugs
　vs. cosmetics, 2–3
　defined, 2
Dry skin, 30
　in aging, 25
　causes of, 25
　characteristics of, 25–26
　criteria for using moisturizers, 31
　microscopic structure of, 26
　overview, 24
Dyes/fragrances in shampoo, 232

E

Eccrine sweat gland, 12
Echinacea, 136
Eczema.
　hands, 110
　see also Dermatitis
Eflornithine cream, 247–248
Elastin
　fibers in skin structure, 9
　in cosmetic preparations, 132
　skin aging and degeneration of, 46
Electric cautery with needle for telangiectasia, 93
Electrolysis for permanent removal of hair
　advantage of, 250
　complications from
　　infection, 255
　　inflammatory reaction and scarring, 254
　contraindications, 254
　effectiveness of, 255
　equipment needed for
　　direct electrolysis, 250
　　electrocoagulation, 251
　　instruments for home use, 251
　　needle, 251–252

instructions for performing, 252
minimizing pain associated with, 253
mode of action of, 249
reappearance of hair, 255–256
EMLA cream, 253, 276
Emulsifier, 19
Emulsion, liquid, 19, 22
Enzymes, hair removal, 247
Epidermal cells, 8
Epidermis
 basal layer of, 7
 increased turnover of cells in, 7
 long-term effects of sun exposure on, 80
 structure of, 7–8
 thickness of, 6
 tumors of, 118
Epilation, 242
Erythema, 79
 minimal erythema dose, 85
Excisional biopsy, 129–130
Exfoliants, 155
Exotic facial masks, 45
Exotic ingredients in moisturizers, 32
Eye creams, 20
Eye irritation
 sunscreens and, 85
Eyelid ptosis, 206

F

Facial aging, 193
Facial cleansing
 abrasive cleansers for, 42
 creams and liquid emulsions vs. soaps for, 41
 for acne, 65–66
 masks, *see* Facial masks
 overview, 41
Facial expressions, skin aging and, 54
Facial hair, 241
Facial masks
 effects of, 45
 exotic, 45
 functions of, 43
 overview, 43
 peeled off, 44
 rinsed off, 43
Facial volume loss, 194
Famciclovir, 185
Fat, 15
Fatty bases
 in cosmetics, 15–17
  animal-derived, 15–16
  derived from minerals, 16
  ointments, 16–17
  plant-derived, 16
Fatty tissue,
 in cellulite, 99
 sub-cutis, 13
Fillers
 biodegradable
  general, 194
  collagen-based, 197
  hyaluronic acid, 197–198

PLLA, 198–199
Radiesse®, 198
nonbiodegradable
 general, 194
 Artefill® and Artecoll®, 199
 polyacrilamide gels, 200
 silicone, 199
 correction of changes due to aging, 194–195
 correction of facial defects due to trauma/disease, 196
Finger tip unit, 171
5-Fluorouracil, solar keratosis, 121
Foaming agents in shampoo, 232
Folliculitis, 243, 277
Foods sensitivity, acne and, 65
Formaldehyde, 262
Foundation creams, 20, 27, 215, 325
Fractional photothermolysis, 189
Fragrances and perfumes in soaps, 38–39
Freckles, 159
Furocoumarins, 161

G

γ-Linoleic acid, 137
Gels
 in cosmetics preparations, 22
 for hair, 240
Gentian violet, 170
Glabridin, 164
Glossary of terms, 273–282
Gloves, rubber, 110
Glycerine, 29
Glycolic acid, 148
 see also α-Hydroxy acids
 application to sun-damaged skin, 150
 as humectant, 149
Glycosaminoglycans, 29
Green tea, 164
Gum tragacanth, 236

H

Hair, 10–11
 bleaching, 248
 causes of excess, 241
 color, 223
 damage
  to external surface, 238
  to growth, 227–228
 formation of, 222
 growth rate, 226–227
 removal
  permanent, *see* Electrolysis, for permanent removal of hair
  temporary, *see* Temporary hair removal methods
 shampooing, 229, 233
 structure of, 10–11
  hair shaft, 221
  sebaceous glands and papilla, 222
 styling, 240
 types of, 221
 washing, 236

Hair conditioners, 237
   methods of using, 240
   mode of action of, 238
   types of
      cationic surfactants and cationic polymers, 239
      protein conditioners, 240
Hair follicle
   number, 221
   acne lesions and structure of, 60
   definition, 220
   general, 10–11, 221–222
   hard keratin in, 222
Hair growth
   aging, 48
   factors affecting, 227–228
   hair life cycle
      general, 224–226
      catagen phase, 224
      telogen phase, 224
   rate, 226–7
Hair loss
   baldness, 228
   normal and abnormal, 226
Hair removal
   hair removal, permanent (electrolysis), 249–256
   laser treatment, 190–191
   hair removal, temporary
      chemical depilatories, 246–247
      epilation/depilation, 242
      general, 241–248
      plucking, 243–244
      scraping, 243
      shaving, 242–243
Hair root cells, 10
Hair shaft, 10
   cuticle, 237
   layers of, 223–224
   microscopic structure of, 223
   with early signs of damage, 237
Hair structure
   general, 10–11, 221–222
   transverse section, 255–256
Hair types, vellus/terminal, 220
Hamamelis virginiana, 166
Hand eczema, 110
Hard keratin, 10
Hard soap, 34
Hexachlorophene, 169
Hirsutism, 254
   in corticosteroid use, 171
Histamines in dermatitis, 113
Honey, 141
Hormones
   in acne, 72–73
   estrogen, replacement therapy, 56–57
   Hormone Replacement Therapy (HRT), 56–57
Human collagen products, 197
Humectants, 28–30
   subtypes of, 29–30
Hyaluronic acid
   chemical structure of, 197
   cross-linking of, 198
   in dermis, 132

Hyaluronic acid dermal fillers
   chemical structure of, 197
   cross-linking of, 198
Hyaluronidase, 136
Hydrogen peroxide, 170
Hydroquinone, 162
Hydroquinone monobenzyl ether (HMBE), 163
Hypercarotenaemia, 90
Hyperpigmented skin lesions
   camouflage, 213–214
   definition of, 159
   post-inflammatory, 161
   treatment of
      α-hydroxy compounds for, 153
      bleaching preparations for, 161, 164
   types, 159–161
Hypoallergenic preparations, 112
Hypoallergenic soaps, 40
Hypopigmented lesion, defined, 158–159

I

Infection of skin, 107–108
Inflammation of skin
   acute, 106–107
   causes and types, 106, 107
   defined, 106
   characterization of, 106
   chronic, 107
   diagnosis of, 112–113
   post-inflammatory pigmentation, 161
   treatment of, 113–114
   types of, 107–108
Inflammatory lesions of acne, 63–64
Injection lipolysis
   for cellulite, 101
   for eliminating double chin, 104
   for eliminating undesirable accumulation of fat in back, 104
   overview, 102
   procedure for, 102–105
   side effects of, 105
   substance used in, 102
   use of phosphatidylcholine in, 102–103
Intense pulsed light (IPL), 191
Intra-hypodermic injection, 209
Intra-epidermal technique, 208
Iodine-based solutions, 170
Iodoform, 170
Irritant contact dermatitis, 109
Isotretinoin for acne, 73–75
   course of, 75
   during pregnancy, 74–75
   precautions for patients taking, 74
   recommended dosage of, 75
   side effects of, 73–74

J

Jessner's solution in chemical skin peeling, 179, 181
Jojoba oil, 137

K

Kaolin, 44
Keratin
  general, 7, 10
  of hair, 222
  of nails, 257
Keratinocytes
  general, 7
  tumors originating from, 119–123
Keratinous layer, 4,7
Keratolytic products
  in acne, 70
  allantoin as, 137
  defined, 278
  for dandruff, 235
  in hair removal, 246–247
Keratosis, 119, 278
  solar, 119–120
Kligman's formula, 163, 183
Kojic acid, 164

L

Lactic acid, 29, 40, 148,
Langerhans cells, of epidermis, 8
Lanolin, in cosmetics preparation, 15
Laser instruments
  for sun spots treatment, 191
  for tattoo removal, 187–188
  for treating blood vessels, 188
  hair removal using, 190–191
  skin peeling using, 188–189
  for telangiectasia, 94
  types of, 187
Lasers
  noninvasive, 189
  properties of, 187
  uses of, 187
Latex in facial cleansing masks, 44
Lavender, 134
Lavendula officinalis, 172
Lentigines, solar, 80
Leukocytes, 9, 106
Light-colored skin lesions, 213
Lines of expression in skin aging, 51, 202
Lipid film, 26–28
Liposomes, 175
  efficacy of, 178
  fusion with membrane, 177
  unilamellar/multilamellar, 176
  uses in cosmetics industry, 177
Liposomes in cosmetics, 30
Liposuction, 101
Liquid emulsion
  defined, 19
  facial cleansing, 41
  general, 19, 22
Liquid nitrogen, bleaching, 164
Liquid silicone, 194, 199
Lotions 21, 278
Lunula (nail), 258

M

Magnesium polysilicate, see Talc
Make-up
  causes acne, 66–67
  for telangiectasia, 95
Malic acid, 148
  see also α-Hydroxy acids
Malignant melanoma, 124
  characterization of, 125–125
  incidence of, 124
  management, 128–130
  self-examination of
    in front of mirror, 126–127
    with help of second person, 127
  vs. nevi, changes suggesting malignancy, 124–126
Malignant tumor
  benign vs., 116
  progress of, 117
Manicure, 260–261
Masks, see Facial cleansing masks
Matricaria chamomilla (chamomile), 135
Mechanical scraping of hair, 243
Medulla, hair, 223–224, 278
Melaleuca alternifolia, 136
Melanin
  eumelanin, 223
  general, 8, 78
  factors influencing production of, 158
  pheomelanin, 223
Melanocytes, 8, 78
  hair follicle, 223
  loss in aging, 48
  suntanning, 78
Melanocytic nevi
  growth of, 123
  types of, 124
  changes suggesting malignancy, 124–126
Melanoma, see Malignant melanoma
Melasma, 160, 214
Menthol
  in aromatic oils, 138
  in astringents, 166
Mephisto sign, 206
Mesogun, 208
Mesolift, 210–211
Mesolipotherapy, 211
Mesotherapy
  basic principle of, 207
  conditions to avoid, 211
  cosmetic uses of, 207
  history of, 207
  preparations prior to, 208
  side effects of, 211
  site of injection, 209
  techniques of
    intra-hypodermic injection, 209
    mesolift, 210–211
    multipricking, 208–209
    point per point injection, 209
    tremor, 208
Metastases, 116
Methylxanthines, for cellulite, 100

Micelles, 34–35
Mild soaps, 40
Miliaria, 91
Milk products,
    and acne, 65
    and tetracyclines, 72
Minipeel method, 150
Moisture content, skin aging and, 48
Moisturizers
    α-hydroxy acids as, 149, 150
    beneficial effects of, 26
    body vs. face, 32
    guidelines for using, 32
    for hands, 33
    humecatants, 28–30
    natural moisturizing factor (NMF), 27
    non-oily, 29
    occlusives, 28
    selection of, 30
    in shampoo, 231
    in soap, 38
Moisturizing creams, 20
Mole, *see* Melanocytic nevi
Mousses for hair, 240
Multipricking methods, *see* Superficial intradermic methods

N

Nail disorders, 272
Nail hardeners, 262
Nail moisturizers, 262–263
Nail polish removers, 263
Nail polishes
    application of, 262
    constituent of, 261
    side effects of, 262
Nail sculpturing, 264
Nail structure
    general, 258–259
    nail bed and cuticle, 259
    lunula, 258
    matrix, 257–258
    nail plate, 257
Nail tips, plastic, 263
Nails
    artificial, 266
    brittle, 260, 271–272
    growth, 258–9
    composition of, 257
    cosmetic treatment of
        manicure, 260–261
        moisturizers, 262
        nail hardeners, 262
        nail polish, 261–262
    cutting, 259, 260
    fragility of
        external causes of, 272
        local and systemic treatment for, 273
        skin diseases and, 272–273
Natural moisturizing factor (NMF), 27
    components of, 29–30
Natural skin lines, 268

Networks of blood vessels
    on face, 92–93
    on legs, 94–95
    on skin, 95
Nevi (melanocytic)
    growth of, 123
    types of, 124
    changes suggesting malignancy, 124–126
Neoplasms, *see* Tumors
New Fill®, 199
Nickel in contact dermatitis, 109
Night creams, 19–20
Niosomes, 177
Nitrocellulose, 261
Nodules, 59, 64, 279
    treatment by cosmetician, 69
Nonbiodegradable fillers, *see* Fillers
Non-oily moisturizers, 29
Nucleic acids, 132
Nylon fibers (for nails), 261

O

Occlusives, 28
Ochronosis, 162
Oil, 15
    aromatic, 138
Oily skin, 30
    criteria for using moisturizers, 31
    soaps use on, 38
Ointments, 16–17
Onychodystrophy, 265
Onycholysis, 265
Open comedones (blackheads), 58, 62
    release of contents of, treatment by cosmetician, 68
Orally administered medications for acne
    antibiotics, 72
    hormonal preparations, 72–73
    isotretinoin, 73–75
        course of, 75
        during pregnancy, 74–75
        precautions for patients taking, 74
        side effects of, 73–74
    tetracyclines, 72
Organic cosmetic preparations, 23
Outer layer of skin, *see* Epidermis
Oxybenzone in sunscreens, 84
Oxygen free radicals, 138, 279
    role in skin aging, 56

P

Panthenol (provitamin B), 140
Papules, 58, 63
    treatment by cosmetician, 69
Para-aminobenzoic acid (PABA), 84
Paraffins, 16, 279
Paronychia, 265
Pastes in cosmetics, 21
Patch test, 112–113, 280
Pearlescents, 232, 236, 261
Pedicure, 260
Peel-off facial masks, 44

Peeling, *see* Chemical skin peeling
Peeling agents, 181
Pellagra, 55
Petroleum jelly, 280
pH, 35–36
pH scale, 36
Phenol in chemical skin peeling, 181, 185, 280
Phosphatidylcholine in injection lipolysis, 102–103
Phospholipids, 29, 142, 175, 280
Photoaging of skin, 49–50
    characteristics of, 49
    vs. chronological aging, 49
Physical activity to control skin aging, 55
Physical exercise for cellulite, 100
Phytodermatitis, 110–111
Phytophotodermatitis, 111
Phytosterols, 137
Pigments, 158
Pigmentation
    hyperpigmented lesions
        camouflage, 213–214
        post-inflammatory, 161
        treatment of
            α-hydroxy compounds for, 153
            bleaching preparations for, 161, 164
        types, 158–161
    hypopigmentation, post-inflammatory, camouflage, 212–213
Piroctine olamine, 235
Pityrosporum ovale, 234
Placental extracts, 132
Plant extracts, 131
    allantoin, 137
    aloe vera, 133–134
    aromatic oils, 138
    chamomile and calendula, 135
    echinacea, 136
    for cellulite, 100
    γ-linoleic acid, 137
    jojoba oil, 137
    lavender, 134
    oil of Australian tea tree, 136
Plant oils, 16
Plant-derived fatty bases, 16
Plucking of hair
    advantages and disadvantages of, 244
    using
        cold wax, 246
        tweezers, 244
        warm melted sugar, 245–246
        warm wax, 245
Point per point injection technique, 209
Poly-L-lactic acid, 198–199
Polyacrilamide gels, 199, 200
Polyhydroxy acid, 156
Postmenopausal women, HRT for, 56–57
Potassium permanganate, weak solutions of, 170
Povidone iodine, 170
Powders, in cosmetics preparation, 17
Pregnancy mask (melasma)
    camouflage, 213–214
    general, 214
    treatment, 161–164

Pregnancy
    and isotretinoin, 74
    and retinoic acid, 146–147
    and tetracyclines, 72
Preparations for external use for acne
    α-hydroxy acids, 70
    adapalene, 71
    antibiotics, 70–71
    azelaic acid, 71–72
    benzoyl peroxide, 70
    containing salicylic acid, sulfur, or resorcinol, 70
    retinoic acid for, 71
Preservatives
    in cosmetics preparations, 22
    in shampoo, 232
    in soaps, 38–39
Prickly heat, 91
Primula obconica, 111
Propionbacterion acne, 75
Propolis, 141
Propylene glycol, 29
Protective layer of skin, 6
Protein conditioners, 240
Proteins
    in cosmetic preparations, 132
    in hair conditioners, 240
Provitamin B, 140
Psoralens, 90
Ptosis of brow, 205–206
Pulsed-dye lasers, 187
Pumice stone, 243
Purpura, 171, 280
Pustules, 58, 63–64
    treatment by cosmetician, 69
Pyrithione and pyridine derivatives, 235

Q

Quaternary ammonium surfactants, 235

R

Radiesse®, 198
Rebound effect, 172
Resorcinol for acne, 70
Retinoic acid
    for acne treatment, 143
    beneficial effects on skin aging, 143–145
    bleaching effects, 163
    guidelines for using, 145–146
    mechanism of action of, 145
    precautions for using, 146–147
    pregnancy, 185–186
    side effects of, 146
    warnings, 146–147
Retinoic acid for acne, 71
Retinoids, 147
    for cellulite, 100
Retinol, 147
Rinse-off facial masks, 43
Roaccutane®, *see* Isotretinoin
Rosacea, 93
Royal bee jelly, 141
Ruby lasers, 187

S

Salicylic acid
  dermatological uses of, 156
  for acne, 70
Scalp
  heating of, 228
  local pressure on, 228
Scars
  camouflage, 214
  scarring risk with peeling, 185
Scurvy, 55
Sebaceous glands
  anatomy, 10
  in acne, 61–63
  in aging, 48–49
Sebum, 10, 61–62
  acne lesions and structure of, 60
  enlargement, skin aging and, 48–49
Seborrhea, 234
Seborrheic dermatitis, 108, 234
Sebum, 10, 60, 222, 229
Selenium disulfide, 235
Senile lentigenes, see Solar lentigenes
Shampoo
  components of, 236
    antidandruff ingredients, 235
    chelating agents, 232
    conditioners, 231–232
    dyes/fragrances, 232
    foaming agents, 232
    moisturizing agents, 231
    preservatives, 232
    surfactants, 230, 231
    thickeners, 232
    vitamins, 232–233
  principle of action of, 229
Shaving of hair, 242–243
Silicone
  in fillers, 199
  in moisturizers, 33, 110
Silver sulfadiazine, 79
Skin
  ability to retain moisture, 25
  and age, see Skin aging
  applying foundation cream to, 215
  cover cream application method for, 219
  facial masks for moisturizing/cleansing of, 43
  function
    production of vitamin D, 7
    protective layer, 6
    social interaction, 7
    temperature regulation, 6
    transmission of sensations, 6
  penetration of substances into, 142, 175
  preferable directions for applying preparations to, 267
  prolonged soaking, 27
  repeated placing of damp cloth, 27
  types of
    by color, 82
    by lipid content, 30
  water content of, 24
  wetting of, 27
Skin acidity, protection against infections, 35
Skin aging
  α-hydroxy acids preparations role in, 148
  chronological aging
    changes appear with, 48–49
    degeneration of elastin/collagen fibers, 46
    thinning of skin, 47–48
  control of
    avoid smoking, 52–53
    avoid sun exposure, 52
    avoid unnecessary stretching of the skin, 53–54
    healthy lifestyle to, 55–56
    topical products for, 54–55
  major characteristics of
    fine wrinkles, 51
    pronounced lines of expression, 51
    skin sagging, 52
  overview, 46
  photoaging, 49–50
    characteristics of, 49
    vs. chronological aging, 49
  retinoic acid effect on, 163
Skin care, cosmetic preparations, 2
Skin cleansing, 34
Skin color
  factors influencing, 158
  oral medications alters, 90–91
Skin damage,
  due to smoking, 52–53
  due to sun exposure, 80–82
  telangiectasia, 69, 121–127
Skin dryness
  causes, 25
  factors in prevention of, 26–27
Skin irritation
  due to α-hydroxy acids, 154
  due to β-hydroxy acids, 155
  sunscreens and, 85
Skin lesions
  camouflaging, types of
    light-colored lesions, 213
    melasma and scars, 214
    pink-to-red lesions, 212–213
    transient injuries, 214
  freckles, 159
  melasma, 160
  nutritional deficiencies and, 55–56
  postinflammatory pigmented lesions, 161
  sun spots, 159–160
  technique for camouflaging, 214
    cover creams, see Cover creams
    foundation creams, 215
Skin peeling, see Chemical skin peeling
Skin pH, 39–40
  alteration by soaps, 40
  substances alter, 40
Skin protection, cosmetic preparations, 2
Skin resurfacing
  basic principle of, 188
  beneficial effect of, 189
  fractional ablative, 189–190
  laser instruments for, 189

Skin sagging, 52
Skin structure
  dermis, 8–12
    blood vessels in, 6
    collagen and elastin fibers, 9
    dermal cells, 9
    eccrine sweat gland, 12
    hair, 10–11
    sebaceous glands, 10
  epidermis, 7–8
    basal layer of, 7
    increased turnover of cells in, 7
  overview, 4
Skin thickness, 4–6
Skin tumors
  frequent checkups of, 128
  in dermis, 119
  in epidermis, 118
  originating in keratinocytes
    basal cell carcinoma, 122–123
    solar keratosis, 119–121
    squamous cell carcinoma, 121–122
  originating in melanocytes
    malignant melanoma, 124–126
    melanocytic nevi, 123–124
  self-examination of
    hands and soles, 128
    in front of mirror, 126–127
    with help of second person, 127
Skin types
  by color, 82
  by lipid content, 30
Sleep and skin aging, 55
Smoking causes skin aging, 52–53
Soapless soap, *see* Synthetic soaps
Soaps
  for acne, 40, 65–66
  additives, 38–40
  advantages of, 37
  antibacterial, 39
  fatty acids in, 34
  fragrances and perfumes, 38–39
  hypoallergenic, 40
  intermediate group of, 37
  liquid emulsion and cleansing creams vs., 41
  micelles, 34–35
  mode of action, 34–35
  moisturizers in, 38
  pH factors, 35–36
  possible disadvantages, 35
  preservatives and coloring agents in, 38–39
  synthetic, 36–37
  transparent, 38
  use on oily skin, 38
  washing body and face with, 40
  with antibacterial properties, 39–40
Social interaction, skin, 7
Sodium laureth sulfate, 230
Sodium lauryl sulfate, 230
Soft tissue augmentation
  fillers for, *see* Fillers
  indications for, 194–196
  patient selection for, 196

Solar keratosis
  clinical features of, 119
  treatment of, 121
Solar lentigines (sun spots)
  general, 49, 80
  cause of, 159
  laser treatment for, 191
Solar radiation, 77–78
  effects on skin, 78
  spectrum of wavelengths, 77
Solariums, 90–91
Solution, 28
Sorbitol, 29
Soy, 164
Spermaceti in cosmetic preparations, 16, 28
Spider telangiectasia, 95–96
Squamous cell carcinoma, 121–122
Starch used in powder, 17
Stasis dermatitis, 96
Steroids, *see* Corticosteroids
Stretching of skin causes skin aging, 53–54
Strontium sulfide in hair removal, 246
Subcutaneous fat in cellulite, 98, 99
Subcutis, 4
  cellulite and, 98
  structure of, 13
Sulfur for acne, 70
Sulfides in hair removal, 246
Sulfur preparations
  in acne, 70
  in shampoo, 235
Sun exposure
  acne and, 66
  advantages of, 89
  and prolonged use of α-hydroxy acids, 153
  changes in skin pigmentation due to, 185
  hyperpigmentation due to, 161
  immediate complications of excessive, 79
  long-term effects
    effects on dermis, 81–82
    effects on epidermis, 80
  protection from, 82–89
    enhancing skin endurance, 85
    minimize sun exposure, 83
    sunscreens for, 84–87
  short-term effects of, 78–80
    sunburn, 79
    suntanning, 78–79
  skin aging and, 52
  skin damage by, 80–82
  tips for protection from, 87–88
  vitamin D, 6–7, 79–80
Sun protection factor (SPF), 85–86, 87
Sun spots, *see* Solar lentigines
Sunburn, 79
Sunscreens
  chemical, 84
  considerations for using, 84–86
  for sun exposure, 84–87
  in moisturizer, 32
  physical, 84
  recommendation for using, 86

Suntanning, 78–79, 158
  prevention from, 87
    advice on minimizing damage, 88
    artificial, 89–90
Superficial intradermic methods, 208–209
Surfactants
  in soaps and shampoos, health hazard and, 37–38
  in synthetic soaps, 36–37
  in shampoo, 230
Suspensions in cosmetics, 20–21
Sweat glands
  apocrine, 13
  eccrine, 12
Synthetic dyes, 170
Synthetic soaps, 36–37

T

T-zone, 30–31
Talc used in powder, 17
Tanning, *see* Suntanning
Tanning oils, 91
Tar for dandruff, 235
Tattoo removal using lasers, 187–188
Tea-tree oil, 136
Telangiectases/Telangiectasia
  arborizing, 95
  camouflage, 212
  corticosteroid use, 171
  general, 92–93
  spider, 95–96
  solar damage, 49–50, 81
  treatment, 93–94
  venous insufficiency, 96
Telogen phase, hair growth, 224, 226
Temperature regulation by skin, 6
Temporary hair removal methods
  bleaching, 248
  chemical depilatories, 246–247
  cold wax, 246
  eflornithine cream, 247–248
  mechanical scraping, 243
  plucking, 243–244
  shaving, 242–243
  warm melted sugar, 245–246
  warm wax treatment, 245
Terminal hair, 241
Tetracyclines for acne, 72
Theophylline, 100
Thickeners in shampoo, 232
Thioglycolates, 246
Thinning of skin, 47–48
Tinctures, 17, 20
Tissue expanders, skin aging, 53–54
Titanium dioxide
  in absorbent masks, 44
  used in powder, 17
  in sunscreens, 84
Toilet soap, 34
Toners, 166–167
Topical corticosteroids, *see* Corticosteroids
  preparations, types of, 172–174
  side effects of, 171–172
  uses of, 171

Topical products for skin aging, 54–55
Topical retinoids for acne, 71
Tragacanth, 236
Transmission of sensations, skin, 6
Transparent soap, 38
Trichloroacetic acid, 181–182, 185
Triclocarban, 39
Triclosan, 39
Tumor
  formation of, 115
  malignant, 116
  source in human body, 117
Tumors of skin
  frequent checkups of, 128
  in dermis, 119
  in epidermis, 118
  originating in keratinocytes
    basal cell carcinoma, 122–123
    solar keratosis, 119–121
    squamous cell carcinoma, 121–122
  originating in melanocytes
    malignant melanoma, 124–126
    melanocytic nevi, 123–124
  self-examination of
    hands and soles, 128
    in front of mirror, 126–127
    with help of second person, 127
Tyrosine, 90

U

U.S. Food, Drug and Cosmetic (FDC) Act, 1
Ultraviolet-A (UVA) radiation, 78
Ultraviolet-B (UVB) radiation, 78

V

Valciclovir, 185
Vanishing creams, 19
Varicose veins, 96
Vellus hair, 220
Venous insufficiency, 94
  in legs, 96
  alleviation of, 97
  venous lake 187
Vitamins
  anti-oxidants, 138–139
  general, 138
  panthenol, 140
  penetration of epidermis, 177
  used as preservatives in cosmetics, 22
  in shampoo, 232
  in skin preparations, 139
  vitamin A derivates, for cellulite, 100
  vitamin C and provitamin A, 140
  vitamin D
    production by skin, 7
    sun exposure and, 79–80
  vitamin E, 78–9
Vitiligo, 163, 212–213

W

Warm wax treatment, 245
Washing
  body and face with soap, 40

dry skin, 25
   repeated, 27
Water content of skin, 24
Water-absorbing substances, in keratinous layer, 29
Water-repellent layer of silicone, over keratinous layer, 33
Wax
   defined, 15
   for hair removal, 245–246
Weight gain avoidance for cellulite, 99
Wetting of skin, 27
Whiteheads, *see* Comedones
Witch hazel extract, 166
Wool alcohols in cosmetic preparations, 16

Wrinkles
   facial expressions and, 54
   skin aging and fine, 51

X

Xerosis, 25, 48

Y

Yeasts, Pityrosporum ovale, 234

Z

Zinc oxide used in powder, 17
Zinc pyrithione shampoo, 235
Zinc salts, astringents, 166